THE POWER OF PLACEBOS

The Power of Placebos

●

How the Science of
Placebos and Nocebos
Can Improve
Health Care

JEREMY HOWICK

JOHNS HOPKINS UNIVERSITY PRESS | *Baltimore*

© 2023 Johns Hopkins University Press
All rights reserved. Published 2023
Printed in the United States of America on acid-free paper
9 8 7 6 5 4 3 2 1

Johns Hopkins University Press
2715 North Charles Street
Baltimore, Maryland 21218
www.press.jhu.edu

Cataloging-in-Publication Data is available from the Library of Congress.
A catalog record for this book is available from the British Library.

ISBN: 978-1-4214-4638-7 (hardcover)
ISBN: 978-1-4214-4639-4 (ebook)

*Special discounts are available for bulk purchases of this book. For more information,
please contact Special Sales at specialsales@jh.edu.*

For Claire, Sebastian, and Acer

CONTENTS

ACKNOWLEDGMENTS

I have relied heavily on the James Lind Library and the writings of Ted Kaptchuk and Jeffrey K. Aronson for identifying historical studies of placebo and nocebo effects. Many of the early ideas for the book were developed in conversation with my PhD supervisor, John Worrall. I presented drafts of the chapters of this book to a graduate seminar at Oxford University, and many students provided written comments that I used to revise the manuscript (especially Sanjay Ramakrishnan and Lunan Zhao). Other colleagues were kind enough to answer questions, including Giulio Ongaro, Rémy Boussageon, Przemysław Bąbel, and Stephen Senn. I learned a great from Daniel Moerman. He tried (probably, to him, unsuccessfully) to make me write in an even more reader-friendly way and to see more meaning in things. Kerry Hood and the PrinciPIL team helped with much of the groundbreaking work on reducing nocebo effects. I am grateful to Raffaella Campaner for facilitating my sabbatical at the University of Bologna, where I wrote the first draft of this book. Dinesh Palipana has provided general encouragement and gave me useful comments on the last chapter. My wife, Claire, was an inspiration and support, and our wonderful young children, Sebastian and Acer, put a smile on my face even when they interrupted by joining me at the computer to "work" on the book with me.

THE POWER OF PLACEBOS

CHAPTER 1

A Manifesto for the Next Revolution in Nocebo and Placebo Studies

When he had asked me if I knew the cure for headache, I somehow contrived to answer that I knew.

Then what is it? he asked.

So I told him that the thing itself was a certain leaf, but there was a charm to go with the remedy; and if one uttered the charm at the moment of its application, the remedy made one perfectly well; but without the charm there was no efficacy in the leaf.

—PLATO, *Charmides*[1]

Three factors are of major importance in the suffering of badly wounded men [during World War II]: pain; mental distress; and thirst. Therapy has been almost entirely directed to pain, and this usually limited to the administration of morphine in large dosage.

—HENRY KNOWLES BEECHER, "The Relief of Suffering"[2]

Cenobo and Bocepal

Insomnia is a serious chronic disease that affects many people. Treatment often involves sedatives, which have side effects ranging from dependence to overdose and death. A pharmaceutical company called Panycom developed a new drug called Cenobo to treat insomnia. Small trials suggested it worked better than existing sedatives and did not appear to be addictive. Panycom invested in a larger trial with over a thousand patients. The National Institutes of Health sponsored yet another large trial, also with a thousand patients. But before the trials were finished, it became clear that Cenobo caused harms ranging from headaches to nausea in half of the people in the trial. There were also seven reports of serious amnesia. The amnesia was rare, and it couldn't be established whether Cenobo caused the amnesia or whether it would have happened anyway. Yet, because Cenobo seemed likely to play a role in the serious amnesia, Panycom compensated a number of those who suffered from it an undisclosed amount believed to be between 20 million and 30 million dollars in total. Panycom pulled Cenobo from the market and stopped making it.

Luckily for Panycom, the Cenobo disaster didn't sink them because another drug they developed called Bocepal (for treating migraines) fared much better. Migraines are terrible, common, and often treated with drugs that can have serious side effects, including dependence. Like Cenobo, Bocepal showed early promise, so both Panycom and the National Institutes of Health sponsored large trials. Bocepal was a huge success. Not only was it cheap and effective for treating migraines, but the trials also found that the side effects of Bocepal were positive: it reduced other chronic and acute pain, mild depression, and mild anxiety by a small amount. At some of the medical centers that were part of the trial, more dramatic benefits were observed, including people completely coming off their strong pain and depression medications. The dramatic benefits were rare and could have occurred even without the drugs, but some people swore by Bocepal, and it became a blockbuster drug for treating migraines.

Then something strange happened. Some doctors still believed that Cenobo was an excellent treatment for insomnia. Not believing the reports of the serious side effects, they thought Cenobo was the best option for some of their patients. They were able to obtain Cenobo from a rogue pharmaceutical manufacturer in a developing country. When they gave Cenobo to patients, the doctors mentioned the possible harms but emphasized that in their experience, Cenobo was a sound treatment and that the benefits outweighed any harms.

A different set of doctors didn't believe that Bocepal was any good. They said that it couldn't work as well as it appeared to and that the fact it did so many things at once was suspicious. Instead of Bocepal, they prescribed more expensive and more potentially harmful treatments like diclofenac, which causes heart attacks in some people.[3] When their patients asked them about Bocepal, these doctors said that Bocepal was okay but not nearly as strong as diclofenac.

Clearly, the doctors who prescribed Cenobo, and the doctors who *didn't* prescribe Bocepal were acting unethically. Cenobo was harmful, and withholding Bocepal prevented benefits. In ethics-speak, causing harm violates the doctors' duty of non-maleficence (to do no harm), and avoiding likely benefit violates the duty of beneficence (to help whenever they can).

As you may have suspected, "Bocepal" is an anagram of the word "placebo," and "Cenobo" is an anagram of the word "nocebo." Like Cenobo, nocebos are harmful, and like Bocepal, placebos are beneficial for many people. It follows that not prescribing placebos and allowing nocebo effects to thrive is unethical. This conclusion is an oversimplification because it ignores other relevant issues including (a) whether placebos require deception, (b) whether we can generate placebo effects without placebos, and (c) whether it is possible to avoid nocebo effects while being honest to patients. These issues will be examined rigorously in the remainder of this book.

For placebos to be an ethical requirement and for nocebos to be avoided more rigorously, things need to change. Currently, some well-known doctors consider placebos to be unethical. Asbjørn Hróbjartsson, who is the director of Cochrane Denmark (formerly the Nordic Cochrane Centre) wrote a paper titled "Clinical Placebo Interventions Are Unethical, Unnecessary, and Unprofessional."[4] Alain Braillon, a physician and an expert on public health, says that a placebo is "far from benign: it is disease-mongering."[5] In parallel, nocebo effects appear to be widespread. About half of the people in clinical trials *who take placebos* report at least one negative side effect (often a nocebo effect), and it appears that many of them can be avoided.[6-8]

The First Revolution in Placebo Studies

The main message of this book is that placebo studies are ready for their next revolution. The first revolution moved placebo studies from the outside to within successful normal science. Now the knowledge needs to move from inside the walls of academia and into the real world. Anything less forfeits a benefit to patients and harms them. Unfortunately, outdated beliefs about placebos and nocebos, together with the fact that placebo research has become a victim of its own success, are barriers to the next revolution.

Outdated Mistaken Beliefs

The outdated beliefs that hinder the second revolution in placebo studies are that placebos are fake and that they require deception and trickery. These are mistaken. Recent research has shown that placebos do not always require deception to be effective,[9] and more importantly, we don't need sugar pill placebos to invoke placebo effects.[10] An overarching theme of this book is that these outdated beliefs can safely be put to rest and therefore that we need more placebo treatments and fewer nocebos in practice.

The Success of Placebo Researchers

Placebo research has come a long way. In the early days of my PhD research, I was told more than once by senior academics at conferences that placebo research was a fringe activity. Little more than a handful of people had been focusing on placebo research. They included Ted Kaptchuk, Irving Kirsch, Daniel Moerman, Bruce Wampold, Jerome Frank and Julia Frank, Fabrizio Benedetti, George Lewith, Arthur Shapiro and Elaine Shapiro, John Kelley, Harald Walach, and Wayne Jonas. Their interest in placebo studies arose from various sources including interest in non-Western medicine. For example, Jerome and Julia Frank took magical and religious healing seriously.[11] Ted Kaptchuk was an acupuncturist as well as a doctor. George Lewith prescribed homeopathy because of what he believed were its often useful placebo effects. Because of its roots on the fringes of mainstream medicine, placebo research was often lumped together with alternative medicine,[12] and those who studied placebos were sometimes considered to be alternative scientists.[13] Indeed, many early placebo researchers struggled to survive in academia. Daniel Moerman had to establish himself as an ethnobotanist, doing most of his placebo research on the side. Ted Kaptchuk had to fight tooth and nail to be taken seriously at Harvard. Others moved away from placebo research into other more accepted areas.

While united in their interest in placebos and nocebos, they espoused a variety of incompatible theories about placebos. In the last century, Arthur and Elaine Shapiro published a book claiming that placebos were "nonspecific" treatments.[14] Others claimed placebos were "inactive" treatments.[15] Still others called placebos inert, and there were other definitions besides.[10] None of these definitions was satisfactory: placebos have been shown to have specific effects, and inactive or inert things can't have effects, whereas placebo treatments do.

In parallel, there was a debate about how placebos (however they were defined) worked, with some favoring conditioning and others expectancy.[16] Related to the varied theories about what placebos are and how they worked, there was no consensus about whether it was ethically sound for doctors to give placebos to patients, and when they could be used in trials.[17-20] In short, the field lacked the coherence that characterizes many established disciplines. The situation of placebo researchers a few decades ago might be loosely compared to that of the physicists described by Thomas Kuhn before Newton's theory of optics became widely accepted:

> One group took light to be particles emanating from material bodies; for another it was a modification of the medium that intervened between the body and the eye; still another explained light in terms

of an interaction of the medium with an emanation from the eye; and there were other combinations and modifications besides. . . . Those men were scientists. Yet anyone examining a survey of physical optics before Newton may well conclude that, though the field's practitioners were scientists, the net result of their activity was something less than science.[21]

Kuhn was not saying that the earlier physicists lacked scientific ability; it was just that the field was not coherent. Likewise, the early placebo researchers were individually successful yet did not have widely accepted fundamental tenets. In fact, because many were viewed as dabbling in a questionable fringe activity, they arguably had to be *better* than average scientists to survive in academia. The lack of coherence and the association with alternative healing made placebo studies an easy target for skeptics. In 1994, Peter Gøtzsche said that the placebo could not be defined in a logical way.[22] A few years later, with his colleague Asbjørn Hróbjartsson, he published a megastudy in the eminent *New England Journal of Medicine* claiming that placebos didn't have effects. Other skeptics joined in.[23] (Aside: paradoxically, many of these same skeptics invoke the placebo effect as a reason why some people respond well to alternative medicine.)[24] If placebos can't be defined or don't have any effects, then serious scientists would not bother studying them. That was the implication of the skeptics' studies: placebo science was bunk, and those who studied them were not serious scientists.

In response to these skeptics, or perhaps independently, the early placebo researchers doubled down. In 1994, Jos Kleijnen published a paper in the United Kingdom's most eminent medical journal, *The Lancet*, exposing a serious flaw in Gøtzsche and Hróbjartsson's method.[25] In 2001, Zelda Di Blasi and colleagues published a review of "context effects" (which is another word for "placebo effects") in *The Lancet*.[26] In 2002, in a widely read book, Daniel Moerman proposed to overcome the problems with defining the placebo by eliminating the term "placebo effect" in favor of "meaning response."[27] In 2003, Dylan Evans defended the hypothesis that placebo effects were an "acute phase response".[28] Following earlier work by Stewart Wolf and Louis Lasagna, Fabrizio Benedetti conducted a series of studies showing that humans' bodies and brains respond to placebos in much the same way that they respond to pharmacological drugs. Benedetti's research is summarized in a 2009 book, now in its third edition.[29] Also in 2009, Irving Kirsch pioneered research on the size of placebo effects compared with the size of antidepressant drug effects.[30] In 2013 my study was published in which I exposed a fatal flaw in Hróbjartsson and Gøtzsche's method.[31] In 2016, Ian Harris defended the bold view that much of surgery was a placebo.[32] Pekka Louhiala's 2020 book summarizes the advances in the conceptualization of the placebo.[33] Throughout this period, Harvard researchers Ted Kaptchuk and John Kelly published a number of high-quality clinical trials of placebo effects in prestigious journals like the *British Medical Journal*.[34-39]

Meanwhile, other researchers started taking placebo studies more seriously. Benedetti's then junior researchers, Luana Colloca and Martina Amanzio, became eminent in their own right, as did Kaptchuk's junior researchers Alia Crum, Charlotte Blease, and Karin Jensen. Many other eminent researchers also contributed to the growth of placebo studies including Andrea Evers, Jens Gaab, Winfried Rief, Tor Wager, Damien Finniss, Przemysław Bąbel, and Karin Meissner. As a result of the growing cohort of placebo researchers, placebo research has multiplied. Studies with the word "placebo" in the title have doubled in the last 10 years. Researchers in the area have organized themselves into the international Society for Interdisciplinary Placebo Studies (SIPS),[40] whose membership has mushroomed from eight to more than 500 in ten years. The membership includes psychologists, basic scientists, philosophers, medical doctors, and others from over 20 countries, and the society held its third international conference in Baltimore in 2021.

Placebos have also infiltrated popular culture. There have been popular science books,[41-43] a documentary that had a record 2 million viewers in the United Kingdom, and a rock band called Placebo, which has sold over 11 million records. There is also a placebo diet,[44] and I recently discovered that there is even a "Saint Placebo," whose blasphemous website contains information about "how much Saint Placebo loves you."[45]

The placebo research community's accomplishments have led to progress.[46] It's now widely accepted that like drugs, placebos affect our brains and bodies in measurable ways,[26] and placebo and nocebo effects can be studied in the same way "regular" drugs are—namely, in controlled trials.[32] Skeptics can no longer legitimately deny that placebo effects exist, at least for some ailments like pain.[31] There has also been great progress in our understanding of how placebo treatments produce their effects with a peaceful resolution of the dispute between proponents of conditioning and expectancy: both mechanisms are now recognized as playing a role.[29] Studies of how placebos and nocebos affect brains and bodies have also served to demystify the science, making it seem more real, no longer alternative or fluffy.[47] At a sociological level, the fact that many leading placebo researchers come from top academic institutions around the world, including Harvard, Oxford, Stanford, Dartmouth, and Sydney, has contributed to legitimizing studies of placebos and nocebos. The recent knowledge has been organized in several edited volumes.[48-50]

In short, the field of placebos studies has become more coherent, larger, and successful. Uncertainty about the nature, effects, and ethics of placebos has been reduced. Collectively these advances are what I call the first revolution in placebo studies. This first revolution established placebo studies as a legitimate field of inquiry and proved that placebo effects are often like drug effects. The forthcoming chapters in the book expose the resistance to implementing what we know about placebos and nocebos for patient benefit as outdated. Now would be an ideal time to focus on *implementing* what we know about placebos and nocebos to benefit patients, to avoid the metaphorical prescription of Cenobo, and withholding of Bocepals. Yet, as I explained above, there is resistance to implementation, and this is why placebo studies needs a second revolution, one that shifts the focus from basic research to implementation.

The Second Revolution In Placebo Studies

The second revolution in placebo studies is required to stop the unnecessary proliferation of nocebo effects and to ensure that patients benefit from placebo effects. The second revolution is also a necessary part of the solution to the current crisis in healthcare. Currently, 2 in 3 physicians report being burned out,[51] and have higher suicide rates than other professionals.[52] Drowning under paperwork that takes half their time,[53,54] they are leaving the profession in droves.[55,56] In parallel, the cost of health care keeps rising,[57] while the ultimate outcome, life expectancy, is leveling off or dropping for the first time since World War II.[58,59] Many of the things that are part of placebo treatment, including empathic care, have been shown to reduce burnout,[60] and they are mostly free.[61]

Unfortunately, barriers remain to putting the research on placebos into practice. The first barrier is a paradoxical consequence of placebo studies' success. To succeed in academia, one must specialize, and subspecialize. Like other successful academics, placebo researchers have also specialized. The problem is that that specialization encourages separation between disciplines. Research about how placebos work is usually done by psychologists, investigations into the nature of placebos by philosophers, inquiries regarding ethics of placebos and nocebos by ethicists, and analysis on how effective they are by clinical epidemiologists. To be sure, this research often overlaps, and the different researchers have regular contact at conferences. Yet, to make the case for or against using placebos in practice, the specialist research needs to be connected. Otherwise, attempts to measure the size of placebo and nocebo effects risk being (mis)informed by inaccurate conceptualizations of placebos and nocebos. Then, the mistaken conceptualizations of what placebos and nocebos are, combined with the mistaken estimates of how big their effects are, feed into unsound arguments about whether we should use them. Interdisciplinary academic research can facilitate the implementation by bringing all the pieces of placebo and nocebo science together. Yet "interdisciplinary research" is often a well-liked buzzword that is hard to achieve in practice.

Another barrier to the implementation revolution is that putting things into practice requires skills that most researchers don't have. Good academic analysis requires careful thought, considering every angle, being slow, and being skeptical about one's own conclusions. Putting things into practice requires a "just do it" attitude that is more common among entrepreneurs (who themselves, because of the lack of rigor and skepticism in their approach, are usually ill suited to academic research). Because they are so different, academic success and entrepreneurial success rarely occur in the same people. Pharmaceutical companies have huge financial incentives to put their research into practice and spend about as much on marketing as they do on research,[62] and they use almost completely different teams to do each job. Putting placebo and nocebo research into practice may require outsourcing the implementation. This will be challenging because the massive financial incentives and resources available to pharmaceutical companies are not available to placebo researchers.

Combining Placebo and Nocebo in the Same Book

Much of the new research in the area of placebos has been done on nocebo effects, and I have focused on that new research in this book. I also mix placebo research and nocebo research. This is because there often is no intrinsic difference between positive and negative effects. What counts as a negative effect depends on the patient's values, beliefs, background, and desires. For example, a relatively common side effect of selective serotonin reuptake inhibitors is sexual dysfunction.[63] For many, this is a negative effect of these antidepressants. But the very same phenomenon is a positive effect for people with premature ejaculation. Loss of appetite could be a negative effect of a drug for some but a positive effect for those who are trying to lose weight. A placebo treatment that lowers anxiety could be a benefit for an overly anxious patient, but a nocebo effect for a tired student who is about to fall asleep during an exam. Because they are not different, the research about placebos and placebo effects is relevant to the research on nocebos and nocebo effects, and vice versa.

A Caveat (Sort Of)

My claim that we need more placebo treatments and fewer nocebo effects in clinical practice warrants a caveat. My earliest memory is of my baby brother Alexander when I was two years old. I have a vivid memory of him, my mother and I sitting on the kitchen floor. I asked Mom if I could hold him. She said I could if I sat down on the floor and held his head. I sat down and held him, and I remember that he smelled good (the way babies do). He was helpless. For the Christmas holidays, we went to my grandparents' house in Edmonton. Apparently, Mom got up at around 4 a.m. to feed little Alexander, and he seemed happy and healthy. A few hours later, I woke up, and Mom said, "Let's go wake up the baby." The next thing I remember is Mom giving mouth-to-mouth to the baby. The proof I remember is that almost a year later I tried to give Mom mouth-to-mouth. At two years old I had probably never heard the word "tragedy," but even in my little way I understood that something really sad was happening. For years afterward, I reacted viscerally whenever I heard an ambulance, and from time to time I would ask my mom what happened and cry.

Nothing I describe in this book will even come close to bringing Alexander back to life or avoiding the pain my parents felt at losing a baby. It won't cure aggressive metastatic cancer either, and it won't make your leg grow back if it gets blown off by a land mine. Thankfully (very thankfully), such tragedies are rare. Most people, most of the time, do not suffer from serious illness. The vast majority of people suffer from milder things like headaches, back pain, colds, and mild depression. None of these things need drugs, all of which have potentially serious side effects. For these cases, placebo effects help and nocebo effects harm.

Even for the more serious conditions that placebo treatments can't cure, placebos can often be useful add-ons. We'll see in the upcoming chapters that placebo treatments can improve recovery time after surgery, reduce morphine use, and lower pain. Meanwhile, knowledge of nocebo effects can help avoid unnecessary harm to patients in clinical trials and clinical practice. More importantly, even "real" (nonplacebo) treatments have placebo components. Take the story of Ms. B:

> Ms B, a 75-year-old woman with an alcohol use disorder and gastro-esophageal reflux disorder, presented to the oncology clinic following her new (incidental) diagnosis of gastric carcinoma. During the visit, the oncologist explained the importance of assessing the depth of the tumor's invasion into the gastric wall (i.e., to stage the tumor and to decide on treatment options). He noted that if the tumor was confined to the most superficial layer of the stomach, it could be excised during an endoscopy. If the tumor went deeper, Ms B would need radiation and/or chemotherapy or surgery. The oncologist arranged for an immediate visit by the surgeon, who informed her that the cancer would almost certainly be invasive and that he planned to remove a large part of her stomach. He described her surgery as very serious but necessary because her cancer was likely to lead to death. As the surgeon turned to write his note in the electronic medical record, Ms B began to shake her head from side to side and cry.[64]

Ms B's doctors were following what they took to be the best "evidence-based" guidelines and thought they were helping. They saw an acute problem, a tumor, and proceeded to focus on how to get rid of it. They didn't think that communicating in an empathic and compassionate way was worth their time. Ms B is not a real patient, but her experience appears to be common. I witnessed something remarkably similar when I accompanied my mother when she visited her oncologist for her metastatic breast cancer check-up. After making us wait eight hours, his assistant called us into the office, where we waited a further 15 minutes. Eventually, the very important oncologist came in with some notes in his hand, said that everything was okay, then turned to leave. Needless to say, that "okay" in the context of metastatic breast cancer does not mean "okay" in the normal sense, but just that things weren't deteriorating faster than expected. Also, my mother had planned to ask two questions, one about other treatment options and one about the additional medications she was taking.

"I have a few questions," she said. Keeping his hand on the door-handle, the very important oncologist replied, "Yes?"

My mother asked the question about changing her treatment to which the very important oncologist replied, still with his hand on the doorhandle, that he didn't think it was a good idea. She didn't bother asking the second question (instead, we made another appointment to return the next week to ask another doctor). If her oncologist had taken a bit more time and acted a bit more compassionately, it would not have done much to change the course of my mother's illness. However, it would have made her feel better in the moment, and reduced her anxiety after the appointment. Moments are all she and many others have, and the recent research on placebo effects can help enhance those moments even when placebo treatments in and of themselves would obviously be inappropriate.

Who This Book Is For

This book is part of the second revolution in placebo studies. The second revolution requires collaboration between doctors and other health care professionals, health care managers, as well as other groups ranging from hospital designers to patients. Doctors who wish to enhance the care of their patients by taking the science of placebos and nocebos into account can use this book as a manual. Medical researchers who need to make decisions about the ethics of placebo-controlled trials and how to reduce unnecessary nocebo effects can use the book as a guide. Philosophers of medicine and ethicists interested in recent advances in placebo studies can get a grasp of the field in a single, readable volume. Hospital designers who wish to organize their spaces in a way that reinforces what doctors do can be inspired. Policy makers who wish to organize their institutions in a way that promotes patient and practitioner health can find evidence to support initiatives which achieve this. The science in the book can also be used to improve the quality of anyone's interpersonal communication and relationships.

The need to communicate to different groups explains why the book is written in a casual style. Because the book has an interdisciplinary audience, I had to avoid technical terms specific to each discipline. Clinical epidemiologists are very comfortable with terms like P-values, Cohen's d, random effects, and odds ratios that are puzzling to most others. Doctors sometimes communicate to each other with terms such as "upper respiratory tract infection" (instead of "common cold"), "hypertension" (instead of "high blood pressure") and "myocardial infarction" (instead of "heart attack") that most nondoctors don't understand. Philosophers and ethicists often use Latin terms such as *prima facie* (on the first impression), *a fortiori* (all the more so), *ceteris paribus* (all other things being equal), that might as well be Martian to most people. Writing in a jargon-free, casual style was a way to make the book understood by a multidisciplinary audience. Second, much of the book's contents is of potential interest to readers who are not academics, including medical practice and hospital managers, and the lay public. Third, much of my work is publicly funded, paid for by the taxpayer. Public funding bodies are increasingly demanding that academics be accountable to the taxpayers in several ways— including by writing in plain English where possible. I support efforts to make academics more accountable because I take it to be an ethical duty to serve taxpayers who pay my bills. In short, writing in a jargon-free, casual style is a strength of the book.

Making rigorous arguments is often more difficult and riskier when they're presented in a casual style. Blaise Pascal famously said that he wrote a long letter because he didn't have time to write a shorter one. This seems counterintuitive because usually writing more takes longer. However, as Pascal understands, it takes a great deal more time and thought and effort to express things concisely. There is a parallel when it comes to writing in a casual style. It can be difficult to make rigorous arguments and explain technical matters without resorting to technical terms. It is certainly riskier, because books and papers that

Philosophy and Science

Ancient philosophers didn't just walk around in robes arguing with each other (although it seems they did that too). They contemplated in order to live better lives and improve the lives of those around them. Plato developed a theory that was put into practice for government. Aristotle developed a philosophical method for understanding the real world. The Stoic, Epicurean, and Hedonistic philosophies were guides for living well, and they were followed by their adherents. Socrates believed in the supremacy of reason, and he accepted dying for his belief. In the eighteenth century, Jean-Jacques Rousseau's philosophy was integrated into real-life politics. John Stewart Mill's philosophy led him to support the suffragette movement. So intimate was the link between philosophy and the world that science used to be called *natural philosophy*, and Isaac Newton's revolutionary book was titled *Mathematical Principles of Natural Philosophy*. I share the ancient approach to philosophy and use my training to address real-life problems. In this case, it requires combining philosophy (to investigate what placebos and nocebos are), empirical research (to measure their effects), and ethics (to appraise whether they should be used). This book is a case study of merging philosophy with medical science.

are written in an understandable way can be criticized by anyone, whereas highly technical prose is protected from outside critique for the simple reason that few people understand the jargon.

I'm not the only academic who writes in ways that nonacademics can understand. The long tradition of rigorous academic writing that is written in a more casual style includes some of Plato, Thomas Kuhn, Bertrand Russell (sometimes), and, more recently, Bent Flyvbjerg. These examples show that one can be rigorous while writing in a casual style.

What Is to Come

The book is organized into three parts. Part I discusses what placebos and nocebos are, part II reviews how we should (and shouldn't) measure their effects, and part III presents the case for whether we should use them. This order is logical: to know whether we should use them, we need to know whether they are effective, and to measure whether they are effective, we need to know what they are (what we are measuring). Because each part of the book builds on the next, it is preferable to read it in order. However, each chapter, section, subsection, and page can be appreciated independently. So, you can open the book on any page where a new chapter or section begins and enjoy it. By the end of the book, I hope the reader will have learned something while having been entertained and also inspired to join the second revolution in placebo studies.

PART I

THE TROUBLED STORY OF PLACEBOS AND NOCEBOS

The "placebo" terminology, despite its defects, is too engrained in the scientific literature to replace it at this time, especially in the absence of a satisfactory alternative.
—DAMIEN FINNISS ET AL. "Biological, Clinical, and Ethical Advances of Placebo Effects"[1]

To measure how big the effects of placebos and nocebos are and whether we should use them, we need to know *what* we are measuring. In other words, we need to know what placebos and nocebos are. By exploring what they are, part I of this book provides the foundation for the other parts.

A central problem that I will address in this part of the book is countering the claim that placebos or nocebos don't exist.[2,3] If this claim were correct, we would all be better off banishing the words "placebo" and "nocebo" entirely (and I wouldn't be writing this book). Before concluding that there is no such thing as placebos or nocebos, we should at the very least systematically review and critique how the terms are and have been used in the past. I don't believe that any of the "placebo deniers" have done this.

CHAPTER 2

Please Me, Please

Placebos and Nocebos in Practice

One of the most successful physicians I have ever known, has assured me that he used more of bread *pills*, *drops* of coloured water, & *powders* of hiccory ashes, than of all other medecines put together. It was certainly a pious fraud.

—THOMAS JEFFERSON, Letter to Caspar Wistar[1]

The history of medical treatment until relatively recently is the history of the placebo effect.

—ARTHUR SHAPIRO AND ELAINE SHAPIRO, *The Powerful Placebo: From Ancient Priest to Modern Physician*[2]

Dr. Osler

Jennifer Worrall tells a true story of her time as a junior doctor in a central London hospital in the 1980s with a patient I'll call Jane and a senior doctor I'll call Dr. Osler (Worrall does not use names):

> [Jane] was very demanding and difficult to please and claimed to suffer from continuous agony from her ulcer (although there were none of the objective signs of pain, such as sleep disturbance, increased heart rate and blood pressure, pallor and sweating). All of the many mild-to-moderate analgesics were "useless" (according to the patient) and I did not feel opiates were justified, so I asked the advice of my immediate superior. [Dr. Osler] saw the patient, discussed her pain and, with a grave face, said he wanted her to try a "completely different sort of treatment." She agreed. He disappeared into the office, to reappear a few

minutes later, walking slowly down the ward and holding in front of him a pair of tweezers which grasped a large, white tablet, the size of [a] half dollar. As he came nearer, it became clear (to me, at least) that the tablet was none other than effervescent vitamin C. He dropped the tablet into a glass of water which, of course, bubbled and fizzed, and told the patient to sip the water carefully when the fizzing had subsided. It worked—the new medicine completely abolished her pain! [Dr. Osler] has used this method several times, apparently, and it always worked. He felt that the single most important aspect was holding the tablet with tweezers, thereby giving the impression that it was somehow too powerful to be touched with bare hands![3]

Officially recorded stories like Jennifer's are difficult to find because they involve deceiving patients, which is usually unethical. A contemporary doctor who admitted treating a patient in that way would therefore risk being disciplined. But it does happen. After I gave a lecture to a large audience of general practitioners in France, an Italian doctor who shall remain anonymous wrote to me about his experience treating someone in Monaco:

I was called to the bedside of a wealthy 77-year-old Milanese woman whom I knew well. She spent her summers in her mansion in my small village (450 inhabitants) where I am the only doctor. She complained of debilitating lower back pain. However, she was able to move well; she was very flexible. Her ability to move well made me doubt whether the pain was mechanical in origin. I performed a routine examination, and she insisted on receiving an injection. Not wanting to give her unnecessary and potentially harmful pharmacological substances, I administered an injection of distilled water. She was so satisfied that seven days later she called me for the same reason and demanded the same solution, "which had done me so much good."

So, I turned my back to her in order to prepare the injection of distilled water, out of her sight. As I filled my syringe with the water, I heard her calling out, "Doctor, is it a placebo that you are giving me?"

I froze and was plunged into an abyss of perplexity. I was ethically bound to tell her the truth. But, if I did, the placebo injection might not help her, and I was also ethically bound to help the patient. I decided that truth had to prevail.

"Yes, that's right, ma'am," I said.

"Thank goodness. It helped so much last week," she immediately replied.

I proceeded to inject her with the distilled water in silence, feeling quite strange.

Few would deny that Dr. Osler's vitamin C and the Italian doctor's distilled water were placebos. But when we try to pinpoint exactly what placebos are in general, it gets tricky. I'll explain a lot more about why it is tricky below (and provide a solution). For now, consider that vitamin C and water are placebos for pain, but not for treating scurvy or dehydration, respectively. Relatedly, placebos are not "inactive" (vitamin C is not inactive for treating scurvy) or "nonspecific" (vitamin C achieves its effect through concrete mechanisms of action). The fact that placebos and nocebos are hard to define is cited as a barrier to putting placebos to use.[4-6] It is therefore important to come up with a defensible definition of placebos. I'll start to do this by reviewing some key moments in the history of the words "placebo" and "nocebo."

Genesis of the "Placebo"
Early References to "Placebo"

Over two thousand years ago, Plato wrote about a leaf that cured headaches but only if the doctor administered the leaf with a song. To be sure, the leaf was not referred to as a placebo even though we might refer to it as such today. The word "placebo" (as it is currently used in medicine) can be traced to St. Jerome's fourth-century Latin translation of the Bible. He translated verse 9 of Psalm 114 as *placebo Domino in regione vivorum*. "Placebo" means "I will please," and the verse is "I will please the Lord in the land of the living." The fact that the word "placebo" was introduced as part of a prayer, which is related to beliefs, reflects how the word is used today.

Controversy about placebos can be traced to St. Jerome too. Jeffrey Aronson points out that the translation may not be correct.[7] The Hebrew transliteration is *et'halekh liphnay Adonai b'artzot hakhayim*, which means, "I will walk before the Lord in the land of the living." Aronson points out that walking and pleasing are not the same thing. Yet St. Jerome wasn't that far off: why would the omnipotent Lord walk with anyone who didn't please Him?

Psalm 114 was used in prayers at funerals, and at some point, people started referring to the entire prayer as "placebo." At that time, and even today, it was common for the mourning family to provide a feast for those who attended the funeral. After all, many would have traveled from far away, and they would be hungry. Because of the free food offered at funerals, distant relatives—even people who pretended to be relatives—attended the funeral just to enjoy the feast. Yet they seemed to chant the "placebo" prayer in earnest. This deceptive practice led Chaucer to write, "Flatterers are the Devil's chaplains, always singing Placebo" in the fourteenth century.[8] The relationship between placebos and deception persists today, although, as we will see later, placebos can work even if patients know they are placebos.

Chaucer also named one of the characters in his "Merchant's Tale" Placebo. The protagonist of the tale is an old wealthy knight called Januarie. Januarie is lecherous and courts a younger woman called May. To legitimize his desire for recreational sex, he considers marrying her. Before making his decision, he consults two of his friends, Placebo and Justinius. Placebo is eager to gain favor with the knight and only says things that the knight wants to hear. He tells the knight how courageous he must be for considering a young wife and that it's a good idea. Justinius, on the other hand, is more cautious, citing Seneca and Cato, who preached virtue and prudence in the selection of a wife. After listening to them both, Januarie sides with Placebo, saying to Justinius: "I don't give a straw for Seneca, nor for any of your proverbs and school terms. They're not worth a sack of parsley! Placebo—you have the final word."[9] Januarie married the young woman, only to be cuckolded on his wedding day.

Eventually, the term "placebo" was used to describe a medical doctor. In a book published in 1763, Dr. Pierce refers to a physician as "Placebo."[10] Upon visiting a patient one morning, Pierce reports what he observed:

> He boiled his nostrums over the patient's chamber fire; with his own hand, he carefully divided the doses. . . . Calling one morning to visit a Lady, I found him lolling on the bedstead. Asking her how she did, she answered, Pure and well, my old friend the Doctor has been just treating me with some of his good drops. . . . His wig was deeper than mine by two curls, he corresponded with the most eminent, as he reported they prescribed. Was it any wonder that Placebo grew in grace?

This doctor Placebo was kind, impressively dressed, and he sat at the patient's bedside. Recalling Dr. Osler's vitamin C, he also prepared the medicine carefully, so his patients could see what he was doing.

Soon after references to people as placebos began to appear, treatments we would now call placebos were used to describe medical treatments. An early example of this comes from a series of letters between the German philosopher Gottfried Leibniz and his medical doctor friends Christiaan Huygens and Denis Papin. Referring to a method he used to keep sick people happy without hurting them, Papin writes, in 1704, that the solution is "to give them something harmless like pills made of white bread crumbs, that are well cooked so they aren't recognized as such; sick people often report getting much better after taking these; either because they were given just at the time when the sickness was going to subside on its own, or because the force of the imagination contributed to improving things" (author's translation).[11] William Smellie, writing in 1752, is the first person I'm aware of who uses the term "placebo" to describe a medical treatment. He wrote, "it will be convenient to prescribe some innocent Placemus, that she may take between whiles, to beguile the time and please her imagination."[12] ("Placemus" is another form of the word "placebo.") The quotation from Thomas Jefferson at the beginning of this chapter suggests that treatments we would deem to be placebos were commonly prescribed to patients at that time.

The term "placebo" begins to appear in medical dictionaries a few decades later. In the second (but not the first) edition of George Motherby's *New Medical Dictionary* of 1785,[13] "placebo" was defined as "a common place method or medicine." But this won't do: morphine might be common, but it's not a placebo. Jeffrey Aronson surmises that it could be due to *placere*'s secondary meaning of "to be popular," which could be related to "common."[7] A few decades later, "placebo" appeared in Robert Hooper's 1811 *Medical Dictionary* as "any medicine adapted more to please than benefit the patient." Hooper's definition can't be accepted because he implies that pleasing a patient is different from benefiting them. If a patient is depressed, then pleasing them also benefits them medically.

More Recent (and More Confusing) Definitions

The number of definitions of placebos has multiplied over the last hundred years. In a 1955 essay that made placebo studies popular titled "The Powerful Placebo" (much more about this paper in chapter 5), Henry Knowles Beecher referred to placebos as "pharmacologically inert substances," the administration of which, however, has "real therapeutic effects."[14] I like Beecher's study, but his definition isn't quite right: inert substances can't have effects. Moreover, as the philosopher Adolf Grünbaum pointed out,[15] even the proverbial sugar pill is not inert in insulin-dependent patients.

A few decades later, Arthur Shapiro defined the placebo as any therapy or component of therapy that is deliberately used for "its nonspecific, psychological, or psychophysiological effect, or that is used for its presumed specific effect, but is without specific activity for the condition being treated."[16] Shapiro is correct that placebos act in a general (nonspecific) way. Insofar as they please a patient, or make them feel relaxed, their benefits are not specific to a particular condition. But a serious problem with equating nonspecific with placebic is that "nonspecific" is not a very specific word. Lisa Grencavage and John Norcross found that it is used in over 27 ways.[17] One of its meanings is "identifiable" or "operating through a specific mechanism." Yet now we know that placebo analgesia exists and operates through the release of endorphins (natural morphine) into the bloodstream.[18] This is just as "specific" as injecting morphine through a needle. "Specific" is also sometimes used to mean "well defined," or "quantitatively precise." But estimates of placebo effects illustrate that their effects can be quantified in much the same way as the effects of other treatments are quantified.[19,20]

Another problem with Shapiro's definition is that he seems to equate placebos with "psychological" or "psychophysiological" treatments. But it's mistaken to equate placebos with psychological treatments for at least two reasons. First, there is no such thing as something purely psychological. Second, while certain forms of psychological therapy could turn out to be placebos, to classify them all as placebos before defining placebos seems too quick (more about this in chapter 4).

It is also a mistake to include the reasons why a doctor gives a treatment in the definition of placebos (recall that Shapiro says that the placebo is "used for its presumed specific effect, but is without specific activity for the condition being treated").[16] If that were right, then the mere belief that snake oil had a direct physiological effect would render the snake oil a nonplacebo. The intentions of a doctor are one thing; objective facts about whether and how a treatment works are something else.

The *Oxford English Dictionary* defines the placebo as a "drug, medicine, therapy, etc., prescribed more for the psychological benefit to the patient of being given treatment than for any direct physiological effect." By equating placebo effects with psychological effects, this definition suffers from one of the problems with Shapiro's definition. Worse, all treatments that provide "psychological" benefits—including antipsychotic, antidepressant, or psychotropic drugs—automatically count as placebos according to the *Oxford English Dictionary* because they are prescribed "for the psychological benefit." Yet powerful antipsychotic drugs are not placebos.

The American Medical Association defines placebo as a "a substance provided to a patient that the physician believes has no specific pharmacological effect on the condition being treated."[21] This definition is flawed for the same reasons some others already mentioned are flawed. Placebo effects can be specific, and what the physician believes is not the main determinant of whether a treatment is a placebo.

Avoidance and Denial

In view of all this confusion, it shouldn't be a surprise that some have recommended dropping the word "placebo" altogether. After examining the research on placebos until 1994 (much of which is mentioned above), Peter Gøtzsche concluded that "the placebo concept . . . cannot be defined in a logically consistent way and leads to paradoxes."[22] We'll see in chapter 6 that in his widely cited study, he decided to adopt a "practical" approach and define placebos as any intervention labeled as such in the report of a clinical trial. But this approach doesn't work. Suppose someone reported using penicillin as a "placebo" in a trial of some new antibiotic as a treatment for pneumonia. The response will of course be "no one would, and if they did we would not take the trial seriously." But this reaction seems precisely to show that we work with some concept that involves judgments about what placebos are. In fact, Gøtzsche's "practical" approach led to a mistaken estimate of placebo effects.

Worse, he goes back on his stated policy of accepting any treatment labeled as a "placebo" in the report of a clinical trial. For example, he excludes studies in which "it was very likely that the alleged placebo had a clinical benefit not associated with the ritual alone (e.g., movement techniques for postoperative pain)."[23] Here he seems to sneak in a definition of placebos as the effects of "rituals," which is no improvement on earlier definitions. Ritual feasts or fasts are not placebos.

The philosopher of science Robin Nunn is bolder than Gøtzsche. Writing in the *BMJ*, Nunn suggests that the linguistic confusion I have mapped is irredeemable: "every way of looking at the placebo concept invites criticism, because it doesn't make sense."[24] The reason for the confusion, according to Nunn, is that there is no such thing as the placebo. He suggests that medical science would be much improved and clarified if placebo-talk were eliminated.

Others have tried to get away from the problem of defining placebos by using a different word. For example, some use the word "sham" or "dummy." These are problematic because they imply that placebos are fake, which is not always true (see part II).[25] It seems that running away from trying to define placebos causes more problems than it attempts to solve.

Definitions That Others Have Used

Charlotte Blease recommended moving beyond discussing how academics define the term to looking at how it is actually used in medical research and practice.[26] That is a useful part of the solution, but the problem is that the term is used in different ways. Over the last 30 years, several researchers have asked doctors whether they have used placebos. These surveys all imply different definitions of "placebo." For example, Przemysław Bąbel asked doctors in Poland whether they had prescribed placebos. He initially didn't define "placebo," leaving it up to the doctors to define it for themselves. Over half (55%) of doctors admitted to doing so at least once.[27] Bąbel then asked the same doctors whether they prescribed treatments "primarily to enhance patient expectation" (this is his preferred definition of placebos). With the new definition, 80% of the same doctors reported prescribing placebos once. Do 55%, 80%, or some other proportion of doctors prescribe placebos? It depends on what you mean by "placebo." And when it comes to determining whether we should use or avoid them in clinical trials or practice, we need to address what is and what is not a placebo treatment.

Professor Bąbel's survey isn't unique. I systematically searched all the studies of placebo use up to October 2019. I identified 28 surveys (including one that I conducted), and on average, it seems that more than half of doctors admit to prescribing placebos at least once in their careers.[28] Twenty-two of the studies included a definition of placebos. Most defined them as nonspecific or inactive (which I've shown above to be unacceptable), and often distinguished between "pure" and "impure" placebos.[29] Here is a definition of pure and impure placebos that I've used before:

> Pure placebos are interventions such as sugar pills . . . or saline injections without direct pharmacologically active ingredients for the condition being treated. Impure placebos are substances, interventions or 'therapeutic' methods which have known pharmacological, clinical or physical value for some ailments but lack specific therapeutic effects or value for the condition for which they have been prescribed. These may include: nutritional supplements for conditions unlikely to benefit from this therapy; probiotics for diarrhea, peppermint pills for pharyngitis, and antibiotics for suspected viral infection.[30]

The idea is that pure placebos are always placebos, while impure placebos are placebos sometimes. This distinction is only a rough guide. Just as antibiotic treatments can function as treatments (for bacterial infections) or placebos (for viral infections), so sugar pills and saline solutions can be treatments for some conditions and placebos for others. Dr. Osler's vitamin C is a placebo for pain but not for scurvy, sugar is a placebo for some things but not for diabetes, and even saline injections are good for treating unhealthy pressure in the skull.

The difference between pure and impure placebos is therefore probabilistic. Most things such as sugar pills or saline injections that are called pure placebos are placebos for most things. As a result, the surveys were mostly accurate. Still, it would be more accurate to say that what counts as a placebo is relative. Relative to a bacterial infection, antibiotics are not placebos, but relative to viral infections they are. Sugar pills are placebos relative to pain, but not to diabetes. Saying that what counts as a placebo depends on, or is relative to, a certain ailment avoids the need to use the incorrect pure/impure distinction.

A Definition of Placebos at Last

Love is an untamed force. When we try to control it, it destroys us. When we try t
imprison it, it enslaves us. When we try to understand it, it leaves us feeling lost
and confused.

    —PAOLO COELHO, *The Zahir: A Novel of Obsession*[31]

I began this chapter with examples of things I think most of us would
be happy to call placebos. Below are a few facts we can say about placebo treatments that will amount to a definition based on the true
stories of Jennifer and the Italian doctor, as well as the history and
usage of the concept.

1. *Placebos are inert, but only in a relative sense.* The core ingredient
   of Dr. Osler's placebo (vitamin C) was inert for Jane's pain. Yet,
   the very same vitamin C would not be inert for preventing or
   treating scurvy. The vitamin C is only a placebo *relative to* pain.
2. *The patient's knowledge is relevant.* If Dr. Osler had added vitamin C into Jane's food without Jane knowing, the vitamin C
   would not have reduced her pain. This is not true for things
   that are not placebos. If Dr. Osler had somehow given Jane a
   large dose of morphine without her knowing (say, by disguising
   it in her food), Jane's pain would have been reduced.
3. *Placebo treatments are complex.* Dr. Osler's vitamin C was large
   and white. It had other ingredients that made it bubble in
   water. It was not taken alone, but rather with water. On top of
   that, placebos have features like color, size, and perceived or
   actual cost. These other features can influence how people
   respond to them. Placebos also come in different forms including pills, injections, or surgical procedures. When the inert part
   of the placebo is combined with these additional ingredients
   (and other things like the doctor's words and manner), an effect
   can arise.
4. *Placebos are delivered in a social context that matters.* This context
   includes doctors who appear knowledgeable and authoritative,

after a greeting from a receptionist who was or wasn't friendly, and tests taken by a nurse who was or wasn't kind. Dr. Osler's treatment involved a ritual. He gave the patient the placebo cautiously, with tweezers. It came with concrete warnings ("this is a completely different sort of treatment") and instructions ("drink it carefully").

5. *The context (or environment) in which the placebo is administered matters.* No matter how eminent Dr. Osler appeared to Jane, his treatment might not have had the same effect if it had been given in a parking lot. It was given in a hospital in central London that has a heliport.

6. *Placebos are (potentially) beneficial.* Placebos that are harmful are called nocebos, so this is true by definition.

Combining these insights, I can now define placebos.

Placebos are complex treatments whose core components such as (part of) a pill, injection, or even surgical procedure are inert relative to the disorder but when given in a meaningful context can have a beneficial effect.

This definition avoids the problems with previous attempts, while capturing how it has been and is used correctly (fig. 2.1). However, in answering the question of what placebos are, I have raised two other questions. The first is, if the core ingredient of the placebo doesn't have an effect, why bother with it? Why not just have everything that surrounds the placebo—the meaningful context, the confident doctor with encouraging words? To use Plato's example, why not have the charm without the leaf? The answer is that we can and should. However, the placebo combined with everything else is probably more powerful. Placebos are complex treatments that include inert components that are intertwined with other features in meaningful contexts. Also, disentangling all the parts can be misleading (see part II).

A problem with my definition is that in defining placebos, I have used another word that is difficult to define: "meaning." If you ask

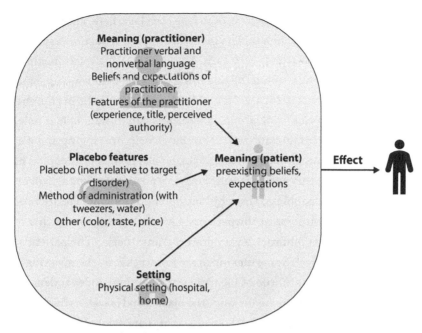

FIG. 2.1. How complex placebo treatments produce their effects

someone what something means, they usually understand what you mean. Outside academia, I'm not aware of anyone having asked, "What do you mean by mean?" This is because we all seem to know what meaning means . . . until we try to define it (try it yourself). To escape from the problem of defining meaning, some of my colleagues have suggested replacing "meaning" with "semiotic."[31] I don't think that is an advance, because the word "semiotic" is obtuse and includes meaning as part of its definition.

Instead of trying to define meaning, I'll recreate how Daniel Moerman (in my correspondence with him, based on his published works) describes it:

> Dr. Pavlov rings the bell then feeds the dog. The dog comes to know that when he hears the bell, he's likely to get some food. Simplifying, the bell means "food is coming; get ready to eat; salivate!" X means some sort of placeholder. Soft voices, champagne, candles, whispered "nothings"

often mean something like love, or maybe even love; here, meaning is rather vague. Little white tablets mean drugs/pain reduction/aspirin. We can learn these things very early. So, a meaning is a relationship between two things, where the one thing ("ringing bell") means something else, in the classic case, "food." But we also ring bells in churches to announce services, or the end of services, or that the couple is now married, or the infant baptized. "The church bells are ringing and it's Tuesday . . . someone must have just gotten married!" This hospital has three heliports; this means it *must* be a very powerful hospital, full of terrific doctors; people go there by helicopter all the time! We are now using fentanyl on some of the patients! I know that this means this patient might get fentanyl, a very powerful anesthetic. (The patient's response increases!) Some meanings are iconic: that is, the meaning is sort of built in. The Statue of Liberty means freedom, independence, autonomy. Black cloud means rain (the black cloud is water which will pour down on us as rain). Some meanings are symbolic, things like "love," "freedom," "happiness." The doctor's white coat means something like "clean, careful, scientist." Meaning is not inherent in things like pills: it is attributed to things by people. This explains why some studies suggest that blue pills seem to have a sedative effect on people . . . unless they are Italian men, in which case the color blue excites them (their football team wears blue).

So, despite the difficulty some people may have defining "meaning," I take meaning to be understandable. Therefore, my definition of placebos seems to be acceptable despite using the potentially vague term.

Nocebos

There are no atheists in foxholes.

—APHORISM

At least in modern Western medicine, there are no nocebos, only negative effects of placebos, which are called nocebo effects. Outside modern Western medicine, however, there are things that we might call "nocebos." These include black magic and voodoo curses. Larry Dossey reports how he and his doctor friend Bill treated a very sick patient in south Texas near the Mexican border, where hexing and spells were part of the culture. The patient revealed that he had recently visited a fortune teller who used nail clippings to reveal his future. When the man refused to pay, the fortune teller used the same nail clippings to hex him. The man knew he had been hexed and became melancholic and stopped eating. Nothing in the conventional medical arsenal seemed to help the poor man. They decided to set modern medicine aside and devised a ritual that he described as follows:

> We concocted an elaborate ritual in an attempt to save the man's life. Late one night, when the moon was full and the hospital wards were deserted, we rolled the victim in a wheelchair into a darkened examination room. Dressed in white coats in the near darkness, we stood silently for a long while, letting the tension build. Then Bill said to the man what we were about to do, assuring him that our magic was more powerful than that of the fortune teller who had cursed him. He then clipped a lock of the man's hair and stated that the hex would be reversed as he burned the hair in the small eerie flame we had made in an ash tray. He added, to my immense relief, that if the victim told anyone we had done this, the curse would return stronger than before. The man was terrified but visibly impressed. When the zany ritual was finished, we whisked him, trembling and speechless, to his bed. . . . The dehexing worked like a charm. The old man awoke the next morning feeling energetic, hungry, and happy, a victim no longer. He was eventually discharged from the hospital in perfect health.[33]

This story suggests that the nail clippings used by the fortune teller were a nocebo. Anecdotes similar to these are more common that you might imagine.[34] In 1929, John Blymyer fought with and killed a man called Nelson Rehmeyer in York, Pennsylvania. Rehmeyer was a renowned black magician who wanted to curse Blymyer. To perform the curse, he needed a lock of Blymyer's hair.[35] Blymyer was defending himself against an attempted curse. Many historical anecdotes describe voodoo curses that have killed people. The phenomenon is common enough to have a name: "psychogenic death."[36]

The exotic stories of voodoo-hexing nocebos may not be as distant from our modern sophisticated experience as we think. When I worked in Rio de Janeiro as a rowing coach, a close friend of mine was a medical student who would take every chance he had to make fun of people who believed in any alternative medicine, especially "macumba," which is a kind of magic practiced in Brazil. "It is so primitive," he would often say. Then, one afternoon we were walking along a very crowded street. Suddenly, we came to a place where the crowd parted, as if Moses himself was clearing space. I thought there must be a great hole in the pavement that people didn't want to fall into. But it wasn't that. It was what looked to me like chicken feathers tied up with a red string on the ground. As soon as my friend saw this he followed the others and made a wide berth around the feathers. I followed him, also making a wide berth. I asked him why people were avoiding the feathers.

"Macumba," he said, in a way that made me feel as if I should have already known.

I was a bit confused. "I thought you didn't believe in that," I said.

He muttered something in Brazilian Portuguese, claiming that it was hard to explain in English. I didn't believe him, because his English was fluent. Yet, secretly, I was happy that I had not accidentally stepped on or over the feathers. Most of us in developed countries are not familiar with the kinds of voodoo nocebos I've just described. However, nocebo effects are common.

Nocebo Effects are Serious and Common

Mr. A

Mr. A was in a clinical trial of a new antidepressant medication. He received a bottle of pills the day before and impulsively took all the remaining 29 pills. He immediately felt that he had made a mistake and asked his neighbor to take him to the hospital. He was very fearful that he would die of the overdose.

He arrived at the hospital saying, "Help me, I took all my pills," and then collapsed. As he fell, he dropped the empty prescription bottle. The doctors read the label, which confirmed it contained pills to be taken as part of a depression trial. But it did not say whether the capsules were the active medication or placebo. His blood pressure was dangerously low at 80/40 and his heart rate dangerously high (110). His breathing was rapid, and he was lethargic. Over four hours, he had to be given six liters of fluid to keep his blood pressure normal.

Then a physician from the clinical trial arrived and determined that Mr. A had taken placebos. When he was told that the pills were placebos, Mr. A expressed surprise then almost cried. Within 15 minutes, he was fully alert, with blood pressure and heart rate back to normal. Mr. A had not overdosed on a new antidepressant drug: he had overdosed on fear. The negative effect was a nocebo effect.[37]

Dramatic experiences like Mr. A's are rare, but less serious negative outcomes following negative expectations are increasingly recognised as common. The first mention of the nocebo-effect concept that I'm aware of appears in a short letter by W. P. Kennedy, published in 1961, titled "The Nocebo Reaction."[38] He chose "nocebo" because it is Latin for "I shall harm," which is the opposite of "placebo," meaning "I shall please." He was inspired by Henry Knowles Beecher, who found that patients who had taken placebos in clinical trials reported drowsiness, headache, nausea, and many other undesirable side effects. For the 30 years following Kennedy's letter, I found only 12 mentions of the word "nocebo" in the medical literature.

Now research on nocebos is blossoming. For example, some great colleagues and I did a megastudy of more than 250,000 patients like Mr. A who had taken placebos in clinical trials.[5] In clinical trials, patients usually don't know whether they are taking the placebo or the real treatment, so they think they might be taking the real drug. Half of them reported some negative side effect, such as diarrhea, rash, asthma, or headache. One in 20 of them had such bad side effects that they dropped out of the trial. These negative side effects were not all nocebo effects (more about measuring nocebo effects in chapter 5). But many of them were, and it's easy to see why. In clinical trials, researchers force people to "understand" everything bad that might happen to them. They make them read a piece of paper that lists all common and uncommon potential harms. Then patients have to sign it to prove that they are aware of all the potential risks. The pieces of paper sometimes do not mention potential benefits at all.[39] Good ethics requires that people know what they are getting into before they sign up for a trial. But this doesn't mean that we shouldn't be careful both to be honest and also to avoid unnecessarily scaring them.

If we read the small print on over-the-counter medications we can buy at the pharmacy, nocebo effects would be even more common. For example, most of us have taken acetaminophen (paracetamol), but we don't look at the paper that comes in the package. If we did, we would learn that acetaminophen might cause serious skin reactions (including fatal ones like toxic epidermal necrolysis), abnormal liver reactions, stomach bleeding, and increase the risk of asthma for children if taken by the mother while pregnant. If that's not enough to scare you, it can also cause stroke, heart attacks, and ulcers. Some readers will feel a bit anxious just reading about those side effects, even if they hadn't taken acetaminophen recently. At least some of the mild side-effects following COVID-19 vaccines were most likely nocebo effects,[40] and this may have contributed to vaccine hesitancy.[41]

The lock of hair, the bone, and the chicken feathers were what we might call nocebos. Nocebos are the same as placebos but have negative effects. Treatment with placebo involves giving a complex intervention such as a pill, injection, or even surgical procedure that is inert (relative to the disorder) on its own but when given with other components in a meaningful context, can have a beneficial effect. When the effect is harmful, it is called a nocebo effect.

CHAPTER 3

Placebo Components and Meaningful Contexts

What Makes Inert Things Effective

In my practice, when I'm working with the patient, I am very careful of what I say, because any negative words could hurt the patient. So, with Western medicine, a doctor could be treating a patient, and he can mention death, and that is sharper than any needle. Therefore, with the tongue that we have, we have to be very careful of what we say at the time and point we're treating the patient.
—LARRY DOSSEY, *Be Careful What You Pray For*[1]

Sopa de Pedra

When combined with other "ingredients" in a meaningful context, inert things mixed can have effects. Consider the story of *sopa de pedra*, or stone soup. The people of Almeirim in Portugal tell the story of a poor monk who many centuries ago passed through the village on a pilgrimage. As was customary at the time, he knocked on someone's door to ask for a place to stay and a meal. The family said he could stay the night. But they were poor and said that they didn't have any food to spare.

"I don't need your food. I will be making a delicious and filling . . . stone soup."

With arched eyebrows and curious looks, the family invited him in, and gave him a large pot full of water and pointed him toward the fire where he could prepare his meal. The monk crouched down next to the pot and slowly reached into his pocket, from which he produced a smooth stone. He dropped the stone into the water and proceeded to watch his "soup" cook. After some time, he took a small sip of the soup with a spoon, licked his lips and said, "It's coming along, but it could use some seasoning." The wife brought him some salt. After watching the soup cook for a few more minutes, he tasted it again, pondered, and said that maybe some scraps of meat they had lying around, like pork belly or a bone, might be better than the salt. The wife graciously obliged and gave him a bone. The monk repeated his ritual of waiting, tasting and pondering, and this time he said that the soup might need something to enrich it, such as leftover potatoes or beans from a previous meal. The wife obliged again and added their leftover beans and potatoes. This continued for a few more rounds before the monk announced that his stone soup was finally ready. They all enjoyed the delicious soup. At the end, the monk reached into the pot to get the stone, washed it off, and put it into his pocket for next time.

We can draw many different messages from the story of stone soup. A simple one is that the poor monk was deceptive. A puritan might even say that he was breaking the ninth commandment, forbidding him to lie. After all, he said it was *stone* soup, and it wasn't (just) stone soup. I think that is too simplistic. The monk wasn't hiding what he was doing; he was doing it in plain sight. In that sense, he wasn't being deceptive. Also, the monk's stone may have had iron in it, which it which actually enriched the soup with important nutrients. Moreover, the ritual of boiling the soup and creating the suspense would have made it taste better (did your mouth water as much as mine as you read the story?). Since mouth-watering is a sign of an active digestive system, the way in which the monk prepared the soup may might have improved the ingested nutritional value of the soup.

Meaningful contexts, or meaningful features of interventions can have effects on their own, and when they are combined with placebos, they probably have even greater effects. The effects can be positive (placebo effects) or negative (nocebo effects). In the rest of this chapter I'll list many of the important meaningful features and contexts that combine with placebos to produce effects.

Placebo Features

Stephen Maturin [made] his medicines more revolting in taste, smell, and texture than any others in the fleet; and he found it answered—his hardy patients knew with their entire beings that they were being physicked.

　—PATRICK O'BRIAN, *Master and Commander*[2]

Saying a placebo is a sugar pill (which usually means a lactose pill) is incomplete and wrong. Placebos have colors, tastes, and smells; they can be expensive or cheap; they can be invasive or not; they can be given by caring or cold practitioners; and they can be delivered in a calm environment or in a hectic hospital. All of these things can influence whether they have a positive or negative effect. The idea that illness and healing in general involve a broad spectrum of factors beyond the simple biomedical ones is not new. In 1977 George Engel proposed the biopsychosocial model of illness (it has since morphed into psychoneuroendocrinoimmunology).[3] Placebo research demonstrates the role of psychological and social factors involved in illness and healing very clearly because the simpler biomedical approach has trouble explaining how placebo effects arise.

Color and Size

Studies suggest that for most patients, pink tablets produce a greater stimulating effect than blue ones,[4,5] with the possible exception that blue tablets seem to stimulate Italian men. For Italian women, blue is the color of the dress of the Virgin Mary (a calm, protective figure). By contrast, for Italian men, blue is the color of their successful national soccer team. For the men, blue means victory and excitement.[6]

Good Branding

A study of 835 women published in 1981 compared the effect of branding on both placebos and painkilling drugs.[7] The placebos and drugs were labeled with a known brand or simply as analgesic tablets. The branded placebos had a greater effect than unbranded placebos. In a more recent study published in 2008, different price tags were placed on the very same placebo pills ($0.10 and $2.50). The "expensive" pills performed better at reducing pain than the "cheaper" pills.[8]

The Wrong Branding Can Induce Nocebo Effects

In 2017 patients on a branded antidepressant called venlafaxine (brand name "Effexor") were switched to a new generic formulation (Enlafax). Other than the fact that it is much cheaper, the generic version is identical to the branded one except for . . . the brand. In 2018 two major media outlets in New Zealand ran stories alleging that the new generic drug was less effective and more harmful. A group of researchers tracked side-effect reports and found that the stories about side effects, including serious side effects such as suicidal thoughts, increased following the news stories.[9] The same group of researchers also surveyed the patients and reported that it wasn't just the news stories which caused the nocebo effects; it was also trust in the brand.[10] The branded version of the drug did not seem to cause as many negative side effects.

Biosimilar drugs are like generics in that they are similar to the patented and approved version of the drugs; unlike generic drugs, however, they are not identical. They can be a bit better or a bit worse, and they are almost always cheaper (being cheaper is the point). Nonetheless, a review published in 2019 found that rates of discontinuation and negative side effects were higher in biosimilars than in branded drugs.[11]

The effect of branding should not be surprising given that more money is spent on marketing and branding than on developing drugs. The reason pharmaceutical companies spend so much money on branding is that it works. For example, the company that developed the antidepressant fluoxetine chose the name Prozac. The name is completely unrelated to the characteristic chemical compound that was supposed to be responsible for the antidepressant effect, whereas before Prozac, drug names were often related to the characteristic chemical. The name was proposed by a marketing company called Interbrand. Apparently, the first three letters, *pro,* were chosen because it sounds professional. The last two letters, *ac,* makes people think about being active, and the *z* in the middle just sounds powerful.[12]

The science of placebos and nocebos can help overcome these problematic responses to generics and biosimilars and save taxpayers a lot of money. In one study, 96 patients who were eligible to switch to a cheaper biosimilar were either given a positive message about the drugs being helpful and effective or not. Those given the positive message were more likely to be willing to switch to the biosimilar.[13]

Even labeling someone with a diagnosis (such as diabetes or autism spectrum disorder) can have an effect that is independent of the disease itself. A review of 146 studies found that the diagnostic label could lead to positive or negative expectations, different levels of support, different plans for the future, and different behavior. All of these could impact the course of whatever disease they had independently of the actual disease and were caused by words. The words used by diagnostic labels need to be chosen carefully to maximize their health-enhancing potential rather than inducing unnecessary nocebo effects.[14]

Size and Invasiveness

The bigger and more invasive the placebo, the more effective it seems to be. Following on their research on the effect of color, L. W. Buckalew and Sherman Ross investigated the effect of size and found that larger capsules have greater effects than smaller ones.[15] Other studies show that two placebos are more effective than one,[16] and a systematic review with data from 3,325 patients found that taking placebo pills four times per day was slightly more effective than taking two placebos per day.[17] The relationship between pill size and quantity is probably more complex than the simple "more and bigger is better." I was told a story about an unpublished experiment that might have been conducted without ethical approval. In the experiment, students were shown pills of different sizes and asked to rate how effective they believed the pills were. Apparently both the large pills and the tiny pills were rated as the most effective. Presumably the large pills were thought to be more effective because they must have lots of medicine in them. The small ones? Perhaps they were so powerful that they could only be given in small doses. Also, while two pills are believed to be more powerful than one, six pills could be worse than one. If the medicine is so powerful, why would I have to take six?

Invasiveness also matters. A megastudy of 22 trials that was published in 2000 compared the effects of placebo pills and placebo injections for migraines. It found that 25.7% (222 of 865 patients) given pills reported almost complete recovery after two hours, yet 32.4% (279 of 862 patients) receiving placebo injections recovered.[18] Other researchers have replicated this and found that placebo injections are more powerful than placebo pills.[18-21] A meta-analysis with 79 trials conducted by Karen Meissner and colleagues showed that sham acupuncture is more effective than placebo pills.[22] Sham surgery is the most invasive and most powerful so-called placebo of all, but it might not be a placebo (see chapter 11).[23]

Communication

Pleasant words are as a honeycomb, sweet to the soul, and health to the bones.
　　—Proverbs 16:24

Verbal and body language matter. For centuries before the dawn of modern medicine, the way in which practitioners communicated was called "bedside manner." Doctors would visit sick patients at home, often sitting at their bedside. The doctor described by Pierce in chapter 2, for example, was found to be "lolling on the bedstead." Nowadays health care practitioners are unlikely to visit patients or sit at their bedsides. In hospitals it might be more common, although the need for the "commit to sit" initiative at a Texas hospital suggests that patients would like practitioners to sit down more often than they currently do.[24] Other forms of body language have also been shown to make a difference, especially looking someone in the eyes and touching.[25.]

Empathy and Understanding

The commitment to good "bedside manner" has been replaced by other initiatives, including Schwartz rounds (addressing patients' emotional and social needs),[26] the Balint method (a method to improve communication with patients),[27] compassionate care,[28] person-centered care,[29] and empathic care.[30] These all differ yet also share the idea that practitioners' verbal and body language matter. I'll limit my remarks to empathic care here because it's what I have studied most and because a number of randomized trials have shown that practitioner empathy improves patient outcomes. Yet most of what I say here and elsewhere about empathy applies to other related aspects of patient-doctor communication.

The term "empathy" was initially used to describe a relationship between an observer and an object such as a painting.[31] More recently, it has been adapted for a clinical setting and is characterized as understanding, communicating this understanding, and therapeutic or caring action.[32] There is an ongoing debate about how therapeutic empathy—specifically understanding—can be achieved, and whether it can be taught. I have discussed these interesting questions elsewhere,[33] and refer readers to Jodi Halpern's wonderful book on the topic.[34] Very briefly, empathic understanding does not require you to completely understand, let alone experience, another's emotions or thoughts. Rather, it requires "emotional curiosity," which involves trying to get a grasp on the patient's inner world by asking questions such as "tell me what I'm missing," and creating a shared space for the patient and doctor to discover the best path of action. Another myth is that empathy can't be taught, with some saying either you have it or you don't. Certainly, people have different baseline abilities to be empathic with others, just like people have different baseline driving abilities. Those who are already amazing at empathy can't be taught much by definition, and those who are bad at it (or don't believe it is important) might be challenging to teach. However, most people are neither exceptionally good nor exceptionally bad at empathy, and many rigorous trials demonstrate that it can be taught.[35]

Not only can empathy be taught, but teaching empathy to doctors improves patient outcomes.[36] Trials that show this involves training one group of practitioners to enhance the way they express empathy and leaving the other group to carry on as usual, without the training. Then, both groups of practitioners treat patients, often with pain-related conditions. Then the improvement in patients treated by practitioners who were trained to enhance empathy is compared with improvements in patients treated by doctors who were not.

In one such trial, Olivier Chassany and colleagues trained 84 general practitioners to enhance the way they expressed empathy.[37] As a control group, they enrolled an additional 96 general practitioners to take part in the study but not be trained. The training involved a four-hour workshop that focused on patient-practitioner communication, evaluating pain, and negotiating a therapeutic contract with a patient. Practitioners in the control group attended a workshop of the same length but that covered recruitment and informed consent in clinical trials. The trained group then treated 414 patients with osteoarthritis, and the untrained group treated 428 patients. They measured the pain of the patients in both groups using a scale ranging from 0 (no pain) to 100 (unbearable pain). Over a two-week period, patients in the trained group had better overall pain relief. I have systematically searched for and analyzed randomized clinical trials like Chassany's, and all but one of them show similar, modest, benefits for patients.

Enhanced empathic care does many other good things beyond improving patient outcomes. Empathic communication is likely to improve medication adherence.[38] Medication adherence, in turn, predicts outcomes in clinical trials whether patients take the placebo or the "real" drug.[39] Empathic care can also lead to better choice of treatment. If patients don't feel that the practitioner is empathic, they may not share the extent of their symptoms or the cause (say they caught a sexually transmitted disease because of an affair), which will make it more difficult for the practitioner to make a diagnosis or recommend a cure. In one more true dramatic case, in 1998 my colleagues reported the death of a woman from smoking-related lung disease.[40] The woman had refused to engage with the health care profession due to what she perceived as a lack of empathy. Whenever she visited her doctors, she claimed that they were very judgmental of her smoking habits. My colleagues believe that had the health care practitioners been more empathic, the woman could have been saved. Finally, practitioners who enhance their empathy are better at putting patients at ease.[41,42] Lowered anxiety, in turn, reduces pain and depression.[43]

Continuity of Care

Communication is easier if you know someone better. When I was a child, I had the same doctor, a pediatrician, until I was a teenager. His name was Dr. Elder, and I can still see his bubbly receptionist's smile. His office was close to where we lived, and he had to walk past our busy street on his way home. People would say hello. When I was a teenager, he even hired me to shovel the snow from the steps in front of his office for a few winters. Now, things are different. I'm registered with a practice, so if I make an appointment, it is not with a specific doctor but with the practice. I see whoever is available on that day. Because I rarely go to the doctor's, it is often the first time we've met, so they have no idea who I am, what I do, or what my hobbies and habits are. It may be easier from a scheduling perspective not to assign individual doctors to individual patients (although I have not seen any evidence to prove this). But the doctor who has never seen me before will have less background information about me, which could be useful for making the right diagnosis and choosing the right treatment. In general, meeting any new person is anxiety-provoking compared with a familiar face and smile. The small talk that might arise with a doctor who knew me (how are your kids/your work/your yoga . . . ?) would make me feel more relaxed. But the continuity of care doesn't just make people feel better in a fuzzy way. A major study showed that having the same doctor over time leads to people living longer.[44] This is probably because knowing someone over time leads to more effective communication, better understanding, more accurate diagnoses, and therefore better, more person-centered treatments.

Positive Words

Positive language also helps. An early trial showing this was inspired by my late friend and colleague George Lewith. George was known for being very empathic and positive with his patients. His colleague Bruce Thomas accused him of wasting time, saying that all the time George spent being empathic and positive might brighten things up a bit, but it didn't really help patients. George challenged Bruce to test his skepticism in a controlled trial. Bruce agreed, hoping to finally prove that George was wasting his time with all that empathy and positivity. For his trial, Dr. Thomas first took some cards and wrote "positive" on half and "negative" on the other half. He then shuffled them up and put them in his drawer. When patients came in, he first checked to see whether they needed urgent care. If so, he gave it to them. If not, he opened his drawer and pulled out a card. If the card had "positive" written on it, he would be more friendly and give them a positive message, saying things like: "you will probably feel much better soon." If the card was negative, he would be his usual grumpy self and say things like, "I'm not sure if you are going to feel better soon." After treating 100 patients with each communication style, he couldn't deny the results. Almost twice as many patients who got positive communication reported getting better compared to patients who got his usual grumpy style (64% versus 39%). He reported his findings in the *BMJ* in a 1987 article titled "Is There Any Point in Being Positive?"[45] Dr. Thomas was not blinded, and the outcome was his patients' self-reported feelings rather than a hard outcome. However, numerous higher-quality studies have subsequently been conducted. I've searched for and identified 22 trials like Bruce Thomas's, many of which had more objective outcomes. It turns out that when doctors use positive language, it can improve patients' lung function, reduce the time they spend in hospital, and lower the amount of morphine they need to reduce their pain.[36] In practice, empathy and positivity are probably combined. A doctor who is empathic will be able to deliver a more believable positive message.[46]

Negative Words

The opposite happens when doctors use negative words. This has been demonstrated in studies of positive and negative framing. In one recent example, 203 healthy adult volunteers were each given a placebo pill described as "a well-known tablet available without prescription." They were randomized to receive information presented in one of two ways. Some were told that side effects were common, affecting 1 in 10 people. The side-effect rates were "positively framed" to the others, who were told that the side effects were uncommon and that 90% of people would not be affected. Those who received the positively framed information reported slightly fewer side effects.[47] A related study published in 2003 looked at what happened to patients who were each hooked up to an intravenous line that was supplying painkilling morphine. When the doctors stopped the morphine, they only told some of the patients. The patients who were told the morphine would stop had a faster onset of pain.[48] Other studies have reported similar findings.[49]

Confidence and Trust

Patients will be more likely to believe a doctor's (positive or negative) words if they trust them. The practitioner's clothing, title, and perceived authority can all affect how empathic they are perceived to be and how believable their messages are.[50] Dr. Osler was a senior clinician. Dr. Placebo had long curls and prepared his drops very carefully (demonstrating how skilled he was). An authoritative and confident manner can make a positive message more believable. Experiments have confirmed that trust increases oxytocin levels, which can make people feel better (see chapter 6).[8] Trust is a double-edged sword, however. A negative message from a trusted doctor will also be more believable, and therefore more damaging.

Time

Empathic communication can be more effective if practitioners take more time with patients. In 2008 Ted Kaptchuk and colleagues published a trial reporting what happened to patients with irritable bowel syndrome who received either a longer (45 minute) or a limited (5 minute) consultation.[51] Both groups also received the same sham acupuncture treatment in addition to the consultations. The longer consultation included discussions about the "cause" and "meaning" of the condition, expressions of understanding, therapeutic touch, and positive messages. Sixty-two percent of the patients in the longer consultation group reported adequate relief, compared with 44% in the limited group. Expressing empathy need not take much more time, however. Other studies have shown that a minute or so will do.[52,53]

Setting and Environment

Placebo treatment effects change depending on the setting and circumstances. Toward the end of World War II, the Allies stormed the beach at Anzio—a marsh—by surprise. However, the Allies didn't capitalize on the surprise and were quickly surrounded by Germans, who were on higher ground and started picking the Allied soldiers off. The Germans also stopped the drainage pumps so that the marsh became flooded with salt water, hoping an epidemic would weaken their opponents. This brutal situation lasted a month, until the Germans retreated to Rome. In 1956, Henry Knowles Beecher published a paper in which he compared soldiers who were injured at and evacuated from Anzio with civilians who had similar wounds.[54] He found that 90% of civilians asked for a narcotic to reduce pain after an operation, but only about a quarter of soldiers at the Anzio beachhead who had similar operations required drugs. Beecher explains this difference by referring to "what the pain means to the patient."[54] To the soldiers, serious injury and the operations meant escape from the brutal and deadly Anzio beachhead. They were so relieved that the pain did not mean that much. The civilians, on the other hand, had no such comfort.

There are less dramatic examples than the one involving injured soldiers. A study published in 2000 found that taking a placebo in a hospital can have a greater effect than taking it at home. In the study, 216 out of 673 patients (32%) given a placebo in a hospital reported recovering from their headaches within two hours, whereas 285 (of 1,054) patients (27%) receiving placebos at home reported that their headaches had gone away within two hours.[22] Presumably, the more serious hospital setting and the treatment being administered by hospital staff led to greater expectations of recovery than self-administration at home.

Even within the same hospital or home, the décor can have an effect. Having a window in a hospital room seems to speed up recovery from surgery,[55] waiting rooms that are in gardens lower doctor stress,[56] and people who live in "green" areas recover faster from surgery.[57] Sometimes, just having "green-ness" in the imagination can help. A randomized control trial of 46 healthy volunteers found that participants who had just watched a video of a natural scene had a significantly higher pain threshold and tolerance than participants who had watched a blank screen.[58] A related trial of adults undergoing a painful procedure called bronchoscopy (putting a tube down the throat into the lungs) found that participants who viewed a natural scene reported significantly less pain.[59]

The evidence in this area does not always point in the same direction. One trial of physiotherapy for middle-aged patients with osteoarthritis compared an "enhanced environment" with a "standard environment." The enhanced environment was on the second-floor room of a new building with nice views, pictures of landscapes, and rubberized floors. The standard room was in the basement of an older building. It had wooden floors, no windows, and looked generally worn. Contrary to the researchers' hypothesis, the outcomes were slightly worse in the enhanced environment. Qualitative interviews suggested that the patients felt more "at home" in the standard environment.[60] This suggests that the enhancements of the environment need to be relevant to patients in order to enhance recovery. On balance, however, enhanced environments seem to promote healing. A summary of the studies in this area published in 2018 found that healing environments—those that contain windows, pleasant music, good temperature and air quality—can reduce pain, risk of infection, stress, depression, length of stay in hospital, and mortality.[61]

I'm unaware of studies that link physical surroundings to nocebo effects, but I've witnessed them myself. I spent a night in the hospital with my mother when she was being treated for cancer, and it was unpleasant. There were sounds of agony, beeping, and emergency alarms. At the very least it disturbed sleep, and it doesn't take a rocket scientist to figure out that a good night's sleep is needed for good health, recovery, happiness, and wellbeing.

Beliefs
Patient Beliefs

Patients visit their doctors with different beliefs about what good doctors look and sound like, what kind of environment makes them feel relaxed, and how much they expect medical treatments to make them better. Most people appreciate a bit of extra time with the doctor, but some might think that if the doctor can't make up their mind quickly, they don't know what they are doing. A confident, authoritative doctor makes many people feel like they are in safe hands, but skeptics may have a negative reaction to authority. No single recipe will benefit all patients. This is why Andrew Herxheimer and D. Mark Chaput de Saintonge say that doctors need to take a "placebo history" to find out how patients have reacted to treatments and doctors in the past.

The history can help the doctor moderate their behavior and treatments to maximize the benefit to the patients.

Certainly, beliefs about how effective medical treatments are can often affect how effective they are. Andreas Eklund and colleagues examined 593 patients from a clinical trial for a chiropractic treatment of lower back pain.[62] They divided the patients into those that had high expectations of improvement and those that had low expectations. They found that patients with a higher expectation had a 58% greater chance of reporting an improvement.[62] Other trials have manipulated the beliefs and expectations of patients, usually by having health care professionals deliver positive messages.[33] A recent example was the PSY-HEART trial conducted by Winfried Rief and colleagues in Germany.[63] They randomized patients who were scheduled to undergo coronary artery bypass surgery into three groups: usual care, "support," and "expect." Patients in the "support" group received additional psychological support but were not encouraged to have positive expectations about a fast recovery. Patients in the "expect" group. were encouraged to develop personal ideas and images about their future after surgery, including plans about activities and how they might enjoy their life afterward."[63] Compared with usual care, the expect group had better function, less anxiety, and higher quality of life, and they went back to work sooner. The average improved functioning in the group that was encouraged to think positively about recovery was about 20%, whereas the control group had a reduction in disability of about 10%. The "expect" group also had more robust immune systems, shown by decreased interleukin-8 levels (a marker of inflammation) in their blood after surgery.

Negative Beliefs

Prior beliefs can also lead to negative effects. Patients might have learned to fear people wearing white coats, needles, or hospitals. For example, they might believe (consciously or subconsciously) that needles are for addicts. The mere sight of a needle could cause anxiety and nausea. No matter how beneficial the substance in the needle is, they might experience a negative side effect—a nocebo effect—because of their beliefs about needles.

Doctors' Beliefs

Doctors, nurses, and physiotherapists also have expectations that can influence whether a treatment works. A classic, nonmedical example demonstrating this is the "Pygmalion experiment," carried out in the 1960s. Pygmalion was a Greek artist who sculpted a statue out of ivory. He fell in love with the statue, and through his love and attention the statue came to life. That story is a myth of course.

In a real public (state-funded) elementary school that Robert Rosenthal and Lenore Jacobson call the "Oak School" (the real name is withheld), experimenters administered the "Harvard Test of Inflected Acquisition" to all (over 500) students in grades 1 to 5. Teachers were told that the test "predicts the likelihood that a child will show an inflection point or "spurt" (improve rapidly) within the near future."[64] Then the teachers were given names of the students who were most likely to "spurt." Rosenthal and Jacobson said that the teachers might like to keep an eye out for the children who were about to bloom. They were also cautioned not to discuss the test findings with their pupils or the children's parents.

At the end of the year, they tested the students again. It turned out that the "spurters" improved more than the others. The top 20% of the students named by the test improved in English and math, and teachers reported that their behavior improved more than that of the "nonspurters."

The problem was that there was no such thing as the "Harvard Test of Inflected Acquisition." The test they gave at the beginning and at the end was the standard IQ test, and the 20% of students who were predicted to "spurt" were chosen at random. (Aside: this experiment also shows how bad the IQ test is as a test of "innate" intelligence. The

IQ test is supposed to be independent of the environment and teachers' beliefs.)

The Oak School experiment suggests that teachers' expectations can have objective effects on student performance. More generally, it suggests that "one person's expectation for another person's behavior can quite unwittingly become a more accurate prediction simply for its having been made."[64] The mechanism of Pygmalion effects is not mysterious. A teacher, believing that a student was ready to "spurt" might pay special attention to that student which could easily translate into accelerated rates of improvement, whereas a "nonspurter" who didn't do that well might be ignored: they weren't going to spurt anyway.

Patients who have doctors that believe in the treatments they give have better outcomes. In one study that was published in 1985, 60 patients who just had their molars removed were divided into two groups.[65] The first group were given one of three injections: placebo (saline solution), naloxone (an opioid antagonist), or fentanyl (a powerful painkiller). The injections were all blinded so patients didn't know which was which. These patients were told that the injection would make their pain get better, worse, or stay the same. The second group were also told that the injection would make their pain get better, worse, or stay the same. However, the second group were given one of two treatments: placebo injection or naloxone. That is, the second group was given a placebo or something that would make the pain get worse, and no powerful painkiller.

Patients in the first group who took placebos had four times greater reduction in pain than the patients in the second group who had the same placebos. How could this be? The patients' beliefs were all the same: they were told the same thing about the treatments. The difference was that the doctors knew that the first group might receive a powerful painkiller and that the second group would not. It seems that the doctors gave the patients in the first group more optimistic messages. Recent studies conducted by a lab at Dartmouth College replicated this finding and called the phenomenon of placebo effects transmitted from the doctor to the patient "socially transmitted placebo effects."[66] It seems that when doctors don't believe that a treatment will help, it may not help as much, and if they believe it will harm, it might cause more harm.

Placebo Effects of Active Treatments

Even if a treatment is not a placebo, its effects are often partly placebo effects. For example, the morphine in one of Fabrizio Benedetti's studies was more powerful when patients were told by hospital doctors that the painkiller was powerful.[48] Calling that additional effect a placebo effect might seem odd because there is no placebo. But in reality, nonplacebo treatments are part placebo. For example, when you inject morphine, it's not pure morphine. If it's injected, it contains, in addition to the morphine itself, edetate disodium and citric acid (two preservatives). Manufacturers call these ingredients "inactive," which is true only with respect to pain. If morphine comes in pill form, the pill has additives like cetostearyl alcohol, hydroxyethyl cellulose, hypromellose, magnesium stearate, polyethylene glycol, talc, and titanium dioxide. These additives are used to bulk up the pill, make it taste okay, coat it so it goes down easier, and hold it together. They are also only "inactive" with respect to pain. Hypromellose is used to bulk up the pills, but it is also used in eye drops; magnesium stearate can be used as a laxative; polyethylene glycol is used as a skin cream and used in printer ink; talc is a food additive; and titanium dioxide is a pigment and used in varnishes. Depending on the dose, pills include other ingredients besides.[67] Many of these other things that accompany the drugs like morphine are the placebo part of the treatment. The placebo part of the treatment, together with the meaningful context and the drug itself, are responsible as a whole for the treatment effect. This is an important point because it means that the research on placebos applies to *all* treatments, and can be used to enhance the benefits of all treatments. For similar reasons, failure to pay attention to the placebo part of the treatment can lead to unintended nocebo effects that can be avoided.

Side Effects of Placebo and Nocebo Treatments for Practitioners

When doctors take more time to induce placebo effects in patients, it benefits them as well by reducing burnout.[68] Doctor burnout has been called a global crisis that affects about half of medical practitioners, sometimes leading to suicide.[69,70] Not only is it bad for the practitioners, but a study published in 2008 found that burned-out doctors are six times more likely to make errors.[71] Many of those who are not taking time off due to burnout or getting seriously ill are leaving the profession to work elsewhere. Losing doctors isn't just bad for patients; it's bad for governments and universities that invest thousands of dollars in medical students' education.[69,72]

Placebo Effects without Placebo

To revisit a question from last chapter: If positive language, warm atmosphere, high price tag and everything surrounding the sugar pill placebo works, why bother with the sugar pill placebo at all? The answer is that we can and should use all those other things without placebos. However, we can't assume that the placebo effect will be as strong without the relatively inert pill, injection, or procedure (I explain why in chapter 7).

Relatedly, if we can have placebo effects without placebos, why should we call them placebo effects? This question has led some to suggest replacing the term "placebo effect" with "context effect" or "meaning response." There is nothing wrong with using those other terms, but I don't believe that either term (or any other related one I've seen) works. Consider this passage in which Zelda Di Blasi and colleagues promote using "context effects," instead of "placebo effects." They state: "Such debates [about placebo effects] are understandable given the conceptual and operational difficulties associated with the term 'placebo effect.' In this study, we use the neutral and broader term 'context effects' to refer to placebo effects deriving from patient-practitioner relationships."[72] But if "context effect" is intended to replace "placebo effect," and the definition of "context effect" includes the word "placebo," we end up running in circles. Another problem is that the authors don't account for the additional effect of placebo treatments (like sugar pills) over and above the context effect. So, while contexts are important, the term "context effect" just won't do as a replacement for placebo effect.

Daniel Moerman proposes that we replace "placebo effects" with "meaning responses." He claims that it is *just* the meaning which has the effect and defines the meaning response as "the psychological and physiological effects of meaning in the treatment of illness."[74] I like Moerman's project and adopt many of his views in this book, but I'm not sure that it is just the meaning that is responsible for the response. If a pill is large and blue and expensive and has an effect, it's not just the meaningful features of the pill that have the effect: it's the meaningful features combined with the actual pill that has the effect in the same way that the stone soup without the stone wouldn't be quite the same.

Also, the effects of other features of placebo treatments and meaningful contexts are still referred to as "placebo effects" by most people who have studied them.[75] This is a good reason to keep calling them placebo effects even if placebos are not used. It is okay to replace commonly used terms. But replacing a commonly used term with an equally confusing but less commonly used term is not an advance.

CHAPTER 4

It Depends

The Relativity of Placebos and Nocebos in Clinical Trials

In modern medical research placebos constitute an important methodological tool.
   —ANTON DE CRAEN ET AL. "Placebo and Placebo Effects in Medicine:
Historical Overview"[1]

Placebo Controls as the Standard for Proving Treatments Work (or Don't)

For doctors treating patients in the real world, placebo effects are a good thing. In clinical trials they are treated as just the opposite. In trials, placebo controls are considered to be a nuisance that must be tamed. Placebo-controlled trials, in which a new treatment is compared with a placebo control lie at the heart of modern medicine. Every time your doctor tells you that the drug you take is "proven" to work, they mean it's proven to work better than a placebo control. Every time you pay for a medical treatment (either out of your pocket, through insurance premiums, or taxes), you are paying for something that is supposed to be proven to work . . . better than a placebo control. If a treatment proves to be better than a placebo control, then it is believed to work.[2,3] The opposite is also true: treatments that fail to outperform placebo controls are usually deemed to be useless. (Note that a treatment can prove that it is superior to a placebo indirectly, by demonstrating it is at least as good as another treatment that has proved to be superior to a placebo control.)

Because placebo-controlled trials play such a central role in modern medicine, it is very worrying that the placebo controls used in trials are often inappropriate. Mistaken placebo controls then lead to unfair comparisons and mistaken estimates of the benefits and harms of active treatments.

Digested History of Placebo Controls

Placebo controls and blinding were initially introduced to evaluate what we might now call alternative medicine. The earliest example of a placebo-controlled trial I'm aware of that was not done to debunk or defend what we now would call complementary or alternative medicine is Austin Flint's 1863 trial of 13 people to whom he gave highly diluted "tincture of quissia" (an herb) for treating rheumatism, or joint pain.[4] He found that this placebo control had the same effect as drugs commonly used at the time. Another early example involved a trial of a dubious medical device. In the late eighteenth century, an American doctor, Elisha Perkins, claimed to be able to direct pathogenic "electric" fluid away from the body by using two metal rods. He received the first medical patent issued under the Constitution of the United States for his device in 1796. What became known as Perkins Tractors were very popular in America, and even George Washington is said to have bought a set.[5] They reached Britain in 1799 and became fashionable immediately, especially in Bath, where Dr. John Haygarth was based. Haygarth thought the tractors were a quack remedy and proposed to test their effects in a placebo-controlled trial (although he did not describe it as such).[6] Haygarth designed tractors made of wood, which doesn't conduct electricity, and painted to appear identical to Perkins's metal tractors. He and his colleagues then tested metal tractors on five patients who were in pain. Four out of five reported that their pain had subsided. The next day, they treated five similar patients with the wooden tractors, and again, four out of five reported that their pain subsided. Because the fake tractors worked as well as the real ones, Haygarth and his skeptical friends concluded that the Perkins Tractors did not work.

With contemporary knowledge of methodology, it's easy to poke holes in Haygarth's test. It was very small, the doctors were not blinded, and nothing close to randomization was used. But Haygarth didn't know what we know today about large randomized trials, and his experiment was both pioneering and rigorous by the standards at the time.

What's remarkable is that Haygarth's trial didn't show that the tractors didn't help people, but rather that they didn't help people more than fake tractors. In fact, the success rate of both the fake and the real tractors was 80%, which is very high. After Haygarth, several other doctors investigated whether the fake tractors worked, and they did. Hospital doctors used tractors made of wood, wax, bone, and all of them led to apparently rather dramatic effects.[6] Robert Thomas, age 43, had such bad rheumatoid arthritis that he could not use his arm; fake tractors cured him. Thomas Ellis could not walk without support; fake tractors cured him too. James Prior was paralyzed in both hands; fake tractors cured one of them.

The fact that the fake tractors seemed to work presents a bit of a paradox. On the one hand, they showed that the theory related to electricity could not possibly be true. On the other, the fact that they seemed to produce quite strong effects in many people suggests that both the real and fake tractors worked. Haygarth was aware of this paradox and claimed that it was *faith* in the tractors (fake or real) that caused them to work. He said: "I have long been aware of the great importance of medical faith. Daily experience has constantly confirmed and increased my opinion of its efficacy."

Other early examples of placebo controls tested the effects of homeopathy tablets compared with bread pills. In one of these, the homeopathy outperformed placebos;[7] in another, the patients in untreated groups fared better than those who received both homeopathy and allopathy;[8] and in a number of others homeopathy did not outperform placebo controls.[9,10] By the middle of the twentieth century, placebo-controlled trials were prevalent enough for Henry Knowles Beecher to produce one of the earliest examples of a systematic review of their effects (more about this in chapter 6). (Aside: the fact that one of the earliest examples of a systematic review was related to placebo research is one example of how placebos have played a central role in the development of evidence-based medicine methodology.)

Misleading Placebo-Control Treatments

If I'm doing a placebo-controlled trial of fluoxetine hydrochloride (the main ingredient in Prozac), then the placebo pills must be the same size, taste, and smell as the "real" fluoxetine hydrochloride pills but not contain any fluoxetine hydrochloride. As simple as this sounds, it is often not achieved, and there are no enforced standards to help ensure that it is. Extensive research has identified that the components of placebo treatments are rarely described, and, when they are, their components are often both surprising and clearly lead to mistaken estimates of benefits or harms.[11-13]

Here is another example. In some COVID-19 vaccine trials, participants in the control group (the group receiving a placebo) were injected with a saline solution. In other trials, they received an actual treatment. For example, for the COVID-19 vaccine developed by the University of Oxford, the control group received a meningitis and septicemia vaccine as a placebo.[14] The good thing about using an actual vaccine as the placebo control is that it will cause a reaction, such as muscle pain and soreness, at the site of the injection similar to that of the COVID-19 vaccine. This prevents most patients from guessing correctly whether they are getting the placebo or the real treatment. The scientific term for hiding knowledge of who received what treatment is "blinding." Blinding is often important because if patients know that they are getting the treatment, they may expect to get better, and their expectations can make them get better a bit faster. And if they know they are getting the placebo, they might drop out of the trial because they know they aren't getting the actual treatment (more on this in chapter 8). Adding an actual vaccine to the placebo control helps the trial remain blinded and so prevents expectations and dropouts from confounding the trial.

Placebos that have an ingredient that mimics some of the side effects of the active treatments are called active placebo controls. This can be confusing because they are different from what are called active treatments, but I'll stick with the term because it is entrenched. The COVID-19 placebo was an active placebo because it contained another vaccine. Active placebos are probably much more common than we think. Consider tricyclic antidepressants. Tricyclic antidepressants have been shown to be more effective than placebos in trials described as double-blind.[15] Patients in such trials are warned in advance that the drugs might have side effects such as dry mouth. Patients in a trial who get a dry mouth will then believe that they are getting the "real" antidepressant as opposed to the mere placebo, which could subsequently lead to the tricyclic antidepressant appearing to be more effective than it actually is. To stop side effects from helping people figure out whether they are getting the real drug or the placebo, researchers put ingredients in the placebo that cause the side effect (we saw this with the vaccine placebo example above). Then people who get the placebo and have a dry mouth (for example) also believe they are getting the real drug and have the same expectations. This makes the test fairer. In extensive tests, it has been shown that for many people, the real drugs barely show any benefit over and above "active placebos."[16] This suggests that much of the apparent benefit of tricyclic antidepressants is caused by unblinding and differential expectations.

While active placebos are good for preserving blinding, they can generate mistaken estimates of side effects. We calculate an active treatment's side effect, such as redness and swelling at the site where the needle went in, by comparing it with what happened to people who got the placebo. What researchers are looking for is a difference. If the active vaccine causes more numbness at the site of injection than the placebo, we can conclude that numbness is a side effect of the active vaccine. But if the placebo is designed to cause the side effect (like redness and swelling), then looking for a difference in redness and swelling is pointless. This might have been a price worth paying to keep the trial blinded, but it needs to be considered when determining whether the COVID vaccine (or another trial that used an active placebo) causes that side effect.

When I talk about the examples of the COVID-19 vaccine and antidepressants, people sometimes say that examples like that are not common. They are mistaken. In some trials of oseltamivir (Tamiflu) the active placebo contained dehydrocholic acid and dibasic calcium phosphate dihydrate. This was presumably done to mimic the bitter taste of the active treatment (oseltamivir powder). Making sure the placebo controls were bitter, like the active pills, helped blind the trial. However, dehydrocholic acid can cause stomach aches,[17] and stomach aches are a side effect of oseltamivir. In the trials, oseltamivir didn't cause *more* stomach aches than the placebo, so the researchers concluded that oseltamivir did not cause stomach aches. This inference is mistaken because of the unfair comparison: the oseltamivir probably did cause stomach aches.

In another example, olive oil was once used in so called placebo-control capsules for trials of cholesterol-lowering agents before there was evidence that olive oil reduced cholesterol.[18] We don't know whether the small quantities of olive oil in the "placebo" controls had a cholesterol-lowering effect, but researchers found that the response to olive oil placebos was higher than expected,[18] and olive oil is no longer used in placebo controls for cholesterol-lowering drugs. The olive oil in the placebo control gave the placebo an unfair advantage, making the comparison with the active drugs unfair.

The ingredients used to coat pills can also have surprising effects. Cellulose acetate phthalate is typically used as a coating for placebo pills; it can help the pills go down more smoothly, but cellulose acetate phthalate has also been found to help cure sexually transmitted diseases like herpes.[19,20] If cellulose acetate were used to coat the placebo pills in trials of drugs to treat sexually transmitted diseases, the comparison wouldn't be fair. I don't know whether trials of treatments for sexually transmitted diseases use cellulose acetate phthalate, and this is hard to ascertain because placebo control ingredients are rarely described.

In yet another example, an appetite stimulant called megestrol acetate for anorexia associated with cancer was compared with a lactose (a kind of sugar) placebo.[21] A problem here is that lactose intolerance is common in cancer patients, [22] so the lactose "placebo" controls caused stomach problems among many of the people in the placebo group. This handicapped the placebo control and made the drug look better than it was. A systematic review of 216 trials that used placebos containing maltodextrin (another kind of sugar used in sugar pill placebos) found that a quarter of the trials documented effects of the maltodextrin on immunological and inflammatory markers as well as gut function.[23]

Nobody knows why inappropriate placebo controls are as common as they are, but I hypothesize that there are the following two reasons. First, the mistaken idea that placebos are "inert" makes careful examination of what's in placebo controls appear to be a waste of time. One inert thing is the same as another, so why bother looking carefully at what's in them? The second is that it can be in the interest of someone who is invested (financially or otherwise) in making a drug look effective to choose a placebo that will make the drug look safer or better than it actually is.

Misguided Placebo-Controlled Treatments in Trials of Complex Interventions

So-called placebo-controlled trials of non-drug interventions are even more confused. In placebo-controlled trials of surgery, knee arthroscopy has been defined both as a sham intervention[24] and as an "active" intervention.[25] Unless it is a very strange set of trials, it simply can't be that knee arthroscopy is both a placebo and an active intervention. Trials of breathing meditation for reducing anxiety have also used a variety of purported placebo-control interventions, including audiobook listening[26] and progressive muscle relaxation.[27] Breathing meditation was more effective than the former but not the latter. What are we to say, then, about the effects of breathing meditation to reduce anxiety? The answer, according to the trials, is that it depends on the placebo, which doesn't help patients who want to know whether it "works."

I'll describe so-called placebo-controlled trials of exercise, acupuncture, and psychotherapy in a bit more detail. I've chosen exercise because of a paradox. Nobody who has tried exercise can deny that it has an effect. Unless done in an unsafe way, it makes people feel better immediately. Some of the reasons why it makes us feel better are known. Exercise leads to increased levels of dopamine and endorphins in the body. Large studies have also shown that exercise makes people live longer and better and does many other good things.[18] In spite of its obvious benefits, some evidence nerds say *there is no good evidence for exercise*. They say that the trials of exercise have a "high risk of bias"[28] and that there is therefore no good evidence that exercise is effective.[29] One reason they are mistaken is that they have ignored the problems with placebo-control treatments of exercise.

Exercise

Exercise for treating depression is complex and includes at least the features listed below:

a. Belief that one is being treated with exercise
b. (If done with a trainer) interaction between patient and trainer
c. Other "psychological" benefits of exercise (distraction from daily routine and worry, the sense of achievement, and social interactions)
d. Increased metabolic rate
e. Increased body temperature
f. Increased heart rate for some prolonged period
g. Increased endorphin and adrenaline levels caused by exercise[30,31]

The first problem in constructing a good placebo control for exercise is figuring out which of the features above are the core features, so that we can remove them to construct a placebo control. It's tempting to identify increased endorphin and adrenaline levels (factor g) as the most important for the treatment of depression. But how do you extract those to create a placebo control? How can you make someone run, have higher heart rate, increased body temperature, and so on without also generating higher levels of endorphins and dopamine?

In theory, I suppose one could try injecting chemicals that neutralized endorphins and adrenaline into a control group that was taking exercise. For example, they might get an injection that contains naloxone (a drug that blocks the effects of endorphins), and beta-blockers (a drug that blocks the effects of adrenaline). If you did that, then the placebo control could be exercise plus the injection of the naloxone and beta-blockers. Then, if exercise without the injections did better, you could say it worked. But even a superficial examination of that option reveals its many flaws. For one, the people getting the injection would know they are in the control group because they would be the only ones getting the injection. This problem could be solved by giving the people in the regular placebo group an injection too, but a placebo injection (this is called a "double dummy" design). Then, neither group would know if they were getting the placebo injection or the injection with naloxone and beta-blockers. But the act of injecting someone who is doing exercise itself raises endorphin levels, introducing potential unfairness into the trial. Another problem is that both naloxone and beta-blockers might affect depression too, which makes them ineligible as a standard against which to measure the effects of exercise.

Yet another problem is ethical. We shouldn't harm people in trials, yet both naloxone and beta-blockers can have serious side effects including dizziness, sickness, shivering, and worse. In short, injecting people with naloxone and beta-blockers as part of a so-called placebo control won't do. A clever reader might say that we could find other drugs that block endorphins and adrenaline that don't have effects on depression or negative side effects that could be used to construct a good placebo control for exercise. My answer is: how do you know? You would have to do another trial. A placebo-controlled trial. And even then, you wouldn't solve the problem that injections themselves produce endorphins.

Also, there is no evidence that increased endorphins and adrenaline are the only cause of the antidepressant effects of exercise. What if the really important factor is distraction from daily routine? Focus? Social interactions? More likely, it's a mixture of all these factors that can't be picked apart—the overall effect may exceed (or be less than) the sum of the effects of the parts. Given the difficulties in designing placebo-controlled trials of exercise in theory, it should not surprise us that in practice things go wrong. Some actual placebo-controlled trials of exercise use supervised relaxation[32] and others use supervised flexibility[33] as placebo controls. But neither of these will do. Those controls do not permit the trial to remain blinded, which can make the trial unfair.

Supervised relaxation and supervised flexibility are inappropriate "placebo" controls for exercise trials because they can reduce depression too. Herbert Benson's bestseller, *The Relaxation Response,* first published in 1975, claims that relaxing for as little as 10 minutes per day can have a positive impact on depression.[34] This has been confirmed in a systematic review of randomized trials which showed that relaxation reduces depression by at least a bit.[35] The same is true for flexibility exercises. Yoga, which is sometimes little more than flexibility exercises, has been shown in dozens of studies to have a small antidepressant effect.[36] In brief, the so-called placebo or sham controls used in trials of exercise are not fit for the purpose and lead to underestimates of the apparent effects of exercise.

We'd be considered crazy if we were to do something similar to using supervised relaxation or flexibility as "placebo" in drug trials. Consider the drug called co-amilofruse, which is the generic name for a drug that contains two drugs that are known to reduce high blood pressure and edema: amiloride and furosemide. Say I removed just one of those drugs—the furosemide—but left in the amiloride. That single drug (amiloride) could be a great test to check how much better furosemide was in a blinded trial. But it is obvious that amilofruse is not a placebo, and it should be equally obvious that supervised relaxation or flexibility are not appropriate placebos for exercise trials.

At this stage, the response I often get from skeptics is that we should pick apart all the different features of exercise, test them in separate trials, and then add up the effects of all the different parts. Yet, given that the different parts could interact, we would have to do more than just separate each individual factor. We would also have to isolate groups of factors. We would have to separate groups of two, three, four, and five (remember that there are at least six in total) to test them in different trials too. This would require doing dozens of separate trials. All this additional effort and expense might be justified if there were no other way to test exercise rigorously, but there is. Instead of using mistaken placebo-controlled trials, we can use active controlled trials, which I will describe after showing how confused trials of acupuncture and psychotherapy are.

Acupuncture

So-called placebo-controlled trials of acupuncture face a slightly less daunting problem than those of exercise. Acupuncture is a form of treatment for various disorders that involves insertion of fine needles into "Qi" points. The needles are very thin and usually penetrate to a depth of a quarter to three quarters of an inch (5–40 millimeters) depending on the location. The needle's penetration into the skin is barely perceptible, and acupuncture is widely used. Some researchers advocate a theory involving lines of energy, or "meridians," flowing through the body.[37] However, these theories lack a widely accepted or established empirical base, at least according to conventional science. Moreover, there are different theories about how acupuncture works, and the various theories have led to different so-called placebo controls. Before describing those different controls, below is a list of features of treatment with acupuncture:

a. Patients' and practitioner's beliefs about, attitude toward, and expectations of relief from needling and acupuncture
b. The acupuncture consultation
c. Needle insertion (anywhere in the body, not at the "acupuncture" points indicated by the relevant theory of acupuncture)
d. Needle stimulation (of acupuncture points) at what the relevant theory sees as the correct location
e. Pressure at any point on the body
f. Pressure *at what the relevant theory sees as the correct location.*

A device touted as a "placebo" or "sham" acupuncture procedure is treatment with an ingenious device called the Streitberger needle.[38] This is a blunt needle embedded in a moveable shaft (fig. 4.1). When the device is pressed on the skin, the shaft moves and gives the appearance of penetrating the skin. To hold the device in place, plastic rings are taped to the patient's skin at the acupuncture points. To maintain the deception, the rings are also used for the real acupuncture in those trials. Some researchers claim that the sham needle is "validated," by which they mean that patients supposedly can't tell the difference between real acupuncture and acupuncture with the Streitberger needle. I'll provisionally accept (although it's not quite true—you'll see why in chapter 8) that patients can't tell the differ-

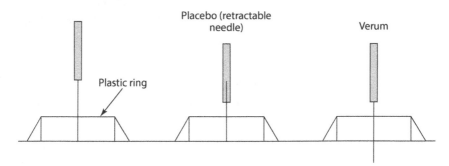

FIG. 4.1. The Streitberger needle (simplified model) from Howick J. The relativity of placebos: Defending a modified version of Grünbaum's scheme. *Synthese.* 2017;194(4):1363–1396. https://doi.org/10.1007/s11229-015-1001-0.

ence between the real acupuncture treatment and treatment with the Streitberger needle.

However, the fact that Streitberger needles might allow trials to be blinded does not mean that they are appropriate placebo controls. The antidepressant sertraline could be used as a control in a test of fluoxetine (another antidepressant), and such a control would be useful for keeping the trial successfully blinded. But sertraline is not a placebo relative to depression.

Trials comparing real acupuncture with acupuncture involving the Streitberger needle typically show very small benefits of real acupuncture.[39] At the same time, evidence suggests that treatment involving the Streitberger needle is more effective than placebo pills,[40] while both real and sham acupuncture seem to be more effective than conventional treatment for back pain.[41] The larger effects of the Streitberger needle compared with those of conventional pill placebos can be interpreted in two ways: either treatment with the Streitberger needle produces an especially large placebo effect,[42] or it is not an appropriate placebo control.[43]

There are many reasons why treatment with the Streitberger needle is not an appropriate placebo control. For one, there is independent evidence that acupressure (which is part of treatment with the Streitberger needle) is effective for treating pain.[44] To be sure, the pressure exerted by real or Streitberger acupuncture needles *might* be less intense than the pressure exerted as part of clinical acupressure, but without a proper trial we don't know. Moreover, the acupuncture consultation (which is often much longer than a conventional consultation) is more effective than standard consultations.[45] In addition to being longer, the consultations also have a specific structure that relies on a theory about health and disease.

Because I've heard the following objections a dozen times, I will clarify them here. First, some say, "but treatment with the Streitberger needle does not penetrate the skin. Acupuncture is all about penetrating the skin, and if penetrating the skin doesn't work, then acupuncture doesn't work." This objection is based on two mistaken assumptions. The main mistake is the idea that we can *separate* all the different parts of acupuncture. If they combine in a way that can't be added like 2 + 2 (most things in biology and chemistry can't), it might be that the effects of acupuncture treatment arise from a combination of needle penetration, the pressure, the consultation, the beliefs, and so on. And the effect of the individual parts might not add up (more on that in chapter 7). The fact is that we simply don't know how the different features of treatment with acupuncture combine to produce an overall effect.

Second, some say that the theory of acupuncture, which involves concepts such as intangible "Qi" points is so much hocus pocus. Therefore, they say, acupuncture can't possibly work. The answer is that the theory is less important than the observed effects. The theory about how acupuncture works could be wrong even if acupuncture itself works. The theory about how or why apples fell from trees was mistaken before Newton, yet the observations that apples fell from trees were accurate. Because of this, historians of science have called the history of science a graveyard of dead theories.[44]

Perhaps more importantly, most patients in pain don't care about whether the Streitberger needle is a "real" treatment or especially powerful placebo: they want to know what will help them move around without pain.

Psychotherapy

Despite decades of effort, no one has shown convincingly that one therapeutic method is more effective than any other for the majority of psychological illnesses.

—JEROME FRANK AND JULIA FRANK, *Persuasion and Healing*[45]

Mistaken placebo controls are also responsible for confusion about the relationship between psychotherapy and placebos. Irving Kirsch spells this confused relationship out in his paper "Placebo Psychotherapy: Synonym or Oxymoron?"[46] Kirsch notes that if we try to apply the drug model to the psychotherapeutic context, we get into quite a tangle. Kirsch defines drug placebos as those with no chemically active ingredients. Since there are no chemically active ingredients in psychotherapy itself, this definition makes psychotherapy itself a placebo. Kirsch then notes that placebo psychotherapy is an oxymoron because it is impossible to design an appropriate placebo control for psychotherapeutic interventions. Setting aside that his provisional definition is problematic (drug placebos do have chemically active ingredients), he is correct to point out the muddle caused by trying to design psychotherapy placebos.

So-called placebos for psychotherapy are often called attention controls and usually involve spending time with a therapist (or some other person). However, the conversations with the therapist in the attention control group avoid topics that are related to the theory of psychotherapy under test. For example, an attention control of psychoanalysis might avoid speaking about childhood experiences or dreams. Other attention controls used in trials of psychotherapeutic techniques have involved stretching, general health education, or receiving a brochure.[47–49]

Because of the problems with attention controls, it should not be surprising that attention controls perform almost as well as real psychotherapy in some trials.[50,51] In one trial investigating whether counseling could reduce the risk of stroke, patients in the "attention" control group were given a brochure and a list of stroke risk factors.[52] Yet, as the authors of the study later point out, "the simple act of giving the brochure and list of stroke risk factors to the attention control group may have resulted in improved knowledge and initiated behavior change for some."[47] It may come as a surprise that some attention controls can cause harm. In a trial published in 2013, the researchers compared counseling with usual care and an attention control in 355 patients. The counseling involved eight sessions in which a trained psychologist educated patients about the benefits of lowering their cholesterol levels. The attention control also involved eight sessions, but the sessions were shorter, and the patients discussed more general topics. The usual care group was not given any additional treatment. After 12 months, it became clear that the outcome in the attention control was worse than doing nothing for some of the outcomes.[53] We don't know why this attention control seemed to have a detrimental effect. The authors hypothesize that the attention control may have undermined the care the patients received outside the trial. The point is the attention control is not an inert intervention and we don't know what its effects are.

Despite the problems with attention controls, psychotherapy often outperforms attention controls in trials. For example, in 1978 Jerome Frank and Julia Frank found that both individual therapy and group therapy were better than minimal contact with therapists that consisted of half an hour every two weeks.[54] An overview of systematic reviews published in 1993 found that when large samples were taken, psychotherapy seemed to outperform both no treatment and attention controls.[55]

The fact that attention controls may be inappropriate for testing the effects of psychotherapy does not mean that all psychotherapeutic techniques are better than placebos either. Indeed, some forms of psychotherapy might be placebos. The use of inappropriate attention controls in psychotherapeutic techniques simply means that the effects of psychotherapeutic techniques, relative to placebo, cannot be inferred from the trials with these attention controls. We will see later how we can rigorously evaluate psychotherapeutic techniques without using inappropriate controls.

How Typical Are Exercise, Acupuncture, and Psychotherapy "Placebo" Controls?

At this stage of the debate, skeptics sometimes say that the problems I've described with mistaken placebo controls are very rare and not worth discussing. I take this to be admission of defeat on the main points I've made, and even then, they are mistaken. The fact is that we don't know how common inappropriate placebo controls are because most researchers don't bother telling us what's in the placebos in their trials. My review published in 2010 found that disclosing placebo/sham ingredients is rare: 8.2% for pills, and 26.7% for injections.[56] My updated review found that this has improved only slightly.[57]

We do know, however, that mistaken placebo control treatments are probably far more common than we think. In 2016 some researchers sought to ascertain whether the physical properties of placebo controls were matched with the treatment. Among the 1,973 trials reviewed, they found that 64% of placebo control interventions were *not* matched in terms of physical properties.[58] Lack of matching makes it hard to keep the trial blinded, rendering the test unfair. In short, lots of mistakes are made when designing placebo controls, and these mistakes lead to mistaken estimates of how effective or harmful are the treatments our doctors prescribe to us. As a prelude to proposing a solution, I'll review the history and usage of placebo controls. This is because the history of placebo controls points towards a solution.

There Is No Placebo Control

There are two related objections regarding the need to define placebo controls. One was recently published by Iain Chalmers and Stephen Senn, who say that we should focus on *what we are withholding from patients*.[54] They claim to be able to do this without referring to placebo controls at all. For example, in a trial comparing vitamin C with a placebo, we should focus on the fact that we are withholding ascorbic acid from those getting the placebo vitamin C. I agree that we should be clear about what we are withholding. To know whether the test is fair, we also need to know what the active substance within the placebo is replaced with. So, a sole focus on what is being withheld will not do.

Andrew Turner goes further than Chalmers and Senn and states that we would be better off dropping the term "placebo control" in favor of extensive descriptions.[55] Turner argues—correctly—that the *purpose* of placebo-controlled trials is to create trials with two groups that are treated the same way *apart* from the fact that one receives an experimental intervention while the other does not. There is no need, according to Turner, to call one of the interventions a "placebo control." Instead, we simply need to stipulate what we intend to control for and then design an appropriate trial, with all the interventions described adequately. Turner is correct insofar as he advocates for adequate descriptions, and I have lobbied for better descriptions of "placebo" or "sham" treatments.[11,12] However, it does not follow that there is no such thing as a placebo control or that we should drop the term. By throwing the term "placebo control" away, we miss an opportunity to distinguish trials that compare trials of morphine and diclofenac (two powerful analgesics) and trials of morphine versus a sugar pill. Surely there is a difference between those two types of trials, and the common way of distinguishing the two types of trials is to state that one of them is a placebo-controlled trial and the other is not. Likewise, Chalmers and Senn are correct to draw our attention to which features are withheld. That is compatible with the (desirable) aim of retaining the term "placebo control" because such controls represent an important subset of potential control treatments.

With the historical prelude and dismissal of the skeptical objections to definitions aside I will now define placebo controls in a way that will help us out of the conundrums described with exercise, acupuncture, psychotherapy, and other placebo controls.

Grünbaum's Definition of Placebos as Relative

The person who has probably done the best job at fixing the problems with defining placebo controls is Adolf Grünbaum. Even critics noted that Grünbaum's conceptualization is the best on offer but didn't like the fact that Grünbaum didn't explain what a "therapeutic theory," which is part of his definition, was (I'll get to that).[56] Most nihilists about placebos and placebo controls don't show any evidence that they've read Grünbaum carefully, and some philosophers of science have criticized what I think are nit-picky and nonessential details of his scheme (see appendix 1). To be fair to these critics, Grünbaum is not easy to read, often writing in tedious detail and even inventing

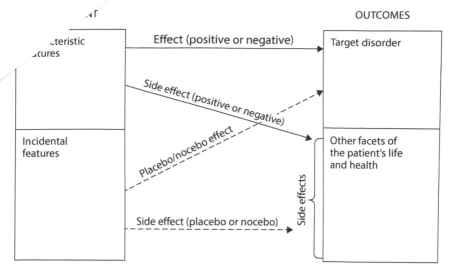

FIG. 4.2. Simplified version of Grünbaum's model from Howick J. The relativity of placebos: Defending a modified version of Grünbaum's scheme. *Synthese*. 2017;194(4):1363–1396. https://doi.org/10.1007/s11229-015-1001-0.

his own words like "placebic." To overcome those problems, I'll explain Grünbaum's main ideas in plain English, leaving the technical details in appendix 1. Most of Grünbaum's innovations can be explained with the diagram (fig. 4.2) that he developed (and that I and many others have adapted).

Beginning with the left-hand box in the figure, the treatment is divided into characteristic and noncharacteristic features (Grünbaum calls the latter "incidental," and to simplify I did not use a new term). As I've mentioned before, even treatments that are considered simple have several components. For example, treatment of depression with Prozac includes fluoxetine hydrochloride as well as several other features such as pill-bulking agents, the potential disruption to the patient's life (they must take time every day to consume the pills), ingredients in the pill casing, the liquid with which the pills are swallowed, and, perhaps most importantly, expectations about the potential effects of fluoxetine hydrochloride and the patient/doctor interaction. Only the fluoxetine hydrochloride is what Grünbaum would call characteristic.

The effects of the treatment with Prozac can be on depression (the target disorder) as well as other things (it might dull your senses). The same goes for the effects of the features that are not core features. They can affect depression and other things (side effects). All the effects can be beneficial or harmful. The harmful effects of the characteristic or core features are toxic effects. Some of the negative effects of the incidental features are nocebo effects, but not all of them are. If someone has a bad tummy reaction because of the bulking agent in the pill, it is not a nocebo effect, but rather a toxic effect of the non-characteristic features.

Grünbaum's figure is remarkable for two reasons. First, it emphasizes that treatments and treatment effects are complex. Not only are treatments complex, but the effects on the patient are complex, affecting the target disorder and other conditions. Second, it illustrates how even treatments that are not placebos are partly placebos. This second fact explains why placebo research is relevant to all treatments. The figure lends itself to a definition of placebo controls as treatments whose characteristic features don't have any effects on the target disorder. That is just another way of saying what I said in chapter 2, namely, that placebos are inert *relative to* a certain disorder.

One element of Grünbaum's theory that cannot be explained with the figure is his emphasis that what counts as a placebo is not absolute or universal. It depends on what disease we are talking about and what patients we are talking about. He uses the well-worn example of a sugar pill to make this point: "none other than the much-maligned . . . sugar pill furnishes a reductio ad absurdum of the notion that a medication can be generically a placebo . . . without relativization to a target disorder. For even a lay person knows that the glucose in the sugar pill is anything but a . . . placebo if given to a victim of diabetes who is in a state of insulin shock, or to someone suffering from hypoglycaemia."[57] In short, whether something is a placebo or a placebo control depends on what it is used for and who it is used on.

While placebo controls are used for different purposes than placebos in practice, they share the same definition. Placebo controls are treatments that do not have characteristic (or core) features that are effective for the target disorder. The noncharacteristic features are inert relative to the target disorder if they are given alone. However, if they are part of the meaningful context the combined treatment can have an effect. The main difference between placebo controls and placebos in practice is that the placebo control has to be the same as the active treatment *apart from* the core (characteristic) features. A placebo in practice is not being compared with anything so its noncharacteristic features do not have to be similar to the noncharacteristic features of anything else in particular. With this definition in hand, I'll revisit the thorny examples of exercise, acupuncture, and psychotherapy placebos. Armed with the right definitions, we can get out of the tangle.

A Solution to the Thorny Cases of Exercise, Acupuncture, and Psychotherapy "Placebo" Control Treatments

Since it's impossible to separate the core feature of exercise from the other parts, it's impossible to design a placebo control for exercise that doesn't have the core feature. This makes a placebo-controlled trial of exercise a nonstarter. In the case of acupuncture and psychotherapy, the core features are separable in principle, but there is currently insufficient evidence to decide which features are the core or characteristic ones, and they may also interact with others. So again, it's a nonstarter. In all these cases, the best thing is to not try to put a square peg into a round hole. Instead of using "placebo" controls, we should compare exercise or acupuncture with other available established treatments. The same thing applies to most complex treatments. Instead of botched placebo-controlled trials, other trial designs that are equally rigorous should be used such as "active" controlled trials. Briefly (I'll explain more in chapter 10), in an "active" controlled trial, the experimental treatment (like exercise or acupuncture) is compared with an established treatment. An advantage of active controlled trials is that they give us information that is more useful. If your goal is to relieve a headache or back pain, it is more important to know which treatment is best, not whether a treatment is better than a placebo.

Active controlled trials are not the only other option. It is also often possible to compare different doses of complex treatments. For example, a study with 80 people compared low and high "doses" of exercise, or supervised flexibility exercises (they called this a placebo control) for 12 weeks.[58] The primary outcome measure was a change in depression. Blind assessors measured the depression scores each week. At the end of the 12-week trial, all groups had some improvement. A high dose of exercise reduced the scores on the scale by 47%. The low dose reduced the scores by an average of 30%, which was similar to the so-called placebo treatment. A trial comparing a high dose of exercise with a lower dose avoids the problems caused by inappropriate placebo controls, while using all the methods, such as randomization and blinding, that make tests fair.

Implications

Botched placebo controls are more common than many believe, and they lead to unfair tests of treatment benefits and harms. Those who question the ability to define placebo controls are not only wrong but avoid solving most of the problems with botched placebo controls. Simply put, proper placebo controls cannot contain any core (characteristic) features, and they need to be otherwise very similar to the active treatment in the test. This definition of placebo controls can be used to evaluate how effective placebos and nocebos are. Research into the effects of complex treatments such as exercise, acupuncture, and psychotherapy need to take this into account.

- PART II

HOW BIG ARE PLACEBO
AND NOCEBO EFFECTS?

For centuries in the Western world, physicians have been aware of the fact that
sick people get better after taking inert drugs. And, it should be clear that they
were then (and are now) somewhat ambivalent about this. Although the reasons
are complex, it must seem odd to a person who has spent twenty years learning
to be a physician, studying the hundreds of medications available, to find that
patients get better just because they have been in a doctor's office for a few
minutes.

—DANIEL MOERMAN, "Meaning, Medicine, and the 'Placebo Effect'"[1]

To determine whether we should use or avoid placebos and nocebos,
we need to know what they are and how large their effects are. I
covered what they are in part I; part II of the book is about measuring the size of placebo and nocebo effects. Problems have plagued
attempts to determine the extent of placebo and nocebo effects for
decades. Take the case of Mr. Wright (a pseudonym). Mr. Wright was
found to have cancer in 1957 and was given days to live.[2] Hospital-
ized in Long Beach, California, with tumors the size of oranges, he
heard that scientists had discovered a horse serum, krebiozen, that
appeared to be effective against cancer. He begged for it. His physician, Philip West, gave Mr. Wright an injection Friday afternoon.
The following Monday, the astonished doctor found his patient out
of his death bed joking with the nurses.

The tumors, the doctor wrote later, "had melted like snowballs on a
hot stove." However, the doctor had injected Mr. Wright with water.
Two months later, Mr. Wright read medical reports that the horse
serum was a quack remedy. He suffered an immediate relapse.

"Don't believe what you read in the papers," Dr. West told Mr. Wright. Then he injected him with what he said was "a new super-refined double-strength" version of the drug. In fact, it was water, but again, the tumor masses melted. Mr. Wright was "the picture of health" for two more months—until he read a definitive report stating that krebiozen was worthless. He died two days later.

The story of Mr. Wright appears to be a dramatic example of a very large placebo effect. However, without properly controlled studies, we cannot rule out a range of other, more "normal," explanations for Mr. Wright's recovery. These include possible misdiagnosis (his tumor might not have been that bad after all), "natural history" (the tumor may have waxed and waned coincidentally with Mr. Wright's consumption of krebiozen), and lack of replication (the story of Mr. Wright has not been verified independently).[3]

Other problems with measuring placebo effects that I'll explore in the next few chapters include those listed below.

1. Just being watched by a doctor (without any placebo treatment) can have an effect.
2. Like "real" treatments, different placebos have different effects for different problems.
3. It is nearly impossible to measure placebo effects using "gold standard" (blinded) trials.
4. We probably can't measure placebo effects separately from the effects of the meaningful context.

All these problems apply to measuring nocebo effects too. To measure placebo and nocebo effects accurately, we need to begin by recognizing the problems. The solution I propose is to take treatment with placebos as a package and measure their overall effects.

I've relegated the more technical aspects of this part of the book to the appendixes. At the same time, the topics are fundamentally a bit technical. While I've done my best to write them in plain English with interesting stories, readers who are not interested in technical matters may wish to browse or skip this part altogether and go straight to chapter 9.

CHAPTER 5

How (Not) to Measure Nocebo and Placebo Effects

More placebos have been administered to research participants than any single experimental drug. Thus, one would expect sufficient data to have accumulated for the acquisition of substantial knowledge of the parameters of placebo effects. However, although almost everyone controls for placebo effects, almost no one evaluates them.

—IRVING KIRSCH, "Listening to Prozac but Hearing Placebo: A Meta-Analysis of Antidepressant Medication"[1]

Beecher's Powerful Placebos

The first attempt to systematically quantify the size of placebo effects was made by the American anaesthetist Henry Knowles Beecher. Beecher put his academic career on hold to serve in the US Army during World War II. While working on the front line in southern Italy, he reportedly saw something extraordinary. With supplies of morphine running out, a nurse injected a wounded soldier with saltwater instead of morphine before an operation. The soldier thought it was real morphine, and it seemed to work: he didn't appear to feel any pain. Beecher is said to have continued the practice whenever supplies of morphine waned, and he became convinced of the power of placebos.

While there are no historical records to confirm this often-repeated account, Beecher *does* report noticing that two soldiers with similar injuries would express pain very differently. Some would scream; others would appear to be in not much pain at all. This led him to the hypothesis that other factors must play a role in the apparent experience of pain.

When he returned to the United States, he did a study that was immortalized in his article "The Powerful Placebo" (1955). He looked for all the placebo-controlled trials he could find, and eventually found 15 studies of treatments for a number of conditions (postoperative pain, cough, pain from angina pectoris, headache, seasickness, and anxiety). The studies had a total of 1,082 patients. He found that overall, 35% (±2.2%) of the patients' symptoms were relieved by placebo alone.[2] His study is still cited as evidence that placebos cause a third of people to get better.

Beecher made a huge advance over and above the anecdotes by quantifying the controlled experiments that included patients treated with placebos. This reduced the chances that the results arose from measurement error. Yet there was a major flaw in Beecher's study: the people who got better after taking a placebo might have recovered even if they had not taken a placebo. People often forget that human diseases and treatments only work in a probabilistic sense. So when Mr. Wright was diagnosed with terrible cancer and was predicted to have a few days to live, what doctors meant (or what they should have meant) is that he *probably* had a few days to live. Even predictions that seem certain are usually just almost certain.[3] For example, Banu Symington reports the case of Robert, an 82-year-old man with stage 4 (the worst stage) of blood vessel cancer called angiosarcoma. Robert was not comfortable with the side effects of chemotherapy, so he and his doctors decided to watch and wait. Most patients with stage 4 angiosarcoma do not survive very long because the cancer has already spread too much. Yet in Robert's case, the cancer went away on its own within half a year.[4] It's hard to tell how exceptional Robert's case is because it's hard to find people with serious cancer who don't get any treatment. Some estimate that 1 in 100,000 people with cancer, including serious cancer, will get better without any treatment.[5] Since almost 20 million people get cancer every year worldwide, it means there could be 200 potential new cases like Robert's every year. Two hundred is a minuscule number by global standards, but it can appear miraculous given the serious nature of the diseases they recover from.

In general, human beings are far better at recovering on their own from illnesses than action-oriented doctors and patients believe. Archie Cochrane was a pioneer of what we now call evidence-based medicine, and he discovered the amazing ability of the body to heal when he was the only doctor in a prisoner-of-war camp during World War II. His camp had 20,000 prisoners living on 600 calories a day. There were epidemics of diarrhea, typhoid, diphtheria, infections, jaundice, and sand-fly fever. There was almost no medicine: just a bit of aspirin, some antacid, and some skin antiseptic. Cochrane expected many hundreds of patients to die, but in fact only four died, and three of the four were shot while trying to escape. Cochrane concluded that his observations demonstrated "very clearly the relative unimportance of therapy in comparison with the recuperative power of the human body."[6] The ability of the human body to heal itself makes it difficult to tell whether a treatment (including a placebo treatment) caused a cure or whether the person would have recovered on their own without treatment. Beecher's study did not control for spontaneous remission or what is sometimes called "natural history."

More recently, Gunver Kienle and Helmut Kiene listed 26 factors ranging from measurement error and false reporting to natural history that can give false impressions of placebo effects.[7] In his defense, Beecher certainly knew about the possibility of spontaneous remission; it's just that the studies available to him didn't allow him to control for it. To test whether placebos really make people get better, we must compare people who take placebos with people who take no treatment at all. Then we can say that there are placebo effects if patients taking the placebo fare better than those left untreated.

Adding to this debate, a distinction is sometimes made between a placebo response and a placebo effect. The placebo response is anything than happens to someone after taking a placebo (including regression to the mean and spontaneous remission).[8] By comparison, a placebo effect is something caused by the placebo treatment. The idea is that not everything that happens after someone takes a placebo should be called a placebo effect. And that is why we need to have no treatment controls to measure placebo effects.

Hróbjartsson and Gøtzsche's Power*less* Placebos

Attempting to correct Beecher's error, Asbjørn Hróbjartsson and Peter Gøtzsche looked at three-armed trials that included experimental, placebo control, and so-called untreated groups (fig. 5.1). Then they compared what happened to patients in the placebo group with what happened to patients who were not treated.

They were eventually able to include 114 trials in their statistical analysis. Typical pill placebos in the studies they analyzed were lactose pills, and typical physical placebos were procedures performed with the machine turned off (such as sham transcutaneous electrical nerve stimulation). A typical psychological placebo was a theoretically

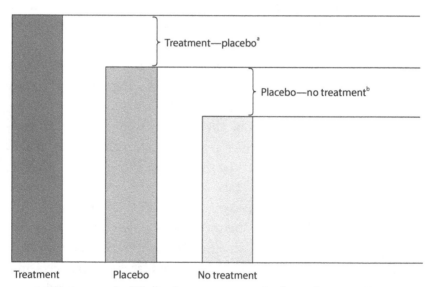

FIG. 5.1. Three-armed trials that have treatment, placebo, and no-treatment groups. Hróbjartsson and Gøtzsche ignored the treatment group to focus on the difference in outcomes between placebo and untreated groups.

neutral discussion, like an attention control, between participant and dispenser. Over 40 clinical conditions were included in the analysis, ranging from hypertension and compulsive nail biting to fecal soiling and marital discord.

Hróbjartsson and Gøtzsche classified the trials according to whether the outcomes were binary or continuous. Binary outcomes don't have shades of gray: either the patient experienced the outcome (for example, their pain was reduced by 50%) or they didn't. (Appendix 2 goes into detail about the difference between continuous and binary outcomes.) Continuous outcomes, on the other hand, come on a continuum. An example of a continuous outcome would be a pain scale where 0 represented no pain, and 10 was the worst pain imaginable. Hróbjartsson and Gøtzsche also divided up the studies according to whether the outcomes were patient-reported (such as pain) or more objective (observer-reported).

They found a small benefit of placebo compared with no treatment. The benefit was "statistically significant" for many outcomes, which means that the results are unlikely to have arisen due to chance. The most common single condition treated in the included trials was pain. Placebos appeared to reduce pain by an average of one or two points on a 10-point scale. So, if someone initially rated their pain at 6, it might be reduced to 5 or 4. However, Hróbjartsson and Gøtzsche question whether the small average placebo effect was real, and they cite two main potential biases that might have confounded their estimate.

1. The trials were not blinded. Patients in an untreated group knew they were not being treated, and patients in a placebo group thought they were being treated. This might have skewed the result. Patients who got no treatment might have had low expectations about the prospects of getting better, and this could have made the placebo seem to be relatively more effective. I discuss this in greater detail in chapter 8.

2. Subjective outcomes might have been biased. A subjective outcome is one for which you must take the patient's word. For example, if the outcome is whether the patient feels happier, you need to ask the patient whether they feel happy, and there is no way to independently verify whether the patient is actually happy. An objective outcome is something you measure and that doesn't depend on accepting someone's word for it. Hróbjartsson and Gøtzsche worry that patients in the placebo group might have told the doctors in the trial that they were happier in order to please the doctors, when in fact they weren't happier. Supporting this hypothesis, the placebo effects were larger when outcomes were subjective and thus susceptible to this kind of reporting bias.[9]

Based on these potential biases, Hróbjartsson and Gøtzsche concluded that "there is little evidence that placebos in general have powerful clinical effects."[9] The title of their paper that published these results was "Is the Placebo Powerless? An Analysis of Clinical Trials Comparing Placebo with No Treatment," which was chosen to be diametrically opposed to the title of Beecher's paper.

Hróbjartsson and Gøtzsche subsequently updated their initial systematic review with and additional 42 studies (for a total of 156) in 2004,[10] and an additional 98 studies in 2010 (for a total of 202 trials).[11] The effect sizes in the updated analyses remained roughly the same, but more of the outcomes were statistically significant, which means that it was less likely that any of the small apparent benefits of placebos arose due to chance. In spite of the improved evidence for placebo effects, Hróbjartsson and Gøtzsche did not modify their skeptical conclusions.

There's no doubt that Hróbjartsson and Gøtzsche corrected an important mistake in Beecher's study by comparing what happens after taking a placebo with what happens when a placebo is not taken. However, in correcting one mistake they introduced several of their own.[12–15]

The First Problem with Hróbjartsson and Gøtzsche's Review: Failure to Define Placebos

Initially Hróbjartsson and Gøtzsche skirted the thorny issue of defining placebos and adopted what they call a "practical" approach, characterizing placebos "practically as an intervention labeled as such in the report of a clinical trial." But this doesn't stand up to scrutiny. Suppose that someone reported using penicillin as a placebo in a trial of some new antibiotic as a treatment for pneumonia. The response would be, "no one would, and if they did, we would not take the trial seriously." But Hróbjartsson and Gøtzsche open themselves up to just that kind of attack. Worse, they go back on their purported policy of accepting any treatment labeled as a placebo. They excluded studies where "it was very likely that the alleged placebo had a clinical benefit not associated with the ritual alone (for example, movement techniques for postoperative pain)." Here they seem to sneak in a definition of placebos as the effects of "rituals," which is no improvement on earlier definitions. Ritual feasting, fasting, or human sacrifice are not placebos. Another problem with their failure to define placebos was the hodgepodge of "placebos" in their review. Along with placebo pills and injections, they jumbled relaxation (described as a placebo in some studies and a treatment in others); leisure reading; answering questions about hobbies, newspapers, magazines, favorite foods, and sports teams; talking about daily events; family activities; football; vacation activities; pets; books; movies; and television shows as placebos. These treatments didn't just look different on paper. The statistical tests for heterogeneity confirmed that their effects varied so much that many researchers would have refused to take an average, insisting that to do so would be combining apples and oranges. The *Cochrane Handbook for Systematic Reviews of Interventions*, which is the methodological Bible for producing the type of study Hróbjartsson and Gøtzsche did, recommends *not* pooling results if heterogeneity is high.[16] The heterogeneity has important implications for what conclusions we can draw from their analysis. Just because the average effect of apples and oranges is small, it doesn't mean that both apples and oranges have small effects. A small average effect is compatible with some placebos having no effects and others having larger ones.

Taking up the problem with the heterogeneity, Irving Kirsch asks us to imagine a trial of all *treatments*.

> Imagine reading, in a prestigious medical journal, an article bearing the provocative title, "Is Medicine Powerless? An Analysis of Clinical Trials Comparing Medical Treatment with No Treatment." Suppose that the authors of this meta-analysis had "conducted a systematic review of clinical trials in which patients were randomly assigned to either medical treatment or no treatment" and had identified 130 trials that met their inclusion criteria. These included clinical trials of medical treatments for the common cold, alcohol abuse, smoking, poor oral hygiene, herpes simplex infection, infertility, mental retardation, marital discord, faecal soiling, Alzheimer's disease, carpal tunnel syndrome, and "undiagnosed ailments." Noting that medical treatment "is difficult to define satisfactorily," the authors "defined medical treatment practically as an intervention labelled as such in the report of a clinical trial." Besides drugs and surgery, the medical treatments in the clinical trials they identified include psychotherapy, homeopathy, acupuncture, meditation, chiropractic, and faith healing. Finding a small but significant treatment effect, along with significant heterogeneity of outcomes, the authors concluded that they had "found little evidence in general that medicine had powerful clinical effects."[17]

Kirsch notes that just because average treatment effects are tiny does not mean that all treatment effects are tiny. Indeed, Bruce Wampold and colleagues divided up the trials in Hróbjartsson and Gøtzsche's review according to different types of conditions and found placebo treatments to be moderately effective in many cases.[15]

Inspired by Kirsch, I turned his imaginary example into a real study. Starting with the same trials that Hróbjartsson and Gøtzsche used, I added an analysis of the difference between treatment and placebo groups. This gave me the average effect of all treatments compared with the average effects of all placebos. I found that the average treatment effect was also small, and that it was smaller than the size of the placebo effect in some cases! Of course, the treatment effect includes the placebo effect, and just because the effect of any treatment (for any disorder) is small, it doesn't mean that all treatment effects are small. In fact, we know that many medical treatments are very effective. Polio vaccines, adrenaline for anaphylactic shock, and antibiotics for sepsis are all dramatically effective and save lives. By using Hróbjartsson and Gøtzsche's method to derive an absurd conclusion, I showed that the method itself was flawed. Philosophers call what I did a *reductio ad absurdum*, or "reduction to the absurd."

The Second Problem with Hróbjartsson and Gøtzsche's Review: The Myth of No Treatment and Underestimated Placebo Effects

Comparing what happens in placebo-treated patients with patients who are untreated corrects Beecher's error but has a major flaw. Patients who are "untreated" usually respond to an ad (which has a meaning to them). They make an appointment (easily with a friendly researcher, or maybe, more taxingly, with a surly attendant). A qualified health care professional asks them questions and gets them to consent to the trial. They often have diagnostic tests to be sure they are fit to be treated with the new wonder drug or intervention. They usually hear from the staff that the intervention is really terrific—that it melts away tumors (or whatever). They may learn that their diagnosis is not as grave as they had imagined (from Dr. Google). Then they learn that they have been randomized to the "no treatment" group. Their disappointment must hurt. They might even seek treatment outside the trial, though they aren't supposed to. Because many get paid to be in the trial, they might not want to give up the money and not even disclose that they have taken other treatments.

To show that this is more than a theoretical problem, I looked more closely at a few of the larger trials included in Hróbjartsson and Gøtzsche's review. In one of these, Hanns-Peter Scharf and colleagues' 2006 trial compared real acupuncture, placebo acupuncture, and so-called no treatment for treating knee osteoarthritis.[18] The patients in the so-called no-treatment group had 10 physician visits within six weeks. In Jean-François Etter and colleagues' 2002 trial, the so-called no-treatment group received a 20-page information booklet covering "reasons for reducing cigarette consumption and advice on how to reduce and included addresses of smoking cessation clinics."[19] In Blaine Ditto and colleagues' 2003 trial, the untreated patients completed numerous questionnaires, had their blood pressure and heart rate measured twice, and then underwent a "typical blood collection process."[20] Ten visits with a doctor in a six-week period, receiving booklets with instructions about how to quit smoking, filling out questionnaires in a refreshment area are not really "no treatment."

As further evidence that the so-called untreated groups were in fact treated, an analysis of the "untreated" groups within Hróbjartsson and Gøtzsche's review found that patients in these groups improved by 24%, all while they were being "untreated."[21] In theory, the 24% improvement could have happened even if they weren't in the trial, but at least part of this impressive change was undoubtedly due to the treatment given to the patients in the so-called untreated groups.

It is nearly impossible to leave patients alone in a trial. If they are left completely alone, you can't gather data from them. And as soon as you start doing something, they are no longer untreated. The treatment they receive improves outcomes in the "untreated" groups and as a consequence makes the additional benefit of the placebo treatment artificially smaller. Hróbjartsson and Gøtzsche acknowledge this problem when they say, "Patients in a no-treatment group also interact with treatment providers, and the patients are therefore only truly untreated with respect to receiving a placebo intervention."[22] However, they do not use this information to temper their skeptical conclusions. In fact, "Hawthorne Effects" (which should be called "John Henry Effects") are well known in medical research.

The Hawthorne Effect and the John Henry Effect

If being observed made people more productive, East Germany, as the most surveyed country ever, would have been a miracle of productivity.

—MILES MORLAND, personal communication

Simply knowing that one is in a trial could have an effect. Many researchers refer to the effects of simply being observed in a trial as a Hawthorne Effect. However, a more accurate term is the "John Henry Effect." The term "John Henry Effect" was introduced by Gary Saretsky in 1972 to describe a legendary American steel driver in the 1870s. When John Henry heard his output was being compared to that of a steam drill, he literally worked himself to death.[23] The John Henry Effect seems to apply to some social experiments, and something parallel might happen in clinical trials. Say someone with a similar disposition to John Henry was involved in a trial to increase how much exercise they do or quit smoking. Knowing that they are being measured and tested, they might do more exercise or push through the pain of quitting cold turkey even if they were in the so-called untreated group. This would lead to an inflated outcome in the so-called untreated group, and a consequent underestimate of any effect in a placebo group.

What should be called the John Henry Effect is often called the Hawthorne Effect. The Hawthorne Effect is named after a series of experiments in the Hawthorne plant of the Western Electric Company in Chicago between 1924 and 1933. The studies were supervised by renowned psychologist and industrial theorist Elton Mayo. His graduate assistant Fritz Roethlisberger. William J. Dickson, head of the Department of Employee Relations at Western Electric, did most of the actual experiments.

In one study the lighting remained stable for the control group and was slowly raised for the experimental group. Productivity increased equally in both groups. In another study, lighting was stable in the control group but was slowly lowered in the other group. Productivity increased steadily and equally in both groups until the lights were so low in the experimental groups that the experimental workers protested and production fell off.[24] In my previous publications, I have mistakenly followed popular convention, and taken the Hawthorne Effect to mean the positive effect of being observed in a trial.[3]

However, the common understanding of what happened during the Hawthorne experiments is largely mythical. At least as far back as 1978, Richard Franke and James Kaul did a statistical analysis of the results of the experiments and found that statistical chance variation could account for 90% of the apparent effect.[25] A paper published in 1992 by Stephen Jones did more extensive statistical analyses and again found no evidence of Hawthorne Effects. In 2014 a systematic review of studies measuring Hawthorne Effects was published by a team in Scandinavia.[26] The authors found that there did seem to be effects of being investigated, but they were tiny.

Even Elton Mayo, who designed the experiments, didn't believe there was an effect of being observed. Instead, he wrote that the improved productivity arose from a feeling that the employee was cared for, from collaboration between workers, and from encouraging social interchange among workers in such a way that made them feel important. In Mayo's words: "The consequence [of employees forming a team] was that they felt themselves to be participating freely . . . and were happy in the knowledge that they were working without coercion from above or limitation from below."[27] To be sure, patients in many clinical trials do not have bosses and are often not socially organized. However, patient support groups are becoming increasingly common and could produce the same type of effect of free participation and autonomy that Mayo claimed to observe. Still, the Hawthorne Effect, if understood in its historical context, is not an effect of being observed, but rather an effect of the feeling of encouraging collaboration and free autonomous participation.

The Third Problem: Failure to Blind Doesn't Do What Hróbjartsson and Gøtzsche Say It Does

Hróbjartsson and Gøtzsche claim that the lack of blinding may have led to an overestimate of placebo effect sizes. I will discuss the issue of blinding in much more detail in chapter 8. Suffice it to say that when participants think they are getting no treatment, they will not have positive expectations about their recovery. By contrast, those who are getting a placebo that they think could be the fancy new treatment will be more likely to have positive expectations. These expectations can influence how effective the placebo appears to be compared with no treatment. This is an interesting hypothesis, but it is not borne out by the evidence. Many patients who take a placebo know it's a placebo yet it still has an effect (see chapter 6).

The Fourth Problem: Biased Authors

In an earlier publication, Peter Gøtzsche recommends blinding manuscript authors.[28] Instead of writing a report comparing a new drug with a placebo (or placebo with "no treatment"), the author would not know which was which. They would only know that there was a comparison between A and B; they wouldn't know what A or B referred to. This would prevent the authors' prejudices from influencing the way they interpreted the results. Gøtzsche would not deny that he is skeptical about anything that is not supported by great evidence, and he is usually correct. At the same time, in several places in his study on placebo effects with Hróbjartsson, the way the authors interpret their results seems to display a lack of neutrality. For example, there was a statistically significant placebo effect in trials with continuous outcomes, and there were more participants in trials with continuous outcomes than in trials with binary outcomes. This would have tempted some authors to claim that there are often significant placebo effects, rather than conclude that there is little evidence for significant placebo effects. Elsewhere, they state that "It surprised us that we found no association between measures of the quality of a trial and [increased] placebo effects."[8] You can only be surprised if you have a preconceived idea of how things should be. One could just as easily be surprised to find no association between measures of the quality of a trial and *decreased* placebo effects. Poor trial quality is usually associated with exaggerated treatment effects. One way to exaggerate treatment effects is for the placebo effect to decrease. On the other hand, increased trial quality could mean that a trial is visibly (to the participant) more tightly controlled. This increase in control could lead to more treatment of the "untreated" groups and hence decreased placebo effects. In short, there is no reason to suppose that there will be a clear relationship between trial quality and the size of apparent placebo effects.

Additional evidence of lack of neutrality arises from Hróbjartsson and Gøtzsche's refusal to update their conclusions even when the data in their updated reviews more strongly supported real placebo effects. In fact, a hallmark of lack of neutrality is the refusal to update one's conclusions based on updated evidence. Yet another way in which their preconceived notions may have influenced them is their decision to lump everything together to get an average result. As mentioned above, this is discouraged by the *Cochrane Handbook*.[16] Had they not been skeptical about placebo effects to begin with, it seems conceivable that they might have cited the handbook and refused to lump all results together.

Recap of Problems with Measuring Placebo Effects

Hróbjartsson and Gøtzsche's systematic review had several problems, especially heterogeneity and the treatment received by "untreated" groups. A more reasonable conclusion to draw from their study is that placebo effects are not as powerful as Henry Beecher's study suggested, and that they vary widely depending on the type of placebo treatment and condition.

The Potential Power of Nocebos

Despite being done a few decades later, studies of nocebo effect sizes have made many of the same mistakes as studies of placebo effect sizes. As with placebo effects, anecdotes like the one about Mr. A (in chapter 2) make them appear large. Here's another reported in the *BMJ* in 1995: "A builder aged 29 came to the accident and emergency department having jumped down on to a 15 cm nail. As the smallest movement of the nail was painful he was sedated with fentanyl and midazolam. The nail was then pulled out from below. When his boot was removed a miraculous cure appeared to have taken place. Despite entering proximal to the steel toecap the nail had penetrated between the toes: the foot was entirely uninjured."[29] The pain and anxiety experienced by the builder had nothing to do with tissue damage caused by the nail but entirely to do with his (self) communication that the nail had penetrated his foot.

In another report, Sam Shoeman (a pseudonym) was told that he had terminal liver cancer and that he only had a few months to live. Sam was desperate to live until Christmas, to celebrate it one last time with his family. He made good progress and celebrated Christmas. A few days after, he was readmitted to the hospital and died within hours. After he died, the specialists discovered that his cancer wasn't that bad after all. One of the doctors suspected that he died because he *expected* to die.[28] Walter Cannon reports numerous cases of voodoo death whereby people wither away and die after they believe they've been cursed. Those are all apparently dramatic nocebo effects. As with stories of dramatic placebo effects, the stories of dramatic nocebo effects cannot be fully trusted. People can die of undiagnosed or misdiagnosed causes, and it could be that the people who seem to die (or even pass out) because of their beliefs would have done so even if they hadn't been cursed or believed something bad would happen. To know whether the effects are nocebo effects, we need to do controlled experiments.

Controlled Studies of Nocebo Effects

At least 20 systematic reviews have investigated adverse event rates within placebo groups within clinical trials.[31] On average, half of placebo treated patients report an adverse event, and 5% drop out due to alleged intervention-induced intolerance.[32] Most of the adverse events were pain-related, but they also include depression, restless leg syndrome, and worsening of symptoms from Parkinson's disease, multiple sclerosis, cardiovascular disease, and, motor neuron disease.[33] Many of these studies refer to adverse event rates within patients who have taken placebos as *nocebo* effects.[34–36]

This is a mistake. Most patients enroll in clinical trials because of an underlying condition that usually has symptoms. Many common symptoms such as mild to moderate pain, nausea, or headaches arise in most people in their daily lives. Such symptoms may be misattributed to the study intervention, including the placebo (fig. 5.2, bottom). To address this, I and a team of researchers used a similar method to the one used by Hróbjartsson and Gøtzsche to measure *nocebo* effects. We compared adverse event rates in placebo groups with adverse event rates in untreated groups.[31] We found that adverse event rates within placebo groups were 53% greater than adverse event rates within untreated groups (6.51% versus 4.25%). The adverse events included diarrhea, headache, nausea, rash, asthma symptoms, bleeding, and upper respiratory tract infection.[31] The additional adverse events measured in the placebo-treated patients were probably nocebo effects.

A slightly different method has recently been used to distinguish between misattributed side effects of statins and nocebo effects. Statins have a small absolute effect (about 1%) for preventing heart disease.[35] Of course, by the time these results reach headlines, the effect size gets exaggerated, with some claiming that statins reduce death by 24%. They derive 24% from 1.1% by calculating the relative risk reduction instead of the absolute risk reduction (a clever marketing trick). This small effect is worthwhile if statins outweigh side effects. This is where things get confusing. On one hand, placebo-controlled trials of statins do not reveal much of a difference in muscle pain between those who take statins and those who take placebo.[36] This suggests that statins do not cause negative side effects. On the other hand, about half of new starters discontinue the medication within the first year.[38] Discontinuation is commonly a result of intolerable adverse effects, primarily muscle pain.[39]

A hypothesis explaining the discrepancy between trials and practice is the *nocebo effect*. To test the hypothesis, some trials (including one I designed) have convinced people who believed they couldn't tolerate statins to alternate between statins and placebos, without knowing which was which. Then the patients were asked to report their side effects daily. It turns out that people report roughly the same number of side effects, such as muscle pain, when they take the statin compared with when they take the placebo. Yet when they know they are taking the statin, they misattribute the muscle pain to the statin. At the end of these trials, when these patients are told that they had as many side effects with the statin as without, they often resume taking the statins. Because the side effects are similar whether the patients are taking statins or not, it seems reasonable to conclude that the side effects are aches and pains that arise naturally but are misattributed to the statins. However, this is not quite right: the trials are all small, and they assume additivity (see appendix 5 for discussion).

There's More

As if all the problems with estimating placebo and nocebo effects described above weren't enough, there's more. In the context of a placebo effect that is combined with a treatment effect, there is no reason to suppose that they add up the way we add $2 + 2$. The placebo or nocebo effect could become bigger or smaller depending on how big the treatment effect is. I'll discuss this in detail in the next chapters.

The Right Way to Measure Placebo and Nocebo Effects

Early estimates of placebo and nocebo effects did not control for natural history and led to an overestimate of placebo effects. Subsequent estimates attempted to control for natural history. However, they introduced several problems of their own, especially heterogeneity. Averaging the effect of any placebo or nocebo for any condition does not tell us whether particular placebos are effective for certain disorders. Moreover, the unrecognized problem of treatment received by "untreated" groups leads to an underestimate of placebo effects. Other problems with measuring placebo effects, including failure to blind, and assuming additivity, will be addressed in more detail in the upcoming chapters. To anticipate, there are no easy solutions to the problems with estimating placebo and nocebo effects. Therefore, despite there

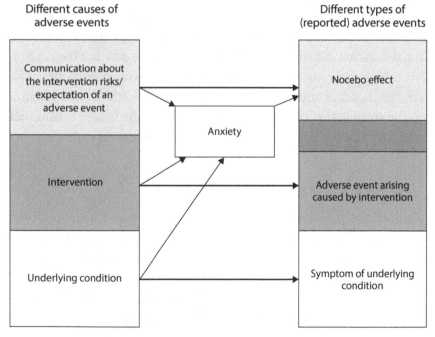

FIG. 5.2. How nocebo effects arise through negative expectations and increased anxiety.

being no doubt that there are placebo and nocebo effects, the exact size of the effects is, and I think will remain, elusive.

Importantly, the fact that a precise estimate remains elusive doesn't mean there are no effects or that we can't gain useful knowledge of the effects. With placebo effects, instead of trying to measure their individual components relative to "no treatment" groups, we should design trials that will provide us with information that is useful to patients. These might involve multicomponent placebo treatment interventions (I describe one of them in chapter 12) that include enhanced communication, calming environment, and expectation management *as a package*. We could then compare the effects of that package in a pragmatic randomized trial with what happens if we provide standard care. If the package is cost-effective, then it should be promoted (I'll say more about these "pragmatic trials" in chapter 10).

CHAPTER 6

Missing the Forest for the Trees

Incomplete Stories about the Inner Workings of Placebos

To us, it seems unlikely that the complexity of human experience can be described in a simple linear model.
— OPHER CASPI AND RICHARD R. BOOTZIN, "Evaluating How Placebos Produce Change"[1]

There are more things in heaven and Earth, Horatio,
Than are dreamt of in your philosophy
— WILLIAM SHAKESPEARE, *Hamlet*, act 1, scene 5

Scientists have been amazingly successful at identifying what happens to our brains and bodies when we experience placebo and nocebo effects.[2-4] An unfortunate consequence of this work on placebo and nocebo inner workings is that we risk missing the forest for the trees. This is a problem because placebo and nocebo effects operate at a global level, yet the individual mechanism studies can give the impression that individual parts operate separately. Moreover, estimating the effects of the individual parts of the placebo effects does not tell us how big placebo effects are as a whole. Relatedly, the studies of individual mechanisms do a good job of explaining *what* happens as we experience placebo effects, yet all largely ignore the *how* and the *why*. After delving into some history of research about how placebos and nocebos work, I'll provide a solution to these problems.

A Digested History of Studying How Placebo and Nocebos Work

Placebo research's journey to credibility began when the physical effects of placebos started to be investigated. This started with Stewart Wolf, who in 1950 reported a study with a single patient (whom he called Tom) in which he investigated the "pharmacology" of placebos.[5] In pharmacology, drugs are known to have a peak effect. That is, they take some time before reaching a maximum effect, after which the effect drops off. For example, if you have a headache and then take an aspirin, it takes some time before the aspirin has its maximum effect, the effect lasts for a while, then it fades away. Wolf found that the time to maximum effect on gastric activity following a saline injection was very similar to that of hydrochloric acid. A few years later, a study with a larger number of patients (23) was done by Louis Lasagna, Victor Laties, and Lawrence Dohan.[6] In addition to finding that the time pattern was similar between placebos and aspirin, they did more research on the pharmacology of the placebo. In addition to identifying peak effects, they found that placebos share other properties with drugs including cumulative effects, and carryover effects.[7]

Twenty years after Lasagna and colleagues did their study, the inner mechanisms of placebos started to be investigated in earnest. Jon Levine and Newton Gordon did a study published in 1978 in which they showed that endorphins (morphine that your body makes) were connected to placebo effects.[8] Their study included 51 patients who had their molar teeth removed. All 51 patients had received a painkiller called mepivacaine after having their teeth removed. Then, three and four hours after the surgery, the patients were given either morphine, a placebo, or naloxone. Naloxone is a drug that prevents morphine from working. All treatments were given in a blind fashion, so the patients didn't know which treatment they were taking. After receiving the injections, most patients who took morphine, and many of those who received the placebo, had less pain. Yet the pain didn't moderate in patients who had received naloxone. This means that naloxone somehow blocked the placebo effect. Since naloxone blocks morphine (and endorphins) from working, and it also blocked placebo effects, the study also suggested that placebo effects are connected to endorphin release. The study has been replicated, and it's clear that treatment with placebo painkillers activates the same parts of the brain that "real" morphine does.[9-12]

The earliest study I'm aware of that investigated mechanisms of *nocebo* effects came almost 20 years later. In 1997, Fabrizio Benedetti and Martina Amanzio published a paper that mimicked Levine and Gordon's but used a different drug. They took 180 patients who had just undergone chest surgery and were experiencing mild pain. All the patients were still in the hospital and hooked up to an intravenous device. The patients gave their informed consent to have their pain *increased* for 30 minutes. Then, some of them were given a placebo (saline) injection and told that the injection would increase pain. The placebo injection increased their pain. Then Benedetti and Amanzio played a trick on the others. Before giving them the saline injection, they gave the patients a drug called proglumide through the intravenous device, without them knowing. Proglumide is a drug that blocks the activity of a stress hormone called cholecystokinin. The patients who were given proglumide did not experience more pain after being given the nocebo saline injection. Since proglumide blocks both the stress hormone and the nocebo effect, they concluded that the stress hormone was responsible for nocebo effects.[13]

You Name It

Levine and Gordon's and Benedetti and Amanzio's early studies were followed by hundreds of others, and the number is growing by the day. It has now reached the point where it seems to be a case of "You name some part of the brain or body, and I'll show you that it changes when placebo treatment is given." Among other findings, studies have shown that following treatment with placebo, oxytocin (the "cuddle molecule") levels,[14] and dopamine (the "happy molecule") levels rise,[15] anxiety is reduced,[16] cannabinoid levels rise,[17] pain messages in the spinal cord get subdued,[18-21] genes change (researchers who study how treatment with placebos changes genetic factors call the genes related to placebo effects the "placebome"),[23-26] and the brain changes.[7,27] Placebo painkillers seem to be associated with less activity in parts of the brain that are associated with pain sensitivity.[28]

Other studies have shown that expecting something bad to happen increases stress hormones like cholecystokinin,[13] which changes the way we perceive touch, pressure, and temperature. It also makes it more likely that we will interpret these things as pain.[28,29] The changed way that we perceive pressure and temperature after believe something bad will happen helps explain expressions like "touchy, and "prickly." People who are touchy or prickly react too strongly to words or indeed touch, perhaps because they expect something bad to happen. It also seems that nocebo effects can be learned when people observe someone else experiencing pain.[30] Many of the studies demonstrating placebo effects are small and have not been replicated, so they cannot be fully trusted. However, the growing number of actual randomized clinical trials demonstrating that there are placebo effects means that many of the claims about placebo effects are very likely to be true.

Related to the fact that it would take volumes to discuss all the placebo mechanisms in detail, it would take volumes to cover all the conditions that placebo effects can allegedly help cure (and that nocebo effects can induce). The most widely studied condition is pain, however, and we have good knowledge about how placebo and nocebo effects arise in a number of other ailments. These include Parkinson's disease (which is related to lower levels of dopamine),[31] anxiety, depression, sleep disorders, irritable bowel syndrome, and sexual dysfunction. Moreover, as I will show below, placebo and nocebo effects almost certainly operate at a global level and affect many systems (and therefore many ailments) at once.

Conscious and Subconscious Expectations
Positive Expectations

When people anticipate that something will happen, it can serve as a self-fulfilling prophecy and arise in part because they expect it to happen. In a study published in 2004, Benedetti and colleagues showed this in a group of 278 patients who had undergone chest surgery for different conditions.[32] The patients were told that they could receive either a painkiller or nothing depending on their postoperative state and that they would not necessarily be informed when the painkilling treatment would be started.[32] All the patients were still in the hospital and hooked up to an intravenous device.

The patients were then randomized into overt and covert groups. The overt group was treated by doctors who "gave the open drug at the bedside, telling the patient that the injection was a powerful analgesic and that the pain was going to subside in a few minutes."[32] Then, one dose of painkiller was administered every 15 minutes, and the patients were asked to rate their pain on a 10-point subjective pain scale in which 0 signaled no pain and 10 unbearable pain. They continued receiving a dose of painkiller every 15 minutes until the patients said that their pain was reduced by 50%.

Patients in the covert group received the same amount of painkiller every 15 minutes and reported how much pain they experienced on the same 10-point scale. But they didn't know they were receiving a painkiller. The painkiller was delivered through a preprogrammed infusion machine (already attached to the patient through the intravenous line) without any doctor or nurse in the room telling them that the powerful drugs would make their pain go away quickly. These covertly treated patients needed 30% *more* drugs to reduce their pain by 50%. The study showed that positive expectations that pain will go away can reduce pain.

Negative Expectations

The opposite is also true. Expecting something bad to happen can increase the chances that it actually happens.[28] In the earliest example of this kind of thing happening I am aware of, a 1968 report describes a study in which 40 asthmatic patients were given a placebo inhaler and told that it contained an irritant that caused asthma attacks.[34,35] Nineteen of the 40 patients reported having asthmatic reactions, and 12 of them developed serious bronchospasms. The 12 patients with strong reactions were cured by giving them another placebo (this time it was a saline injection) that they were told would help. The same study gave a group of 40 non-asthmatic control subjects the same inhaler and told them that it contained an allergen; none of them reported any adverse events. In another example, a 1981 report describes 34 college students who were told that an electric current that might cause a headache was passing through their heads. Over two-thirds of these students reported having a headache, yet there was no electric current—it was a placebo.[36]

In another study published in 2007, patients taking finasteride (a drug to treat enlarged prostates) were told that the drug had a side effect of sexual dysfunction. Compared with other patients who were not told the drug caused sexual dysfunction, the former were three times more likely to report sexual problems compared with patients who were not (43% versus 15%).[37] In an earlier study, published in 2003, patients who were informed about possible sexual dysfunction as a side effect of a drug for cardiac disease were more likely to report experiencing sexual dysfunction than those who were not told (31% versus 16%).[38]

Subconscious Expectations

Linda Buoannono had such bad irritable bowel syndrome that she often couldn't leave the house for weeks on end. She signed up for a trial of "honest" placebos. An honest placebo is a placebo that patients know is a placebo. They are sometimes called open-label placebos. The Harvard doctors in the trial told her that the pills were "placebo pills made of an inert substance, like sugar pills, that have been shown in clinical studies to produce significant improvement in [irritable bowel] symptoms through mind-body self-healing processes."[39] The honest placebos worked better than anything she'd tried in years, and she was able to resume a normal life. Linda wasn't the only person in the trial who benefited from open-label placebos; they had an average beneficial effect as well. Some of the patients might have had a conscious expectation that their symptoms would go away after the placebo (after all, eminent doctors from Harvard told them that placebos might work). However, their recovery was also probably related to their subconscious and prereflective experiences of doctors, hospitals, and taking medicine. We have far less control over our thoughts and beliefs than we believe or think we do, which explains, at least partly, how honest placebos work. If I tell you to *not* think of a red monkey, most of you conjured the image of a red monkey.

Studies which suggest that there can be placebo effects in animals add to the evidence regarding subconscious mechanisms.[40] A study published in 2010 involving 34 dogs with epilepsy found that 79% of the dogs who had received placebo demonstrated a 26% reduction in seizure frequency compared with baseline.[41] While this was a small study that I do not think has been replicated, that placebos seem to work in animals adds to the evidence suggesting that placebos operate at a subconscious level.

A new field of research that I think explains how honest placebos work shows that the brain learns to make predictions based on past experiences. The idea behind "predictive processing" as its proponents insist on calling it (why not just say "learning"?) is that we don't react just to what is out there, to a pill, but to what our brain expects, based on what it has learned in the past.[42] If our brains have learned or been programmed to invoke an immune system response after visiting a doctor, then they might do so even if the treatment received at the doctor's office is a "mere" placebo.

No Classical Conditioning in the Real World

It's tempting to explain how open-label placebos work by appealing to classical conditioning, but I think that's a mistake. Classical conditioning was made famous by Ivan Pavlov who rang a bell and then fed his dogs. The next day he rang the bell again and fed his dogs. After a few repetitions of ringing the bell then feeding the dogs, ringing the bell was enough to cause the dogs to salivate even if there was no food around. The dogs learned to associate something that started off as neutral (the bell) with something they like (food). Some laboratory studies have shown that conditioning works with people too. My favorite is Luana Colloca's study of 46 healthy volunteers who were conditioned to experience a nocebo effect. The volunteers were shown either a flashing green, yellow, or red light. The green flash was followed by a mild, nonpainful electric shock to the ankle, a flashing yellow light was followed by a mild shock, and a flashing red light was followed by a painful shock. After the participants had learned to associate the different colors with no pain, mild pain, or greater pain, Colloca switched things around. Participants received mild shocks following flashing lights of all three colors. But that is not what the patients felt. After a red light flashed, they felt a painful shock although they had received a mild nonpainful shock. This is because they had been conditioned to associate a red light with a painful shock and a green light with a mild shock.

The problem is that real placebo effects do not arise after anything like repeated ringing bells or flashing lights. Sure, patients might have had positive experiences with a particular doctor, hospital, music in the doctor's office, and getting a pill. Seeing that doctor and hospital, hearing that music, or getting a pill may therefore evoke some memories and a reaction of some sort, even if the pill is an open-label placebo. But the combination of factors that people respond to is much more complex than Pavlov's bell. This is why researchers are starting to replace "conditioning" with "learning." People learn to expect something good (or bad) to happen at the doctor's office, or hospital, or when they smell or hear something. Importantly, the learning can be at a conscious or subconscious level.

Overdoing Expectations May Have a Paradoxical Effect

Like many good things in life, overdoing expectations can cause harm. A small study showed that when doctors said that a mildly painful procedure would be *completely* pain-free, it led to lower pain but also undermined trust in the doctor.[43] Presumably, they will be less likely to believe the doctor the next time, so the overly positive suggestion would only work once.

Related to overstating reduction in pain, the act of generating a conscious expectation when it might not be needed can also cause harm. Men with healthy sexual functions who were given a placebo to enhance their performance developed sexual problems.[44] This is probably because it caused the men to pay attention to responses that had previously come naturally, which probably increased their anxiety and deactivated their feed-and-breed responses (see below). However, when placebos were given to men with sexual function problems, their performance improved.

The amazing studies of what happens to our brains and bodies as placebo and nocebo effects are experienced played a key role in the first revolution in placebo studies: they moved the once fluffy field of placebo studies onto firmer, more objective ground. Now, however, the focus on individual mechanisms has several opportunity costs that inhibit putting the knowledge we have into practice.

Placebo Responders

Of course, different people react to drugs, surgery, and placebos in different ways, and a group of studies has investigated whether certain people are more likely than others to respond to placebos. It's tempting to believe that only naïve or gullible people respond to placebos, but that doesn't seem to be quite right. Some studies are starting to show that people who are more suggestible, optimistic, and altruistic respond better to placebo treatments,[45,46] while those who are angrier are more susceptible to nocebo responses.[47] Even more recently, some studies have suggested that brain structure might predict some placebo responses.[48] However, by and large, the research into placebo responders is immature and we can't (for now) predict in advance who will respond to a placebo and who will not. Pharmaceutical companies have a great financial interest in predicting who will respond to placebos yet, they don't even try. Instead, they do this empirically by giving people placebos and seeing who responds. If it were possible to do some preliminary tests to determine who was a placebo responder this would be cheaper than putting them through a placebo run-in period.

The Problem with Placebo Mechanisms Studies: Missing the Forest for the Trees

Recall from chapter 3 that Henry Knowles Beecher found that wounded soldiers evacuated from the Anzio beachhead needed far fewer painkillers than civilians who suffered from the same wounds. This wasn't just because soldiers were tougher (which is no doubt true) but also because, to the soldiers, the wound meant relief from a deadly and brutal battle. He concluded that the amount of pain experienced has little to do with the wound itself. In his words:

> The extent of wound bears only a slight relationship, if any (often none at all), to the pain experienced. This fact fails to support the relevance of experimental [laboratory] pain work to the pathological [real-life] pain experience. The concept underlying all experimental pain methods, that the more severe the stimuli to nerve endings, the more the pain, does not hold for pathological pain. Thus the usefulness of experimental pain methods in man for the purposes to which they have

often been put (evaluation of the analgesic power of narcotic agents) is questionable. Just as the doctrine of specific etiology of disease falls short, so also is the relationship not precise between cause and a symptom of disease (injury) as far as a wound and resulting pain are concerned. The level of anxiety is important in considering the production of pain. The unfortunate and common practice of administering powerful analgesic agents to all injured individuals is clearly unsound. A considerable number of such patients may not have pain. In others alteration of mood, as for example relief of anxiety, can have beneficial effect. In short, even a great wound is not necessarily an "adequate stimulus for pain."[49]

Beecher's point is that the experience of pain is not simple: it depends on additional factors beyond the wound. In the lab, researchers correctly focus on single factors to do tightly controlled experiments. This was necessary to put the field of placebo studies on firm scientific ground. But now that placebo studies have been established, the continued focus on individual and increasingly esoteric mechanisms is getting in the way of gathering more clinically useful data about global placebo and nocebo effects.

Ignoring the Global Placebo and Nocebo Responses

Recall from chapter 3 that the biopsychosocial model considers the interconnections between biology, psychology, and socio-environmental factors of health and disease.[50] It challenges the view that the body is basically a complex machine that has a collection of separate mechanisms. Systems theory extends the biopsychosocial model to emphasize the interconnectedness between components of systems like human beings. Placebo studies can benefit from insights from the biopsychosocial model and systems theory. This is because there are connections between the various activities associated with placebo effects, yet these interactions have been largely ignored. For example, the cannabinoid, endorphin, and dopamine pathways (which have all been shown to be associated with placebo treatment) interact. These internal pathways, in turn, can interact with other systems in the human body as well as the environment. I'll show this by looking at two important and related global responses related to placebo and nocebo effects: the fight-or-flight response and the relaxation (or feed-and-breed) response.

Nocebo, Placebo, Fight or Flight, Feed and Breed

The nocebo effect is associated with stress hormones. We know that the stress response is global. Let me explain with the help of a mythical caveman ancestor.

Imagine a caveman coming home at dusk after a long day hunting. Along the way, he accidentally startles a pack of wild wolves. He freezes in his tracks, yet inside his body things change instantly. Anticipating a brawl or having to run for his life, an almond-sized part of his brain called the amygdala sends signals that result in an orchestrated system of responses to prepare him to run or fight. Adrenaline and cortisol are pumped through his veins to boost energy levels. Blood pressure and heart rate jump to send more oxygen to his muscles. His pupils dilate so that he can see better in the dark. His lung vessels dilate to take in more oxygen. Pancreatic levels adjust to give him more quick-fix sugar energy in his blood. The pain-message system in the brain gets suppressed so that pain will not stop him from running or fighting if he steps on a thorn. If he was hungry, he completely forgets about it because his digestive system gets turned off. If he had a cold, he forgets about that too. It is not in the interest of his survival to worry about a meal or fight off a cold if he needs to fight a hungry wolf.

Our mythical caveman lets out a cry and hurls a stone at the wolves. This time, he is lucky. The wolves weren't hungry, so they slink away. The caveman sighs and walks back to his village, where he relaxes by the campfire, smiling as he reminisces about his adventures. Maybe he has a family who cuddle beside him. What happens *inside* him now is very different. His body changes while happy chemicals like dopamine, endorphins, and oxytocin are released. His digestive system (required for good immune function) also gets into high gear as there is no longer a need to divert all his energy to the muscles needed to run or fight. Our primitive ancestors had physically tough lives, but surprise encounters with wolves were rare, and by most accounts they could relax much of the time.

In our present-day lives, encounters with fierce wolves are rare. But other common life events can trigger similar reactions. Most of us waken with an alarm. Alarms are *designed* to cause some stress, which is a small-scale fight-or-flight response. These alarms are most often on our smart phones, which immediately bombard us with messages, news, alerts, and calendar reminders. Some of these are fun, but many induce more stress. Most often all this happens well before 8 a.m. and continues all day—quite literally until the minute we put our smart phones down and close our eyes. The result is too much fight or flight and not enough relaxation, which contributes to the epidemics of depression, heart disease, and more.[51] This is paradoxical since the fight-or-flight response is amazing for helping us survive acute threats, yet too much of it puts our health at risk, and can make us die younger.

The antidote to too much fight-or-flight stress is the feed-and-breed (or "rest and digest") response. Learning how to relax appropriately has been shown to have a host of health benefits ranging from reduced blood pressure and heart disease to more happiness, better relationships, and longer life.[51] This link between the relaxation response and the immune response is now taken seriously in a relatively new discipline called psychoneuroimmunology, which also has roots in the biopsychosocial model of disease.

Both the fight-or-flight, and the feed, breed, and heal systems are automatic and global. They are automatic because they don't rely on our conscious control. You don't need to say, "go, fight-or-flight response!" if you see a wild wolf. And you don't need to say "go, feed-and-breed system" if you are cuddling by a peaceful campfire with your partner. With the caveat that with rigorous training we can bring them partly within our control, by and large it just happens.

The fight or flight and feed and breed are also global. It is not just that your pupils dilate when there is a hungry wolf eyeing you up as it licks its lips: your heartrate rises too, pancreatic levels are adjusted, adrenaline and cortisol kick in. Setting aside exceptional people who have done a lot of biofeedback or meditation, you can't just have *part* of the fight-or-flight response. It's all or nothing. Ditto for the relaxation response. If your body is feeling relaxed and floppy by a nice campfire in the evening, you will have the happy chemicals like dopamine and endorphins floating around, your digestive system will be up and running, and if you are in an amorous mood, well then. The global nature of the relaxation response explains why studies have shown that relaxing just one part of your body like your jaw can relax your entire body. Try it.

Placebo and nocebo effects are linked to feed-and-breed and fight-or-flight responses. In addition to the direct link between nocebo effects and stress hormones mentioned above, Karin Meissner in Germany has noted numerous experiments demonstrating the relationship between the autonomic nervous system and placebo treatment. These include changes in blood pressure, coronary blood flow, digestion, breathing, and sexual function in both men and women.[37,52] Other studies have found that anxiety decreases following placebo administration.[53-55] In short, placebo and nocebo effects seem to overlap with the relaxation and stress responses, respectively. What seems to be happening is that placebo treatments, together with positively meaningful contexts, induce the relaxation response and therefore can improve immune system function and digestion. And, on the other hand, nocebo effects are an instantiation of a stress response.

At a theoretical level, this implies that placebo effects include improved immune system function, while nocebo effects include suppressed immune system function. Studies are starting to show that this is more than a theoretical prediction.[56] Immune deficiency diseases such as psoriasis,[57] allergic rhinitis,[57] and lupus erythematosus[59,60] seem to respond to placebo treatment. If placebo and nocebo effects are associated with the immune system, it has important implications for our health. This is because our immune systems are incredible. Put simply, and literally, without your immune system you would be dead in a matter of days. My favorite heroes of the immune system (there are too many to mention in this book) are highly trained and very efficient killer white blood cells that specialize in seeking and destroying any cells that have been compromised. A common type of white blood cell that does these seek-and-destroy missions is the natural killer cell. The first time I heard the name "natural killer cell" I thought it was a nickname, and that there was another, more scientific sounding Latin name in textbooks. I was mistaken: "natural killer cell" is the scientific name for these amazing cells.

The link between placebos and nocebos and the immune system may explain some of the dramatic positive and negative responses to placebo treatments like Mr. Wright and Mr. A.

Connections between Patients, Doctors, and Environments

In addition to global systems within individual humans that are associated with placebo responses, interconnections between patients, doctors, and the environment also play a role. I explained in chapter 3 how features of the environment and practitioner can affect healing, and some recent studies have shown that placebo and nocebo effects are contagious. Watching someone else's pain go away can help your own pain go away.[61] Children who watched their mothers exaggerate painful reactions to cold water subsequently had lower pain thresholds.[61,62] The same electric shock will be less painful if we see that it doesn't hurt others around us. If a treatment seems to reduce pain in others, it will be more likely to work for us, even when the treatment is a placebo.[63,64] Even watching a video of someone else being affected positively by a placebo can induce placebo effects in the observer.[64] Studies of individual mechanisms take our eyes away from these connections and focus them on individual parts of one single person's brain or body, which are only part of the placebo story.

Meanwhile, as noted above, doctors who believe their treatments are powerful and effective get better responses from their treatments.[65]

Who Cares about How They Work (As Long as They Work)?

Most proponents of evidence-based medicine believe that while mechanisms are useful for several reasons (generalizing and discovering treatments), they are not useful for confirming whether treatments work.[1-3] This is because, they argue, the mechanisms are not complete, and knowledge of mechanisms can mislead. On the other hand, most philosophers of science who have commented on this issue have argued that mechanisms are far more important, with a dominant view (within philosophy of science) being that we *need* evidence of a mechanism in order to establish that a treatment works.[4] My view is in the middle: understanding mechanisms is more valuable than most within the evidence-based medicine camp believe, but they are not required, as some philosophers of science believe.

References

1. Howick J, Glasziou P, Aronson JK. Evidence-based mechanistic reasoning. *J R Soc Med*. Nov 2010;103(11):433–441. https://doi.org/10.1258/jrsm.2010.100146.

2. Howick J. Exposing the vanities—and a qualified defence—of mechanistic evidence in clinical decision-making. *Philosophy of Science*. 2011;78(5):926–940. https://www.jstor.org/stable/10.1086/662561.

3. Howick, J, Glasziou, P, Aronson, JK. Problems with using mechanisms to solve the problem of extrapolation. *Theor Med Bioeth* 34, 275–291 (2013). https://doi.org/10.1007/s11017-013-9266-0.

4. Russo F, Williamson J. Interpreting causality in the health sciences. *International Studies in the Philosophy of Science*. 2007;21(2):1157–1170. https://doi.org/10.1080/02698590701498084.

Although there seem to be clear connections between different responses that happen in one person, and between one person and the other people and surroundings, few studies that have looked at these things as a whole. We need to know more about how the components of placebo treatments interact to produce an overall, real-world effect.

The Mind/Body Mechanism

The laboratory studies of placebo effects, because they often involve brain scans, imply that all the action is in the brain. The underlying assumption behind this is that the mind is housed exclusively in the brain. Placebo and nocebo effects challenge this view because if minds are exclusively in our skulls, then it is difficult to explain how inert things, even if they are given in meaningful contexts can affect what happens in the brain. How does the mind, which is exclusively in the skull, get affected by nice music or kind words from a physician? The standard answer to this from a "mind just in the brain" perspective is that sounds or colors make it into our brains through our ears, eyes, and other sense organs. Then, the brain interprets it, and poof! We get the different parts of our brains chugging away and doing all the stuff the brain-scan studies show they do to produce placebo effects. That explanation is certainly an important part of the story. But it does not follow that it is the whole story, and the idea that it is the whole story is quite extraordinary. The molecular biologist Francis Crick called it astonishing: "'You', your joys and your sorrows, your memories and your ambitions, your sense of personal identity and free will, are in fact no more than the behaviour of a vast assembly of nerve cells and their associated molecules. . . . This hypothesis is so alien to the ideas of most people alive today that it can truly be called astonishing."[66]

The reason the hypothesis is astonishing is that it conflicts with everyday commonsense experience. To be sure, many things that turned out to be false were accepted based on commonsense experience. It was once common sense to believe that the earth was flat and that the sun rotated around the earth. But just because common sense is not a *definitive* guide to truth, it doesn't mean that commonsense beliefs should be dismissed just because they are common sense. In fact, empiricism, which is a core feature of science, demands that we take (common) sense experience seriously. My experience tells me that when I am watching the sunset, I experience the sun out there, not in my brain. I perceive objects as being out there, where they are. When I meet a friend, my experience of my friend is not in my brain; it is of my friend out there. The astonishing hypothesis dismisses our experiences as completely mistaken.

The astonishing hypothesis is also a dogma because there is no evidence that our minds are restricted exclusively to our brains. While nobody sensible denies that a lot of important activity happens in our brains, the idea that it is *only* there is a hypothesis rather than an established truth. On the other hand, there is no definitive evidence that our minds extend beyond our brains either, but there are good reasons to believe that the mind is not (exclusively) in the brain. For example, the enteric nervous system, which is in the gut, can operate independently of the central nervous system (the brain and spinal cord). When you feel butterflies in your stomach, it is probably the enteric nervous system at work. Those who are in touch with these feelings claim they can "trust their gut instincts." The enteric nervous system plays a key role in digestion and is also connected to the immune system.[67] It also reacts to outside stimuli independently and connects with the brain through a large nerve called the vagus nerve.

The main argument I encounter against the (astonishing) idea that the mind is housed exclusively in the brain is that other explanations are even more astonishing because they involve a religious spirit or God (or something similar) intervening. This is a problem because in some circles *merely raising the question* of whether there is evidence that the mind is exclusively in the brain is enough to get you labeled a quack or pseudoscientist.

One needn't appeal to esoteric ideas to explain how minds could be extended beyond brains. For instance, minds could be properties that emerge from the brain. An example of an emergent property is a crystal. In a sense, there is no more to an ice crystal than H_2O, yet a crystal has properties that are independent of hydrogen and oxygen. Similarly, the activity of the brain might lead to a mind emerging, and the emerged mind might have some properties that cannot be explained by the activity of the brain alone and that could extend beyond the physical limits of the brain. An entire discipline called noogenesis is dedicated to studying and explaining how human minds emerged from brains.[68] The other theory of how the mind could extend beyond the brain involves the idea of perceptual fields that are both in the brain and extend beyond it.[69] Since any moving matter, including the moving matter in our brains, creates electromagnetic fields, the idea that our brain activity could extend beyond our skull should be taken more seriously than it currently is. The Indian science of Vedanta has another explanation about how the phenomenal world of experience arises from an interaction between the subject and object.[70] Certainly, it is dogmatic and unscientific to reject the idea of minds extending beyond the brain or the relationship between an individual's mind and the outside world without proper investigation.

Several experiments have tested the hypothesis of extended minds. For example, tests of telepathy have been done in which people who are physically separated are asked to guess what the other is thinking. Many of these have been conducted and made popular by Rupert Sheldrake.[71-73] Sheldrake describes a number of scientific experiments that seem to support what many people claim to sense, including the sense of being stared at and experiences of dogs who seem to know their owners are coming home.[65] The results of these experiments have not generated a definitive answer to the question of whether minds are extended or trapped in our skulls, but they are suggestive.

The relatively new and growing fields of enactivism and embodied cognition are starting to delve into the connection between our minds and our environments (which includes other people and therefore other minds). The idea behind these new fields is that the distinction between the mind, the body, and the environment is blurry. Promoting the idea of embodied consciousness, Frenkel proposed that the body (and not the "mind") is the primary site for knowing the world.[74] According to this view, if a patient's *body* interacts with a healing context, an appropriate response is generated. The appropriate reaction could include all the responses discussed earlier in this book, ranging from a healing relaxation response, a full immune response, or anything in-between.[75] This theory also holds that our bodies' physical interaction with the world influences or even determines our cognitions.[76] More specifically, sensory signals could evoke different reactions including those involved in positive and negative healing experiences.[77]

The main idea behind enactivism is that our perceptions are not just in the brain but arise (are "enacted") because of an interaction between a person and their environment. A central premise of enactivism is that there is a continuity between life and mind.[78] Empirical support for embodied consciousness and enactivism is emerging. Studies have found that similar areas of the brain that describe certain action verbs such as "walk" are also involved in actual walking, which suggests a connection between the mind (the word) and the body (walking).[79] Embodied cognition and enactivism imply that minds are not housed exclusively in brains. I hope that more research on placebos is done by embodied cognition and enactivist scholars because their research provides more accurate frameworks from which to understand global placebo and nocebo effects. To make their work relevant it has to be accessible whereas it currently is not. The most recent paper I read on the topic had four terms I didn't understand in a single paragraph: metastability, preindividuality, relational-processual, and sensorimotor/psychological. Getting this important knowledge out of the walls of academia will be easier if the knowledge is expressed clearly.

Dissolving Artificial Distinctions between Minds and Bodies
Taking a more global perspective also helps dissolve the artificial distinction between minds and bodies, and between the objective and subjective. Whereas the fact that intangible beliefs can affect our bodies is incontrovertible proof that minds can't be separated from bodies, the near exclusive focus of most placebo studies on body and brain parts gives the impression that humans are just physical machines. David Morris noted that "to most medical people, [the placebo effect] makes as much sense as filling up the gas tank with Earl Grey tea."[80] To which Daniel Moerman adds, "People are not machines, and we shouldn't treat them as such."[81] Relatedly, the science discussed above shows that the distinction between objective and subjective outcomes can get blurry. Sure, death is clearly an objective outcome. But other feelings like pain, depression, and positive outlooks that are viewed as subjective have been shown by placebo researchers to also include

objective changes inside patients' brains and bodies. They are neither just objective nor just subjective, and this artificial distinction fades away if we adopt a more global perspective.

In addition to averting our focus from global effects, the attention on laboratory studies may also have diverted our gaze away from the global "why?" question.

The Big "Why?" Question

From an evolutionary perspective, placebo and nocebo effects don't make much sense. Since we already have immune systems, why should we wait for placebo treatment to boost them? Why doesn't the body just get on with it and heal without the placebo treatment? And on the other end of the spectrum, why would we have evolved to allow negative words from a witch doctor to harm us by suppressing our immune systems?

The first answer to this question is that in most cases our body does simply get on with it. If we get a scratch, our body heals it so that there is no trace; if we get a cold, it goes away within a week; if we have back pain, it usually goes away within three weeks; if we feel down or tired, we usually feel better within hours or days. Our hearts beat over 3 billion times in our lives, and most of us never need to repair any parts because the body heals itself continuously. Our lungs process almost a billion liters of air in a lifetime, usually without needing a check-up or replacing any spare parts. Our skin completely regenerates itself within a few weeks; our stomach linings completely regenerate themselves within a few days. The list goes on. And all this happens whether you get a placebo treatment or not. It's just that studies show that the healing happens a bit better and a bit faster with placebo treatments, and a bit slower with nocebos.[46]

The other answer is a hypothesis from evolutionary biology. The body's amazing innate ability to heal, and the immune system itself, consume a lot of energy. And the more serious the ailment, the more it consumes. Because it's expensive, the wisdom of the body deploys

the immune system wisely. Being chased by a wolf? Not worth spending energy fixing that scratch or fighting that cold; it's better to use
the energy to run. Have an exam upon which (you think) your entire
future depends? Better to ignore the cold so that your energy can focus on studying. Nicholas Humphrey, who suggested this evolutionary idea to me, proposed that there is an inner health governor that
decides when to activate the inner healing and when not to.[82] This
governor decides to activate the inner healing powers when we are
safe. When the caveman is back at the campfire. When the exam is over.
When there is no need to deploy the fight-or-flight response. The
governor also deploys resources if there is a good prospect of getting
social and nutritional support in the future. There is no point evoking
a full-blown immune response in a post-apocalyptic world in which
we and our potential offspring are certain to die of starvation or nu-
clear radiation.

According to the evolutionary view, a treatment with a placebo, from
a trusted health care practitioner (or, for our ancestors, a shaman) of-
fers us an implicit or explicit message: "I'm here to take care of you. It
is safe and I'm going to provide you with whatever you need to get better." Having received this message, the inner governor switches the
inner healing powers on, and our body responds by deploying its full
immune response, natural killer cells and all.

Putting the Basic Science of Placebos to Use

The basic science of placebos has been enormously successful and produced an edifice of knowledge about the detailed mechanisms of
placebo and nocebo effects. For patients to benefit from this knowledge, the knowledge has to be integrated into a search for global mechanisms, global effects, and answers to deeper *how* and *why* questions.

CHAPTER 7

Placebo and Nocebo Effects Don't Add Up

A perturbation in any part of the system shakes the whole.
    —JEROME FRANK AND JULIA FRANK, *Persuasion and Healing*[1]

The power attributed to morphine is then presumably a placebo effect plus its drug effect.
    —HENRY K. BEECHER, "The Powerful Placebo"[2]

Placebo Run-In Periods

Recall from last chapter that many clinical trials have what they call "placebo run-in periods." Before allocating patients to receive the drug or the placebo, they give everyone a placebo for a few weeks. Then, whoever responds to the placebo is excluded from the trial. The reason they do this is that the stronger the placebo response is, the less room there is for the drug to make a difference. By excluding placebo responders, they therefore get an unadulterated estimate of the benefit of the drug.[3] The problem is that if the drug does prove to be superior to the placebo, it is assumed that the drug will have a similar effect in the general population. But ignored interactions can make this assumption a costly mistake. Say that after the placebo run-in period, the difference in outcomes between the drug and the placebo groups was 10%. All the cost-effectiveness calculations, and policy decisions to promote and fund the drug are based on that 10% difference. Yet had they included placebo responders, then the difference between the placebo and the drug would almost certainly have been smaller because the placebo effect would have been bigger. A reason this unfortunate practice continues unchecked is that interactions are all but ignored.

The various features of a placebo or active treatment can either add in a simple way ($2 + 2 = 4$), or they could combine in some way such that the whole is greater ($2 + 2 = 5$) or less than ($2 + 2 = 3$) the sum of the parts. On the face of it, there is no good reason to assume that we can compute the overall effect by adding up the effects of the parts. Most human characteristics don't add up simply. To take a dramatic example, all humans (including me and you) are made up of 11 elements that could be purchased for a few dollars at a pharmacy. These are water (about three quarters) carbon (about a fifth) and some other minerals (about 5% altogether). But nobody would say that they can understand *you* by adding up what they know about these simple elements. The way the properties of the basic elements combine creates something new, the way hydrogen and oxygen create water. Appendix 3 contains a formalization of the assumption that things add up ("additivity"). Although it doesn't seem reasonable to assume additivity, it is assumed more often than it should. When a placebo-controlled trial is conducted, the benefit of the new treatment over and above the placebo control is assumed to remain constant. This assumption—which does not make sense given what we know about human biology and leads to mistaken estimates of treatment effects—is pervasive.

Additivity between Placebo and Active Treatment: Real Examples

The idea that placebo and treatment features interact is not just theoretically plausible. Sigmund Freud often insisted on a hefty fee. But this was not because he needed the money. Instead, he thought that asking people to pay a lot of money would activate his method of psychoanalysis.[4] Paying money by itself has zero effect on curing psychological disorders, and Freudian psychoanalysis has a small average effect.

But (according to Freud) when paying the fee is combined with psychoanalysis, the effect of psychoanalysis increases. We can't add the effect of paying a hefty fee (zero!) to the effect of Freudian psychoanalysis to get the overall effect of receiving psychoanalysis and paying a hefty fee.

Interactions can be formally measured in what is called the "balanced placebo design" (see appendix 4 and appendix 5 for a full explanation). With this design, some patients get a placebo but believe they are getting the real drug ("strong" placebo) and other patients receive the placebo and think they *might* be getting the real drug or the placebo ("weak" placebo). If drug effects add to placebo effects, then the additional benefit of the drug should stay the same whether the placebo effect is strong or weak.

In an example of the balanced placebo design from the late 1980s, John Hughes and colleagues published a paper that compared how good real nicotine gum was for helping people quit smoking compared with placebo nicotine gum.[5] They found 77 regular smokers who were willing to take part in the trial and assigned them to one of six groups.

- Some were told they were receiving real nicotine gum (the left-most columns in figure 7.1). Of those, only half actually got real nicotine gum—the others got a placebo.
- Some were told they were receiving placebo (the middle columns in figure 7.1). Of those, only half actually got real nicotine gum—the others got a placebo.
- Some were delivered the treatment in double-blind conditions—the right-hand columns in figure 7.1—I'll ignore these here.

They then measured how many participants completely quit smoking. They did this by asking, and they confirmed it with a breath test that measured smoking residue.

If we could add the additional effect of the "real" nicotine in the gum to other stuff, then it wouldn't matter whether the person believed it was a placebo or believed it was real nicotine gum. In both cases, the

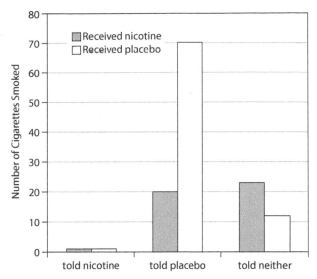

FIG. 7.1. Interaction between placebo and nicotine, showing that there is no drug effect when placebo effects are large

added benefit of the nicotine in the gum should be the same. But that's not what happened. When smokers thought they were taking a placebo, the nicotine in the gum had an added benefit. But when people were told they were getting the real nicotine gum, the nicotine gum didn't have any benefit over and above the placebo at all! What happened in this trial is easy to explain. When the smokers thought that they were getting the real drug, they had strong beliefs and expectations that it would work, and this made the placebo work as well as the real drug. On the other hand, when the smokers knew they were getting the placebo ("just a sugar pill"), they did not believe they would be able to stop and this left room for the drug-induced improvement. It seems that as the strength of the placebo factors moves from weak (they believe the gum is just a placebo) to strong (they believe the gum is a powerful treatment), there is less and less room for the drug to show its effect. The effect of the nicotine in the gum cannot be added to the placebo factors. Whether it has an effect *depends* on how "strong" the placebo is.

In more detail, the way the placebo worked in the nicotine gum example was probably something like the following.[6] The maximum drug response is related to the maximum number of receptors cells have for the drug to attach to. Once the receptors have all been occupied, there is no further room for improvement. If the placebo caused the body to produce enough of its own drugs to occupy all the receptors, then there would be no more room for improvement from the drug. In general, most ailments can only be improved so much. If a strong placebo factor is enough to make your mild pain go away, then adding a drug won't make it go away more.

In another example where things didn't add up, Jean-François Bergmann and his colleagues tested whether a painkiller (naproxen) or placebo reduced pain in cancer patients before French law required researchers to tell patients whether they were getting a placebo. Some of the patients were told they might be getting a placebo (weak placebo factors) and others were told they were getting the powerful painkiller (strong placebo factors). They measured how much pain the patients were in before the treatment, then at 30, 60, 120, and 180 minutes after treatment. They used the visual analogue scale (where 0 is no pain and 10 is maximum pain) to measure the pain. As with the nicotine gum study, they found that the added benefit of the painkiller (naproxen) was smaller when the patients thought they were receiving a powerful painkiller. The effect of the painkiller did not add onto the placebo treatment factors; they interacted in some way.

In a study published in 1966, researchers compared the interactions between a doctor's attitude towards anti-anxiety medicine and the type of clinic. Some of the doctors were instructed to be enthusiastic about the drug's effects, and others were instructed to be skeptical. One of the three clinics was in a particularly wealthy area and attended by people of higher socioeconomic class.[7] Patients were also given either placebos or a real anti-anxiety drug. Among other things, they found that the skepticism of the doctors could either increase or decrease the placebo effect depending on the type of clinic. It seems that the skepticism was interpreted differently by patients with different socioeconomic backgrounds. For some reason, the enthusiastic doctors generated a placebo effect only in the wealthier clinic.

How Common Are Interactions between Placebo and Treatment Features?

With my colleague and friend Rémy Boussageon in France,[8] I did a review of all the studies that have different "strengths" of placebo factors using the balanced placebo design, and over 85% provided evidence of interactions. Sometimes the placebo and active treatments features synergize each other so that the overall effect is greater than the sum of its parts ($2 + 2 = 5$), and at other times they antagonize each other so that the overall effect is smaller than the sum of the parts ($2 + 2 = 3$).

The evidence that placebo effects seem to be getting bigger in the US (but not elsewhere) is also relevant to the additivity versus interactions debate.[9] Simple math means that when the placebo effect is larger, the drug effect is smaller. Related studies suggest that placebo effects are stronger in industry funded trials compared with other trials.[10] The larger placebo effects in the US could be caused by the fact that pharmaceutical companies are allowed to market their products directly to consumers in the US and do this very well. When a patient is in a clinical trial comparing a drug with a placebo (and they are blinded) they will have been exposed to the effective marketing campaigns. This leads to higher expectations regarding their recovery, stronger placebo effects, and smaller drug effects. The benefit of the drug over and above the placebo might be bigger if the marketing were not so effective.

How Do Placebo and Treatment Factors Interact?

We don't know everything about how placebo factors and treatment factors interact. This is because the assumption that they add is so pervasive that few people have tried to figure out why. However, we can make an educated guess. Placebo treatments work by helping the body create its own chemicals like endorphins, dopamine, and oxytocin. These drugs that are produced by the body could interact with the "real" drug. For example, one study of expectations made the surprise discovery that increased expectations (and increased levels of dopamine and oxytocin) led to caffeine being metabolized twice as fast as usual.[11]

Additivity between Placebo Features

The examples so far have shown that placebo treatment features as a whole and treatment features interact more often than is supposed. For similar reasons (biological forces acting in humans usually interact), it is unreasonable to assume that the components of placebo treatments add. Patient beliefs, doctor beliefs, environmental factors, and other components of treatment with placebos almost certainly interact. Unlike the rather strong evidence for interactions between placebo and treatment features, there is less direct evidence for interactions between various features of placebos. It is also more difficult to gather such evidence. One would require trials of two or more different strengths of placebos plus an untreated group, and such trials are rare at best. But there is a great deal of indirect evidence that different placebo features interact. For example, each of the following has been shown to reduce pain by between half and one point on a 10-point pain scale: positive messages, empathic language, doctor pretreatment expectations, calming environment, a brand name, and continuity of care. That means if we were to add these up, we would get a reduction of 6 points on a 10-point pain scale. Such an effect is implausibly large. A reduction of 6 points is more than strong morphine. The chances are that the effects of all these things combine in a way that makes their overall effect smaller. On the other hand, the examples of dramatic recovery following placebo treatment (or dramatic harm following nocebo treatment) could be examples of the whole being greater than the sum of the parts.

Biased Since Mill

Given the theoretical implausibility and evidence against it, why is the assumption of additivity so pervasive? I suspect a lot of it has to do with the materialist world view which amounts to the claim that humans are "lumbering robots" as Richard Dawkins famously said. I also suspect it is because scientists and philosophers—indeed all academics—are trained to isolate single things and analyze them. They are trained to take things apart. Medical scientists take bodies apart. Physicists take atoms apart. Philosophers take arguments apart. The better you are at taking things apart, the better the scientist or academic you are. The skill of taking things apart is important for finding out about parts, for isolating the effective parts of plants to make patented drugs, doing surgery, finding flaws in other people's arguments, and doing other things that make you more successful in academia.

Relatedly, academic disciplines have become increasingly specialized, getting narrower and narrower to create sub-disciplines and sub-sub disciplines. Just a century ago, it was possible for a single person to have state-of-the-art knowledge of all parts of the human body. Now we know so much about feet that an expert in feet will not be an expert in hands; an expert on the liver will not be an expert on lungs; and an expert in eyes will not be an expert in noses.

For the reasons I've listed and no doubt others, it's not surprising that researchers prefer to assume that things add up simply. For example, my colleague Nancy Cartwright, probably the most respected living philosopher of science, states:

> One looks for independent evidence that an interaction is occurring, and some account of why it should occur between these variables and not others, or at these levels and not others. The chemistry examples are a good case. One does not just say the acid and base interact because they behave differently together from the way they behave separately; rather, we understand already a good deal about how the separate

capacities work and why they should interfere with each other in just the way they do.[12]

The emphasis on adding was also propounded almost two hundred years ago by John Stuart Mill, who stated, "Now, if we happen to know what would be the effect of each cause when acting separately from the other, we are often able to arrive deductively, or *a priori*, at a correct prediction of what will arise from their conjunct agency."[13] His statement is curious because Mill was clear that in chemistry, biology and humans, interactions were the norm. In his words:

> The chemical combination of two substances produces, as is well known, a third substance with properties different from those of either of the two substances separately, or of both of them taken together. Not a trace of the properties of hydrogen or oxygen is observable in those of their compound water.
>
> If this be true of chemical combinations, it is still more true of those far more complex combinations of elements which constitute organized bodies; and in which those extraordinary new uniformities arise, which are called the laws of life.[13]

Despite knowing that things don't add simply in biology or chemistry, Mill goes on to say that his Law of Composition of Causes (adding things up) was the general one, with interactions being exceptional. He also states that not being able to easily add up features of things like oxygen and hydrogen is simply because we haven't *yet* figured out how to do it.

Mill may be correct that one day we'll figure out how to add what we know about oxygen to what we know about hydrogen to deduce the properties of water. Ultimately, this claim depends on metaphysical assumptions about holism that I won't get into here. The fact is that now and for the foreseeable future, we don't know nearly enough about hydrogen and oxygen to deduce the properties of water, we don't know enough about the handful of basic elements you are made up of to understand you, and more generally that when it comes to medicine and the human body, there is no reason to assume that the components of complex placebo treatments don't interact.

How to Handle Interactions

Before prescribing, paying for, and using drugs in real life, we need to know whether they have effects in real life. Interactions between placebo and drug effects mean that many placebo-controlled trials do not provide a good estimate of how powerful the drug is in real life. The way to overcome this problem is to use what are called pragmatic clinical trials that mimic the conditions of real life more accurately (more on this in part III). Likewise, if we wish to implement placebo effects in clinical practice (and avoid nocebo effects), we can't assume that adding up the different parts will give us an accurate estimate. We need to look at all the parts of the placebo together in a pragmatic trial. Making interactions rather than additivity the default assumption makes the need for pragmatic trials easy to see. Most importantly, because various placebo or treatment features probably interact, we need to investigate them as a package rather than picking them apart then trying to build them back up to get an overall effect.

CHAPTER 8

Blinding

Stopping People from Peeking through Masks

The patient, treated on the fashionable theory sometimes gets well in spite of the medicine. The medicine therefore restored him, and the young doctor received new courage to proceed in his bold experiments on the lives of his fellow creatures.
—THOMAS JEFFERSON TO CASPAR WISTAR, June 21, 1807[1]

Blinding and Placebos

A blinded trial is one in which knowledge of who got what treatment is hidden. Blinded trials reduce bias arising from expectations, "imagination," or faith. This is why blinding has been trumpeted as being a virtue of medical experiments. Sir Austin Bradford Hill—the godfather of modern medical trials—states: "By the so-called double-blind procedure, when neither patient nor doctor knows the nature of the treatment given to an individual case, it is hoped that unbiased subjective judgements of the course of the illness can be obtained."[2] Similar statements about the benefits of double blinding are affirmed in the official textbook of the evidence-based medicine movement[3] and in many clinical trial textbooks.[4-8]

The fact that blinded trials are often superior is a problem when it comes to measuring placebo effects. To measure placebo effects, we must compare what happens to people who take placebos with people who don't, and people will know if they are taking nothing. Hróbjartsson and Gøtzsche cite lack of blinding in trials that measure placebo effects as a reason to doubt whether they are effective: "Thus, even if there was no true effect of placebo, one would expect to find differences between placebo and untreated groups because of bias associated with a lack of double-blinding."[9] Hróbjartsson and Gøtzsche are correct that lack of blinding can introduce bias but mistaken in the extent to which it is a general problem for measuring placebo and nocebo effect sizes.

Early Examples of Blinded Trials

The term "mesmerize" is derived from a real man's name. Franz Mesmer (1734–1815) believed in something called "animal magnetism," a supposed invisible fluid that ran through peoples' bodies. He became so popular in Paris that he couldn't treat everyone who wanted his therapy individually, so he started treating groups of people at the same time.

Mesmer's group ritual involved placing a large vessel called a "baquet" in the middle of the room. The baquet was large enough for 20 patients to sit around, and it was covered by a lid that had holes in it for each person. The patients held rods that were placed into the holes. The rods were bent at right angles and were pointed toward the part of their bodies that needed healing. In addition to the rods, a rope was attached at one end to the baquet, and then wrapped around the necks or bodies of all the patients. In addition to the baquet, rods, and rope, Mesmer himself was said to be able to convey the magnetism by movements of his eyes and hands. Magnetizing patients also required Mesmer (or one of his disciples) to touch the patients in the lower abdomen. While being mesmerized, many patients experienced a healing crisis, which included fainting, convulsions, spasms, and delirium. Mesmer also warned that magnetizing could be dangerous if not done properly, even causing hemorrhage or stroke.[10,11]

Among Mesmer's many eminent female patients was allegedly the queen of France. There were also scandalous rumours about what happened during Mesmer's healing sessions. Unsurprisingly, King Louis XVI was not impressed with Mesmer and ordered an investigation. The king gathered the great minds in Paris of the time, including Antoine Lavoisier (who identified oxygen), Joseph-Ignace Guillotin, Jean Sylvain Bailly and Benjamin Franklin. They conducted what has become known as the "Royal Commission." (Aside: Guillotin fought against the death penalty, but when his arguments failed, he advocated for what he took to be the most humane form of execution—what we now call a guillotine.)

The experiments involved blindfolding people and telling them they had been magnetized, but not actually magnetizing them. The most striking example involved magnetized trees outside Mesmer's office. Mesmer's assistant, Deslon, was instructed to magnetize one of the five apricot trees in his garden. The assistant touched a tree with his wand and said that anyone who touched the tree would be affected. A susceptible young man who was blindfolded was led to embrace each tree in turn but was not told which one was magnetized. He felt an increasing force of magnetism at each successive tree and finally fell unconscious in a classic mesmeric crisis before the fourth tree. However, it was the fifth tree that Deslon magnetized—the poor young man hadn't even touched it.

Franklin and his friends' blind tests of mesmerism are touted as proof that mesmerism didn't work. The *Skeptic's Dictionary*, for example, states that "Mesmerism is a bit of quackery developed in the 18th century by the German physician Franz Anton Mesmer."[12] After the report, Mesmer left Paris in shame, with his theory of animal magnetism considered debunked.

But the skeptics are wrong: mesmerism *did* work, it's just that it didn't work in the way they thought it did. Reminiscent of John Haygarth's admission that Elisha Perkins's tractors worked because of faith, Franklin and his friends' report admitted that mesmerism had an effect. In their words: "Did any of their patients improve or feel better after taking the cure . . . ? Yes, of course." They then said that it worked because of what they called "imagination" rather than animal magnetism:

No doubt the imagination of patients often has a great influence on the cure of their illnesses. This effect is known only by general experience and has not in the least been determined by positive experiments; but it does not seem that one can doubt it. It is a known adage that faith saves in medicine; this faith is the product of the imagination: thus imagination acts only by gentle means, it acts by spreading calm to all the senses, re-establishing order in the functions and rekindling hope. Hope is the life of man; whoever can give him the one contributes to giving him the other.[11]

A translator of the report interprets what they say about imagination as a premonition that the discovery of the powers of imagination would form the basis for a new science.[11] In a way, the translator was correct because while Mesmer himself was discredited, the practice of mesmerism continued and evolved into what we call hypnosis today.[13] To reiterate, there is a difference between debunking a theory and showing that the treatment (even a treatment based on the wrong theory) didn't have an effect.

Another early example of a blinded trial involved an evaluation of homeopathy conducted in Nuremberg in 1835 by a "society of truth-loving men."[14] Homeopathy had become quite popular among the upper classes in Bavaria, and an argument broke out between a lead homeopathic doctor called Johann Jacob Reuter and a public health official called Friedrich Wilhelm von Hoven. The two men attacked each other in a series of articles in the press, and eventually von Hoven proposed that they do a trial. If the tests showed that homeopathy didn't work, then the government would have to ban it to protect patients. Reuter accepted the challenge and proposed they test the effects of highly diluted salt water.

After a widely publicized invitation, over 120 citizens met in a local tavern. Then, 100 vials were numbered, shuffled and split into two random lots of 50. One lot was filled with distilled snow water, the other with ordinary salt in a homeopathic dilution of distilled snow water. To prepare the homeopathic remedy, a grain of salt was dissolved in

100 drops of distilled snow water and the resulting solution was diluted 29 times at a ratio of 1 to 100, making what is called a "C30" dilution. Next, a list indicating the numbers of the vials with and without the salt dilution was made and placed in a sealed envelope so that nobody who took the vials knew whether it was homeopathy or distilled water: it was blinded. The vials were distributed. At a second meeting three weeks later, those who had taken the vials reported whether they had experienced anything unusual after ingesting the vial's content. Finally, the trial was "unblinded" by opening the sealed envelope containing the code to identify which vials contained distilled water and which ones contained the homeopathic remedy. Five of those who had taken homeopathy and three of those who had taken distilled water reported feeling something unusual. Based on the lack of big difference between homeopathy and distilled water, it was concluded that Reuter was wrong.

Benefits of Double Blinding: Controlling for Beliefs and Expectations

If a patient believes they are getting the latest, newest, shiniest drug that they've read about in the newspaper and that's given to them by a doctor from Harvard or Oxford they are probably more likely to expect that it will work than if they are getting an old, cheap drug, or a sugar pill placebo. In chapter 6 I cited a number of trials showing that when people expect to recover from conditions like pain, they are more likely to recover. When patients have positive expectations about their recovery, they are able to walk sooner after hip or knee surgery; [15,16] return to work more quickly after treatment for low back pain;[17] recover more quickly from whiplash injury;[18] and have higher quality of life following cancer treatment.[19] The young man in the trial of mesmerism had very strong expectations of the power of the mesmerized tree, and his expectations caused him to have a healing crisis even though the trees he touched had not been imbued with animal magnetism.

One trial that compared vitamin C with a placebo for treating the common cold found that vitamin C prevented colds.[20] However, some of the patients were able to tell whether they were getting the real vitamin C because of the sour taste. Other patients were not able to identify the real vitamin C. The patients who could not identify the vitamin C (those who were blinded) did not benefit from the vitamin C compared to the placebo, whereas those who were able to identify the vitamin C did experience a benefit. The best explanation for this is that those who identified the vitamin C *expected* to get better, and these expectations led to a speedier recovery.

Blinding Controls for Patients' Expectations

Recall that so-called active placebos are placebos that contain an ingredient that mimics the side effect of the "real" treatment. These are good because even if we make a placebo pill look like the active drug, the patient will be able to identify the drug if it produces an obvious side effect. Now trials that compare antidepressant drugs with active placebos show very tiny effects. Trials comparing antidepressant drugs with regular placebos show bigger effects. This is almost certainly because the patients in the trials comparing antidepressants with the regular placebos correctly guess which treatment they are taking. If they get a side effect like dry mouth, they say, "Aha! I'm getting that fancy new drug that I've read about in the newspaper. It will probably make me feel better." Their positive expectations about the outcome give them a dopamine or endorphin rush and they feel better. On the other hand, if they don't experience any side effects, they might think, "Oh no. I got the stupid placebo, which is just a sugar pill. It isn't expensive or shiny." They might even develop a negative expectation, which activates nocebo mechanisms and makes them feel worse. This means that the people taking the active drug might feel better because of their expectations, and those taking the placebo might feel worse because of negative expectations. The difference in expectations can make the drug look as if it is better than the placebo, when in fact it is the expectations that account for the difference. Active placebos equalize the expectations and make the test fairer. Trials that use active placebos show *smaller* effects.[21] Using active placebos is a way of ensuring that patients remain blinded and reduces the bias in these trials.

Blinding Controls for Practitioner Expectations

Besides patients, other groups involved in trials can be blinded (see appendix 6). In chapter 3, I cited a study showing that if doctors believe that they are giving the best experimental treatment (as opposed to placebo) to a patient, then their expectations could affect the outcome. In another study that showed this, 63 elderly residents in nursing homes were given a comprehensive check of their mental health and physical abilities. They were then randomly assigned to a "high-expectancy" or "average-expectancy" condition. Nurses were told that the elderly people in the high-expectancy group would recover more quickly and respond better to treatment. After three months, a researcher, who didn't know to which group the participants had been assigned (they were blinded), gave them another check-up. Those in the high-expectancy group did better in three out of the four outcomes measured. They were less depressed, less likely to be admitted to the hospital, and had higher mental status than the average-expectancy group. They only did worse in one of the outcomes: the high-expectancy group needed more assistance from nurses than the other patients. Blinding researchers who assess outcomes can reduce bias. In a trial of cyclophosphamide and plasma exchange to treat multiple sclerosis, neither intervention was superior to placebo when neurologists assessing outcomes were blind.[22] However, when a second nonblinded neurologist completed the same assessments, the results suggested a benefit for one of the two groups.[22]

Extensive research shows that studies that are blinded have different results than those that are not blinded.[23-32] On average, trials described as "double blind" report at least 10% smaller treatment effects than similar trials that are not clearly double blinded.[21,31-34] One study did not find a difference but had serious methodological limitations and should be ignored due to serious methodological problems (see appendix 6).

Successful Blinding Is Not Required in Trials of Dramatically Effective Treatments

Believing that blinding is always virtuous leads to the Philip's paradox.[35] The paradox is that treatments we know are the most effective cannot be tested in blinded trials. In fact, if a treatment demonstrates such noticeable effectiveness that the trial cannot remain blinded, it's not a failure of the trial but a success of the treatment. Stephen Senn uses the famous Tea Lady experiment to illustrate this.[36] Ronald Fisher was one of the main developers of modern statistics (he was also a eugenicist and was paid by the tobacco industry to debunk claims that smoking caused lung cancer, but we'll leave that aside for now). He was invited to a country house where tea was being served, and a guest said that she wanted her milk in the cup before the tea. Or she might have wanted it after. In any case, she was very peculiar about whether the milk was poured first or not. Fisher said the woman wouldn't have been able to tell the difference between milk before tea and milk after tea, but she insisted that she could. They did an experiment with some tea poured after the milk and some milk poured after the tea. The Tea Lady was blinded (she didn't see whether they poured the milk first or not), but she was able to tell the difference. The difference in taste (to her—I don't think I could tell) was enough to unblind her. The fact that she did not remain blind was not a fault of the trial but a testament to the discerning nature of her taste buds.

The fact that trials of dramatically effective treatments cannot remain successfully blinded does not mean the trials are of lower quality. It's just that the success of the blinding is not relevant. However, before the trial starts, we don't know whether the treatment is dramatically effective. If we did, we wouldn't have to do the trial. So, at the beginning of the trial, it is often important to try to blind the trial. If we hadn't kept the Tea Lady blinded, we wouldn't have had a proper trial: she would have seen the milk (or tea) being poured first. This is why it is important for a trial to remain blinded for as long as possible. There is an unfortunate confusion in the recent evidence-based medicine literature about the importance of blinding and the need to report whether blinding is successful. The confusion arises from failing to note the difference between unblinding that arises from the dramatic positive effects of the new treatment (which is extremely rare) and unblinding arising from the side-effects of the new treatment (which is more common).

Why We Need to Know Whether Blinding Is Successful

Blinding is only useful if it works. A mask with holes in it doesn't serve its purpose. Saying a trial is blinded is one thing; making a trial successfully blinded is another. If blinding is not successful, it's like giving someone a mask with holes: their expectations about what is happening will not be controlled for.

Because blinding must be successful to work, evidence-based medicine gurus in the 1990s recommended that trials tell us what the results of tests for success of blinding revealed.[37] There are a few effective ways to measure how effective blinding is (see appendix 6). However, they subsequently dropped that recommendation.[38] Given that blinding is only useful if it works, I don't understand why they removed it.[39] A common thread in all the answers I've seen in print or when I ask people is a speech and a handful of studies by the late and wonderful professor Dave Sackett. I think Sackett would roll in his grave if he knew this because he preferred evidence over expertise. Not only did he write a paper titled "The Sins of Expertness and a Proposal for Redemption,"[40] but he retired (well, sort of) from evidence-based medicine soon after he was acknowledged as an expert. Because of this, I am quite sure Sackett would prefer us to question his arguments rather than blindly appeal to his expertise.

I'll try to recreate Sackett's argument in the best possible light here before showing why it's wrong. First and to reiterate, if the reason for the unblinding is that the treatment was effective, then obviously the failure to keep the trial blind should not count against the methodology of the trial. But in those cases, measuring the success of blinding won't hurt. The fact that trials of dramatically effective treatments cannot remain successfully blinded is not an argument against measuring whether blinding was successful: it's an argument that we should be cautious about how we interpret the results of tests of success of blinding. As one commentator notes, "It seems contrary to an evidence-based approach to avoid obtaining data because we have to struggle with interpretation and measurement."[41]

Moreover, cases of dramatically effective treatments are extremely rare, and when they arise, they are easily identified by the dramatic effects. There's no question that blinding or lack of it gets in the way of identifying dramatically effective treatments. Far more often, though, treatments have very modest effects yet have discernible side effects. In those cases, the small effects can be affected by unblinding, and it is important to measure how successful blinding was. The important difference between unblinding arising from (extremely rare) dramatic effects and (much more common) identifiable side-effects is missing from Sackett's argument against measuring the success of blinding.

Sackett seems to give another reason why we should not test for the success of masking: doctors' wrong guesses. In a study he cites, the doctors thought the placebo (the control treatment) was the treatment, and vice versa.[42] The test for success of blinding failed, but for the wrong reason. He then makes a mistaken inference that because the unblinding arose for the wrong reasons, we shouldn't test for the success of blinding. In fact, his example shows very clearly how the doctors' beliefs corrupted the trial, just not in the anticipated direction. Even though their guesses were incorrect, they could have treated the patients they thought were getting the "more powerful" treatment differently. Then the different treatment could have influenced the results. Far from being an example to support not measuring the success of blinding, it does just the opposite. Besides my colleagues and

I in a recent paper,[43] I'm not aware of any sustained challenges to Sackett's view. Given Sackett's vociferous pleas to *not* trust experts simply because they were experts, I suspect he would have welcomed our challenge. Certainly, he would be rolling in his grave if his successors failed to provide better evidence to explain their views.

Placebo and Nocebo Effects Can't Be Measured in Blinded Trials

Treatments, ranging from most surgical techniques and exercise to placebos, cannot be tested in blinded conditions. If you are in the so-called untreated control group you know you are *not* receiving a treatment or a placebo. This doesn't necessarily mean that exercise or placebo treatments are damned to be supported by substandard evidence. Rather, we could use active controlled pragmatic trials.

Active Controlled Trials

If you are in a trial and someone leaked the information that you were taking a sugar pill, chances are you would have lower expectations about it working than if you knew you were getting the latest wonder drug. But, say the trial compared two different drugs, drug A and drug B in what is called an *active controlled trial*. If someone leaked that you were taking drug A and not drug B, it might not change your expectations too much. For instance, my expectations that aspirin and ibuprofen will alleviate mild headaches are pretty much the same. I almost never take them, but when I do, I anticipate a mild benefit. If I were in a trial comparing aspirin and ibuprofen, it wouldn't really matter if I was blinded or not. My expectations about both are the same. So, in active controlled trials that compare one treatment with another (instead of a treatment with a placebo) blinding patients doesn't matter as much.

For example, say we are measuring the effect of a mega-placebo that includes an open-label sugar pill, administered by an empathic, positive, and authoritative practitioner in a relaxing environment. We could compare that with the effects of a drug (which has already proved superior to a placebo). We could also blind the data collectors, outcome assessors, and statisticians. If the mega-placebo turns out to be cost-effective in a large trial of this type, it would go a long way toward mitigating the inability to blind participants and doctors. I'll discuss such a trial in chapter 12.

Of course, in such a trial, patients might have very different expectations, and those differing expectations might confound the results. To overcome this problem, we could use a patient preference trial.

Patient Preference Trials

A patient preference trial is an active controlled trial that does even more to control for expectations. In trial comparing acupuncture with a drug, here's what would happen.[44] Anyone with a strong preference for acupuncture would be given acupuncture. Anyone with a strong preference for drugs would be given the drugs. Then, only the remaining people (those without strong preferences and expectations) would be randomized to get either acupuncture or the drug. In this way, the preferences and expectations are equalized at the start of the trial. Equalizing the expectations removes the need for blinding, at least to a great degree.

A great benefit of active controlled trials and patient preference trials is that they are closer to real life and are therefore more applicable to real life. In epidemiological terms, these trials have greater external validity. Active-controlled trials also mostly solve problems arising from the fact that we cannot assume additivity (see chapter 7).

Blinding in Estimating the Size of Placebo and Nocebo Effects

Blinding often makes trials more reliable by controlling for patient, practitioner, and others' expectations, beliefs, and (sometimes) prejudices. Just as a transparent blindfold won't stop its wearer from seeing, unsuccessful blinding doesn't achieve its purpose. There are exceptions to this rule, notably trials of dramatically effective treatments where it doesn't matter whether blinding was successful. In estimating placebo or nocebo effects, exercise, and other treatments, blinding patients and practitioners is not possible. In those cases, pragmatic trials and patient preference trials can be used to do some of the work that blinding does, namely, controlling for expectations and beliefs.

WHY EVERY DOCTOR NEEDS TO BE A SHAMAN AND WHY PLACEBO CONTROLS NEED TO BE CONTROLLED

Much of the literature about the placebo effect is, in effect, an effort to debunk, confuse, or minimize it. . . . Efforts to try to actually move forward our understanding of this fundamental human phenomenon are very rare.
   —DANIEL MOERMAN AND WAYNE JONAS, "Deconstructing the Placebo Effect and Finding the Meaning Response"[1]

Armed with knowledge of what placebos and nocebos are, and how big their effects are, we can now make informed arguments about whether we should use them. I argue for two positions that are both almost diametrically opposed to conventional wisdom:

1. It is unethical to *not* use placebos (and to not avoid nocebos) in clinical practice.
2. Placebo *controls* should be avoided in trials much more often than they are.

The Ethical Requirement to Prescribe More Placebos and Avoid Nocebo Effects in Practice

If I'm right . . . then it's medically negligent for any doctor to not also be a shaman—to not also be someone trained in the ritual arts of harnessing the immune and ANS [autonomic nervous system] responses through speaking and dancing the inherent language of the body. Of course, and to some degree, doctors precisely do this—with their array of good potions to put into the body, or operations to take bad things out; with their shaman uniforms of white coats.
—RICHARD GIPPS, "Doctors Should Be Shamans and Perhaps They Are"[1]

Turning the Ethics of Placebos and Nocebos on Its Head

The Hippocratic oath, which has been around since ancient Greece, requires doctors to help their patients and avoid harming them.[2] I started this book with the examples of Bocepal and Cenobo, two imaginary drugs that had been proven to be helpful and harmful, respectively. It is obviously unethical to withhold Bocepal and to prescribe Cenobo. By the same token, since placebo treatments have been proved beyond any doubt to be helpful in many cases, it seems to be an ethical requirement to use them appropriately. However, at the beginning of the book I had not yet cleared up the confusion about what placebos and nocebos are, how effective they are, and whether deception is required for placebo effects to arise. In parts I and II, I established what placebos and nocebos are and that their effects are real. I will now address the last block to using placebos in practice by fully debunking the idea that they require deception.

Why Deception Is Unethical

Lying to patients violates another part of doctors' ethical code, which requires them to respect patients' autonomy. Patients can't make autonomous decisions if they are being lied to. If I lie and say that a new treatment has no negative side effects, you cannot make an autonomous decision about whether it would be a good idea for you to take it. Sadly, until only a few decades ago, such unethical lying happened more often than we might assume with both placebos and active treatments. Sissela Bok reports a horribly unethical case that might make your blood boil as much as it does mine:

> In 1971 a number of Mexican-American women applied to a family-planning clinic for contraceptives. Some of them were given oral contraceptives and others were given placebos, or dummy pills that looked like the real thing. Without knowing it the women were involved in an investigation of the side effects of various contraceptive pills. Those who were given placebos suffered from a predictable side effect: 10 of them became pregnant. Needless to say, the physician in charge did not assume financial responsibility for the babies. Nor did he indicate any concern about having bypassed the "informed consent" that is required in ethical experiments with human beings. He contented himself with the observation that if only the law had permitted it, he could have aborted the pregnant women![3]

The case Bok describes is horrifying, and experiments like it should be condemned. In 1974, when the essay was published, the kind of lying that Bok describes was not restricted to giving placebo treatments. To name just one example from among too many, the Tuskegee Experiment was a study of Black American men with syphilis between 1932 and 1972. The purpose of the study was to observe what happened to people with syphilis if they were not treated. The men were not treated, though from 1947 onward, they could have been cured with penicillin.[4] The men were not told that treatment was available. The Tuskegee Experiment is a terrible stain on the history of medicine and caused mistrust of the medical profession for decades.[5]

Deception can be unethical even if it helps. In one case, a 14-year-old boy was admitted to the hospital with severe migraines.[6] One of the doctors became concerned about the risk of opioid addiction and substituted morphine with placebo (a saline solution) without the patient knowing. The placebo worked, and the risk of opioid dependence was reduced. This seemed like a good result, but when the mother learned of the deception, she complained. A health care practitioner who was aware of the deception was initially disciplined, although the decision to take disciplinary action was reversed when it was clear that the patient was helped.

Why Arguments for Ethical Deception Fail

In a paper published in 2004 David Wendler and Franklin Miller argued that patients can be deceived if they agree to be deceived.[7] They argue that patients might consent to being deceived without being told what they are being deceived about. Patients might be told something like, "You should be aware that the investigators have intentionally left out information about certain aspects of this study."[7] I don't find their argument convincing. To give consent, you must know what you are consenting to. Wendler and Miller respond by noting that patients in these circumstances can only be deceived about matters that would not "affect their willingness to participate."[7] But how can we know in advance whether something would affect patients' willingness to participate without asking them first? Their argument seems to rely on an incorrect and paternalistic premise that doctors can guess what might affect patients' willingness to participate.

Deception Is Not Necessarily Connected to Placebo and Nocebo Treatments

Deception is unethical. However, deception is not strictly confined to placebo treatments. The Tuskegee Experiment shows that it also applies to nonplacebo treatments as well. Likewise, it is unethical to withhold a more effective treatment and give a patient a less effective one whether or not the less effective one is a placebo or something else.

Not only is deception a potential problem with placebo treatments, but placebo treatments do not need to be given deceptively to have their effects. In chapter 6, I described the case of Linda Buannono, whose irritable bowel syndrome was cured by honest placebos.[8] In fact, there have been many studies of honest placebos. In the first one I'm aware of, Baltimore doctors Lee Park and Uno Covi gave honest placebos to 15 neurotic patients.[9] They told the patients: "Many people with your kind of condition have been helped by what are sometimes called 'sugar pills,' and we feel that a so-called sugar pill may help you too."

Many of the patients reported getting "quite a bit better" after getting the placebo, even though they knew it was a placebo. The irony of this study is that after getting better, the patients didn't believe the doctors and thought that the placebos were in fact real drugs (after all, they were neurotic). In a much more recent and rigorous example, 127 patients with chronic back pain (a condition that eats up about 10% of health care budgets in developed nations) were randomized to receive either treatment as usual or honest placebos. They were followed up for three weeks and asked about their pain. Those who received the open-label placebo had less pain than those who received usual treatment. It seems that open-label placebos have effects similar to those of deceptive placebos (placebos that patients think are, or could be, the real treatment).[9-18] The research on open-label placebos is still growing and it may turn out that they are not as effective as deceptive placebos. Still, we've done a systematic review of open-label studies and there is strong evidence that they work,[19] and we know how (see part II). A growing number of examples show how honest placebos could help in practice.

Ethical Honest Placebos
Ethical Placebos: Dr. Osler

Dr. Osler was treating a patient called Robert, who had just broken his arm in a cycling accident. Dr. Osler prescribed morphine to deal with the pain. However, knowing that about 5% of people who are prescribed morphine become addicted, he proposed to replace some of the morphine with some honest placebos. Here's what he said to Robert:

> To deal with your pain, I'm going to follow the evidence-based guidelines and prescribe morphine. It's great in the short term, but about one in 20 people who take it find it difficult to get off the morphine at the end of the prescription and become addicted. Some trials have shown that we can replace some of the morphine pills with placebo pills at random and achieve the same effects as using just morphine. This probably reduces the chances of your becoming dependent and will provide similar painkilling benefits. Would you accept our replacing some of the morphine tablets with placebo tablets? Neither you nor I would know which tablets are the real morphine tablets and which are the placebo tablets. But about a third of the tablets you would be taking would be sugar pill placebos. We would monitor you all along, and if the treatment isn't working, we could switch to morphine alone without the placebos. I think you will respond well to this treatment. Would you like to try this option?

Robert decided to try the placebos, and he didn't need to extend his morphine prescription beyond the post-surgical period. It was a great success.

Ethical Placebos: Real Trials

The example of Robert and Dr. Osler is not real, but real examples show that honest placebos could almost certainly work and reduce the burden of the opioid crisis. In one actual trial, patients who had just undergone spinal surgery were randomized to either receive an honest placebo or usual care. Both groups had access to standard morphine

medication as needed. Patients who received the honest placebo con-
sumed 30% less morphine than the other group.[18] In another actual
trial, patients with abdominal pain or irritable bowel syndrome
were randomized to either receive honest placebos or simply be observed.[17] Both groups were allowed to take a kind of rescue medication
called hyoscyamine which is effective for treating stomach cramps.
Patients taking the honest placebos had less pain and took less
hyoscyamine.

Because they reduce pain and medication use without deception, it
is unethical *not* to use honest placebos in the cases described above.
Yet, current regulations seem to forbid it, or at least are unclear. In the
United Kingdom, the British Medical Association does not mention
how or whether honest placebos can be used outside of clinical
trials.[20,21] The World Medical Association is similarly silent about placebos in practice. As a result, patients suffer because doctors who might
not be aware of the latest evidence regarding the benefits of honest placebo treatments refrain from using them. The American Medical Association allows doctors to use placebos in routine practice as long as
the patient knows that it's a placebo.[22] Other national medical asso-
ciations should follow suit.

Unethical Nocebos: Dr. Ernest

A year later, Robert went to the doctor's office with a mild headache.
Dr. Osler was away on holiday, so Robert had to see Dr. Ernest. Dr. Ernest is a very literal man who interprets his ethical duty to tell patients
his version of the truth, the whole truth, and nothing but the truth.
He examined Robert and decided that acetaminophen was the best
option. As was his habit, he insisted that Robert take the time to understand that while the drug may reduce his pain, it also has several
possible serious side effects.

"Now, Robert," he says, "I know people sometimes don't read the
small print, but I want to be sure that you understand the truth about
this medication. To help you, I've prepared this document that lists all

the small-print side effects in big letters." Dr. Ernest then produced the document.

But Robert wasn't that interested and pushed the document away without reading it.

"Don't worry, doc, I've taken that before and if you think it will do me some good, I'll take it."

"Well, the truth is that I can't say for sure that it will do you good or harm, because almost everything in medicine is uncertain. And even if it helped before, we can't be 100% certain that it will help now. Therefore, I must *insist* that you take the time to carefully study this document. And to be sure that you understand it, I will explain all the medical terms."

Robert shakes his head but doesn't know what to do. Dr. Ernest sees that Robert is not going to read the document of his own free will, so he says, "I see that you are not going to read it. My ethical duty to tell the truth therefore requires that I read these to you aloud. Here they are: 'Side effects of acetaminophen include serious skin reactions, including fatal ones like toxic epidermal necrolysis, abnormal liver reactions, stroke, heart attacks, ulcers, stomach bleeding, and an increased risk of childhood asthma.' Now, do you have any questions?"

After listening to the side effects, Robert got itchy skin, his headache became worse, and he was reluctant to take acetaminophen. He resigned himself to living with the headache and was scared to ask Dr. Ernest about the itchy skin. He said everything was okay and decided to come back to the clinic when Dr. Osler returned from holiday.

The way Dr. Ernest communicated caused some harm. Because it is possible to communicate honestly without causing that harm, it is an ethical requirement to do so. In a less extreme form, Dr. Ernest's behavior is common. My colleague Daniel Moerman reports the following:

> Before I had my first cataract surgery, maybe 15 years ago (not in any sort of trial), I had to read and sign a long, detailed, death-defying statement which was not simply "scary," it was terrifying; among many others, I might go blind. I had nightmares for weeks before the surgery.

Just last week, I had to read and sign a statement that, among other things, stated that extracting an infected tooth from my lower jaw "might break my jaw." I confess that afterwards I felt as if I had been in a serious fist fight, and had lost. But, no broken jaw.[23]

Moerman's nightmares and, most likely, at least part of his jaw pain, were nocebo effects caused by the communication of intervention risks within routine clinical practice.

In discussions, I've heard people argue that Dr. Osler's honest placebos might encourage a pill-popping culture and lead to distrust of the medical profession. If done honestly—and that is what I'm referring to—it would do neither. Not only can placebo effects be induced without pills, but in the example I provided, the idea is to provide less harmful medication and to educate people about their body's innate healing capacity. In fact, the most obviously ethical uses of honest placebos are for cases that help *reduce* the problems associated with too much medicine.[24] For example, they could be used to help cure selective serotonin reuptake inhibitor (SSRI) dependence[25] and to reduce the overprescription of antibiotics.

Deception That Is Not Deception

There are two areas where deception appears to be present, but in fact it is not. First, doctors and patients can come up with a mutually acceptable plan that specifies how much information about harms is provided. Second, doctors can "act" as professionals, and their acting is not deceptive.

Avoiding Nocebo Effects by Not Disclosing Certain Side Effects (with Patient Permission)

I had an experience of a doctor who didn't share all the information about side effects with me, and I think it is an ethically borderline case. As a result of overtraining, I developed a stress fracture in one of my ribs which was so painful that I could barely breathe, let alone train properly. And I had an important race coming up in Boston called the Head of the Charles Regatta. I went to see the team doctor, who prescribed a drug called diclofenac (Voltaren). He told me it was helpful for relieving pain and inflammation, and that it would be safe for me. Like most people, I didn't bother reading the small print that accompanied the prescription, which described all the potential side effects. I just took the pills and felt better quickly. My rib got better, and we won the race. Everyone was happy.

Many years later I looked up the side effects of diclofenac. They included vomiting, diarrhea, headache, constipation, intestinal bleeding, stroke, or fatal heart attack.[26] If the doctor had told me about them, it would have caused great anxiety. I'm naturally somewhat anxious, so just thinking about nausea and headaches could have caused mild nausea or headaches. Then I might have wondered about strokes and heart attacks and been scared to train very hard. The pain in my rib might not have gone away as fast. I might not have won the race, and at that time those races were extremely important to me. The doctor probably knew all that and didn't emphasize the side effects (and, to repeat, he didn't conceal these from me because I could have read the small print yet chose not to). He knew I was young and extremely fit and healthy so much less likely to experience the extremely rare side effects. He was also the team doctor, so he had regular contact with me and could have managed the side effects if they'd arisen.

I don't think that the team doctor behaved unethically. However, my views in this area may not be shared by others, so I don't argue that it is generally ethical for doctors to avoid explicitly discussing drug side effects with patients. It would, however, be ethical to ask patients how much they would like to discuss side effects. For example, my doctor could have said, "I think this drug will help you. There are a number of side effects; some are common and some extremely rare. They're all listed in the leaflet that accompanies the box. I am happy to discuss these with you if you like, and different patients want to know different amounts of information about side effects. I am going to count on you to prompt me if you have any questions."

If he had asked me that, I would have replied, "If it's very rare, I don't need to know about it."

To which he might have replied, "You are young, fit, and healthy. I'm around, and I think it's safe. And you have the leaflet inside the medication box that explains them all should you become curious." Had he done that, it would not have been unethical at all. Asking the patient how much information they want is a way of getting around the problem that some people might consider it ethical to be deceived and others may not. It also avoids the problems arising from Miller and Wendler's paternalism.

My proposal (to ask patients how much they would like to know) happens whenever anyone buys an over the counter medication from the pharmacy. In those cases, nobody forces us to read the small print, and most of us don't. If we can choose whether we read the small print for medications we buy, why can't we have a say in how much scary information our doctors share with us? In fact, if I say that I don't want to know something and the doctor tells me despite my saying that I don't want to know, it is a violation of my autonomy. If patients agree to not discuss certain potential negative side-effects with patients there is no deception involved.

Being a Genki Professional Is Ethically Required

"Genki" is a Japanese word that doesn't have a direct English translation. Roughly, it means energetic or happy. Its characters break down into "original" and "spirit." So *genki* also means "full of spirit"—or something like that. Now I very much enjoy teaching, coaching, and mentoring. I care about those I teach and mentor. When I teach, I like to wear a suit and tie because it helps put me in the right mood, and I also think it shows my students that I care. But sometimes I'm tired— maybe going through a professional or personal issue—and I'm not *genki* on the inside. It also might be hot, and I might not feel like wearing a suit. Unless there's a real emergency that requires me to bow out, I suit up, shine my shoes, snap my heels together, and deliver the teaching or coaching session with a smile. Doing it properly is part of being a professional. Nobody feels *genki* on this inside all the time, but a professional has to play a role. The professional has to fake it a bit to do their job, so that those to whom he or she has a duty—students—benefit. Without using the word *genki*, Hillel Finestone reports doing something like acting *genki*:

> In my practice . . . the speciality of physical medicine and rehabilitation, I frequently treat individuals who are in chronic pain. I find it essential to convey an encouraging, hopeful, often cajoling message to the patient to communicate concern and, more importantly, the need for the patient to work on self-improvement. Moreover, I find that it is often crucial to convey these messages also to the patient's family, support network, and care-givers. These messages are important because they address the emotional needs of the patient and those around him, and I believe they have a clear impact on the patient's quality of life and extent and speed of recovery. However, I am not in the same frame of mind every day. I may be tired, angry, or concerned about an unwell family member. On such occasions, I must, in effect, act to convey the responsiveness and concern that I believe have an important effect on the patient's health.[27]

Finestone states the simple fact that health care practitioners are human and that their moods may vary on different days. Inevitably, on some days, they will not be in the mood that enables them to be. . . . *genki*. On these occasions, Finestone argues, the right thing to do is to fake it. In cases like the one Finestone describes, where the practitioner is *faking* his concern, the patient's autonomy does not seem to be at stake. The fact that the doctor is not in the right frame of mind to feel, let alone to express, empathy, does not impinge on the patient's ability to make an informed decision.

A puritan might say that a doctor who feigns empathy is not acting in accordance with professional standards. They might cite the

American Medical Association,[28] or the UK's General Medical Council,[20] both of which state that doctors must act with honesty and integrity. That would be a radical view because behaving in accordance with the circumstances is part of life. If you were to ask them, I very much doubt that patients or students would mind if they knew you were faking being *genki* when you were feeling tired.

Everyone knows that we don't behave in a church or synagogue or mosque the same way we behave at the pub or the football game. At times, and among certain friend groups, I swear. But I don't swear in front of my immediate family (which includes young children). In the same way, I might not express that I'm a bit tired, and instead fake being *genki* a bit when I'm teaching. Performing different roles is part of being part of society—part of being human. Hence, it is unsurprising that researchers have noted the benefits of acting training,[29] and called for more acting training for health care practitioners.[30,31]

Limits to the Ethical Use of Placebos and Nocebos

Giving someone a placebo when there is a more effective option available is not right. Even if a placebo treatment would reduce a severely depressed person's depression, there are more powerful drugs that will do a better job, and the more powerful drugs should be given. But this isn't an argument against using placebos. It's against using anything less effective when something better is available. Sometimes the placebo treatment is the best option. For example, according to the best and largest studies, most over-the-counter analgesics, like aspirin and ibuprofen, are barely better than placebos for reducing back pain,[32,33] cancer pain,[34] and most chronic pain,[35] yet they can have serious side effects for an important minority of people.[34] So although placebos may not be as effective, they may carry a more favorable benefit/harm ratio. If they can be given honestly, there is no ethical reason to not use them.

The arguments for the ethical use of placebo treatments (and the arguments to avoid unnecessary nocebo effects) extend beyond placebos to nonplacebo treatments. Almost all nonplacebo treatments have a placebo component, so the ethical requirement to exploit placebo effects and avoid nocebo effects applies to almost all treatments. To maximize the patients' response to a treatment, the meaningful contexts should be optimized. Likewise, to reduce the nocebo harms, care should be taken to be honest without scaring patients and increasing the risk of harm.

As with most things in life, this can be taken to ridiculous extremes. There is no need for paramedics rescuing someone from a car crash to spend time communicating with empathy, and surgeons need to focus on the highly technical task of performing surgery once the operation starts. But in most cases, placebo effects benefit patients in some way, and therefore it is unethical not to use them. For example, while surgeons should not occupy their minds with thoughts of good communication skills while they are cutting an anesthetized patient and performing a complex operation, discussions with the patient about the decision to do surgery,[36] encouraging the patient to have reasonably positive expectations about recovery,[37] and having a healing environment (see chapter 3) can all improve surgical outcomes.

When it comes to nocebo effects, the ethics are much clearer. If communicating in an unnecessarily negative or unempathic way increases a patient's experience of pain, anxiety, or depression, doing so violates the ethical requirement of doctors to do no harm.

Why Every Doctor Needs to Be a Shaman

David Newman described what he called the "placebo paradox." The paradox arises from the fact that on the one hand it may be unethical to use a placebo (because it requires deception to be effective).[38] On the other hand, it is unethical for doctors to not use something that heals patients. Yet, this paradox dissolves because placebos do not require deception. For many common ailments, placebos can work even when patients know they are placebos, and sometimes they are the best option. Since doctors are required to help patients, they are also required to prescribe honest placebos in many of these cases. Even when placebos are not the best option and an active treatment is given, taking care to maximize placebo effects is an unadulterated imperative, demanded by doctors' duty to help patients. In parallel, it is unethical to induce nocebo effects when this can be avoided. Because using placebos and avoiding nocebo effects requires excellent communication skills, doctors need to adopt some (not all) of the skills usually attributed to shamans to perform their duties. All regulatory restrictions against the use of ethical placebos should be removed, and regulations should be introduced to prevent unnecessary nocebo effects.

CHAPTER 10

Fewer Placebos and Nocebos in Trials

A Plea to Return to the Original Declaration of Helsinki

The present popularity of placebo-controlled trials is easy to explain by marketing considerations and regulatory needs, but difficult to justify on scientific grounds.
    —MURRAY ENKIN, "Commentary on Howick: Questioning the Methodological Superiority of 'Placebo' over 'Active' Controlled Trials"[1]

The additivity of drug and placebo effects of antidepressant medication needs to be assessed empirically. If these effects are found not to be additive, alternative designs will be needed to assess drug effects.
    —IRVING KIRSCH, "Are Placebo and Drug Effects in Depression Additive?"[2]

Unethical Placebo Controls

Phil drank too much and developed alcoholic liver disease. We've known since the 1990s that steroids prevent death in about 20% of people with this disease.[3] In the early 2000s, a new drug came along for treating alcoholic liver disease. To get it approved, the drug companies had to test it in a trial. The drug company representative paid Phil's doctor to help get patients to enroll in the trial, and Phil's doctor suggested that Phil enroll. Phil had a vague idea of what a clinical trial was, but he trusted his doctor's recommendation and signed up without doing any background research or asking his doctor many questions. The trial compared the new drug against a placebo instead of comparing it against steroids. Phil ended up in the placebo group and died. Had the drug company compared the new drug against steroids, there was a 20% higher chance that he would have lived.

Phil is not a real patient, but the trial of new drug against the placebo was a real trial,[4] and there were real patients like Phil in the trial. Had the drug companies proposed the trial of a new drug against placebo before the year 2000, ethical ethics committees wouldn't have allowed them to proceed. They would have said that the new drug had to be compared with what was proved to work: steroids. Before 2000, the World Medical Association's ethical code (called the Declaration of Helsinki) made it clear that placebos could not be used unless there was no proven treatment: "In any medical study, every patient—including those of a control group, if any—should be assured of the best proven diagnostic and therapeutic method. This does not exclude the use of inert placebo in studies where no proven diagnostic or therapeutic method exists."[5]

This version of the declaration made it easy for doctors to abide by their professional codes of conduct. Ethical codes as old as the Hippocratic oath demand that doctors help their patients as much as they can. Being part of a trial in which patients are not given the best available care is a violation of this ethical code. The earlier version of the declaration also aligns with patients' interests. The most useful trial for patients is one in which a new treatment is compared with the best one we have.

The early version of the declaration also reflects what we would choose to do in any other situation. When I use Google Maps to find out how to get to a nearby restaurant from my office, it provides me with a walking route, a driving route, and a cycling route. I can then make a wise choice about how I'd like to get there. If I feel like a bit of exercise or the parking is notoriously difficult, I might choose to walk or cycle. On the other hand, if I must go somewhere else afterward that is further away, I can choose to drive. If Google Maps didn't provide me with this comparative information, I would not be able to make a wise choice. We do something similar when we buy dishwashers, refrigerators, or most other things. For a dishwasher, we might compare the price, how eco-friendly it is, and how long the warranty lasts for a variety of options. This comparative information is needed to make a wise choice. If I don't have comparative information about walking, cycling, or driving routes, I can't make a wise choice. If I compare the dishwasher to no dishwasher or a fake "placebo" dishwasher I can't make a wise choice. The logic of the need to make a comparison of all available options is obvious.

Despite being good and obvious, in 2004 a new version of the Declaration of Helsinki came out that allowed placebos even if administering them involved withholding a proven therapy. The document states:

> a placebo-controlled trial may be ethically acceptable, even if proven therapy is available, under the following circumstances:
> - Where for compelling and scientifically sound methodological reasons its use is necessary to determine the efficacy or safety of a prophylactic, diagnostic or therapeutic method; or
> - Where a prophylactic, diagnostic or therapeutic method is being investigated for a minor condition and the patients who receive placebo will not be subject to any additional risk of serious or irreversible harm.

Even more recently, the 2013 version of the declaration used very similar language, allowing for placebo-controlled trials even if there is proven therapy when there are "methodological" reasons for doing so. The problem was that these new versions of the declaration didn't tell us what these "compelling and scientifically sound methodological reasons" were. Say it's true that there are "scientifically sound" reasons that make placebo-controlled trials the best option. That means that anything else (such as a trial comparing the proven treatment with the new treatment) is *less* scientifically sound. Any trial that is not sound could be a waste of resources, which is also unethical from a societal point of view.

The new declaration puts doctors who take part in the trials in a bind. On the one hand, they have experts from the World Medical Association telling them that placebo controls are sound practice even if there is a proven treatment (and that anything else would be an unethical waste of money). On the other hand, they have their professional codes of conduct telling them to help patients as much as they can and give them the proven therapy instead of the placebo.

The revised declaration has been used to justify other trials like the one Phil was in. We studied a sample of 70 placebo-controlled trials published in 2015 in the top six medical journals, and found three that used placebos when they could have used a known effective treatment.[6] One of them compared a new antipsychotic drug against placebos,[7] even though we know that other drugs reduce psychosis.[8,9] The next compared a new drug for skin cancer against placebos,[10] even though we've known for more than five years before the trial that other treatments were effective.[11] The third compared steroid injections to a placebo injection for treating severe bruising in patients getting rhinoplasties in Brazil,[12] whereas we already knew that other drugs were effective for treating severe bruising.[13]

The authors of these studies claimed that their trials complied with the World Medical Association's Declaration of Helsinki, which they probably did. If the association doesn't specify *what* counts as a sound scientific reason, then anything goes: smart people can think of reasons to justify pretty much anything. This is why I've drafted an open letter to the World Medical Association asking them to revert to their original, more ethically justified position (see appendix 7).

Placebo Add-On Trials Are Okay

Before exposing the so-called sound scientific principles as unsound, I'll distinguish between ethical and unethical placebo-controlled trials (when we have a proven therapy). So far, I've been discussing the simple case in which a new treatment alone is compared with a placebo. In more complicated cases, everyone in the trial receives the established treatment. Then, some patients get a placebo on top of (as an add-on) the established treatment. The other half get the established treatment plus the new treatment. If Phil had been lucky enough to be in a placebo *add-on* trial, he would have been given steroids plus the placebo, and he might have lived. Placebo add-on trials are sound practice if everyone receives the best available established treatment. The ethical objections to placebo-controlled trials do not (and to my knowledge have not been) used against appropriate placebo add-on trials. This is because, as Stephen Senn and Iain Chalmers have pointed out, placebo add-on trials do not usually involve withholding best established treatment.[14] Unless otherwise specified, I'm referring to standard placebo-controlled trials rather than placebo add-on trials.

Why would anyone enroll in a placebo-controlled trial when they could be in a trial that compares the new treatment with the best established treatment? The first reason is that they might not understand what the trial is about. They might not understand what placebos are, or they might not know about the proven treatments. Another reason is that they might be willing to sacrifice themselves for science. But the idea that one is making a greater sacrifice for science if one enrolls in a placebo-controlled trial (if there is an established treatment) presupposes that placebo-controlled trials are more scientifically sound. This is a big mistake. The mistake is tempting to make for historical reasons that I'll describe below.

The Death of King Charles II

Most medical treatments used until about two hundred years ago were either no better than placebo or positively harmful. Here's an example of how the very best doctors in England treated King Charles II. On the morning of February 2, 1685, the king fell and cried out. The doctors started treating him immediately, by slashing his arm open with a knife to take 16 ounces (about half a liter) of blood. They also gave him enemas and a purgatory syrup to make him throw up. Then, they burned him with hot cups, leaving his body covered with blisters. Then they bled him a bit more. On the next day they bled him from the jugular vein. The king got weaker and weaker, and by the fifth day, he was almost dead. The doctors doubled down, bled him some more, and force-fed him a stronger potion. The potion contained extracts of herbs and animals and even a human skull. They mixed this with some ammonia and forced it down his throat. One of the key ingredients appeared to be bezoar, a stone from the stomach of an eastern goat. The king became almost breathless and asked to see the sun rise one more time and say goodbye to all his children. He then said, "I have suffered much more than you can imagine. . . . You must pardon me, gentlemen, for being a most unconscionable time a-dying," and he died shortly after.[15] These doctors—the best in the land at the time—had tortured the king to death. They had based their treatment choices on the best theories of the time (which is why we shouldn't trust theories).

If King Charles II's doctors had used placebo-controlled trials to test their treatments, they would have quickly realized that most of their treatments were harmful. Even recently, some placebo-controlled trials surprise us by revealing that some widely used treatments are harmful. The most famous recent one I'm aware of is the placebo-controlled trials of antiarrhythmic drugs.[16] People believed that anti-arrhythmic drugs worked because of the theory on which they were based. The drugs were successful at reducing arrhythmias (irregular heartbeats), and arrhythmias were associated with heart attacks and death. Since the drugs stopped the irregular heartbeats, and irregular heartbeats were associated with heart attacks, why wouldn't the drugs work? The answer—which I've provided numerous times in this book—is that the human body is incredibly complex, and those simple theories often don't predict what will happen as often as they should. Eventually, a placebo-controlled trial was conducted and showed that the drugs were more harmful than placebos. It was estimated that the drugs—which had been widely prescribed—had killed more Americans each year than were killed in the entire Vietnam War.[17]

These examples provide a strong historical motivation for encouraging placebo-controlled trials: they help prevent harmful treatments from becoming accepted. But the ethical objection to placebo-controlled trials does not apply in cases like the historical ones. If there is no proven therapy, then it is perfectly acceptable to test a new treatment in a placebo-controlled trial. For example, until recently there was no proven treatment for irritable bowel syndrome, so new treatments were compared with placebos. The objection to placebo-controlled trials does not arise where there is no proven therapy, but rather where there *is* a proven therapy.

Of course, there is some debate about what counts as a proven effective therapy. In 1991, Richard Smith suggested that 80% to 90% of our treatments lacked a sound evidence base.[18] However, he was equating "evidence" with "randomized evidence," which is a mistake. Many treatments, ranging from the Heimlich maneuver to tracheostomies, are effective yet they have not been tested in randomized trials. More recent research indicates that between 76% (pediatric surgery) and 96% (anaesthesia) of our current practice is based on compelling (randomized or nonrandomized) evidence.[19-21] Since most of our current treatments are effective, most trials should compare a new treatment with a *contemporary* established treatment. If there is a debate about whether there is a proven therapy, placebo-controlled trials can be ethically justified. It is worth repeating that the revised Declaration of Helsinki states that placebo-controlled trials are acceptable *when there is a proven therapy.*

In Search of Scientific Justification for the New Declaration of Helsinki

The authors of the Declaration of Helsinki do not tell us what the sound so-called scientific reasons are for allowing placebo-controlled trials even when we have a proven effective treatment. There are no references to the statement. My search revealed three. One is the International Conference on Harmonisation, and the two others were jointly published by Robert Temple and Susan Ellenberg of the US Food and Drug Administration.[22-24] Temple and Ellenberg were also authors of the International Conference on Harmonisation document.

The International Conference on Harmonisation is an organization that brings the pharmaceutical industry together with government agencies from the United States, the European Union, and Japan. They convened a meeting to discuss placebo-controlled trials in the late 1990s and produced a document in 2000. Using complex jargon (which I'll explain below), the conference mentions three reasons for allowing placebo-controlled trials when we have a proven effective treatment:

1. Only placebo-controlled trials have assay sensitivity (the ability to tell a difference).
2. Only placebo-controlled trials produce a measure of absolute effect size.
3. Placebo-controlled trials are cheaper and use fewer patients.

Temple and Ellenberg reiterate the same reasons. None of the reasons stand up to scrutiny.

Problems with the Assay Sensitivity Arguments

The word "assay sensitivity" means "ability to detect a difference." I don't know why Temple, Ellenberg, and the International Conference on Harmonisation chose to use a word most people find confusing when they could have used plain English. I do know that the effect of choosing words like that is that many people don't understand the argument and defer to their authority and simply accept the argument that only placebo-controlled trials possess assay sensitivity. Put simply, the assay sensitivity argument is that only placebo-controlled trials can detect a difference, and trials comparing a new treatment with an established one cannot. A trial can detect (or try to detect) two kinds of differences:

1. A difference between an active treatment and a placebo
2. A difference between any two treatments

Placebo-controlled trials are not better at telling either kind of difference. Let's look at each one in more detail.

Trials Comparing a New Treatment with Proven Treatment *Can* Tell the Difference between an Active Treatment and a Placebo

If King Charles II's doctors had compared ingesting bezoar stones with bloodletting, and bloodletting performed slightly better, this wouldn't tell us whether either procedure is better than a placebo. They were both almost certainly harmful to poor King Charles II. To tell whether one treatment is as good as a proven one, we need the proven treatment to be, well, proven. And when we have proven treatments, trials comparing a new treatment with an established one are quite good at telling differences between placebos and active treatments.

Temple and Ellenberg, admit that their arguments do not apply in many contemporary cases when they say, "in some settings, such as highly responsive cancers, most infectious diseases, and some cardiovascular conditions, [trials that compare a new treatment with an established one] do provide a valid and reliable basis for evaluating new treatments."[23] But they only go into detail about one case: selective serotonin reuptake inhibitors. Their conclusion appears to make the general case that all active controlled trials suffer from difference-telling problems.

Their next move is to use doublespeak. They switch from saying that some *trials* can't tell the difference between a more and less effective treatment to saying that some *treatments* have difference-telling problems (they use the confusing and misleading term "assay sensitivity problems"). Now, if they were saying that some *bad* trials aren't good at detecting effects, they'd be right. Small, biased trials cannot be trusted to detect differences. But that is not what they are saying. They say that the trials are fine but that there are treatments that are *definitely* effective yet have trouble showing their effects in good trials. But it's not the job of the treatment to tell a difference: it's the job of trials. A treatment can't have difference-telling problems any more than humans can have feather-growing problems. Treatments can have trouble demonstrating differences if they aren't that effective, and I think that's what Temple and Ellenberg mean. And if they do, it undermines their claim that some treatments are definitely effective yet don't always demonstrate their effects in good trials.

The main example Temple and Ellenberg use of (supposedly) proven treatments whose effects don't show up in trials are a class of antidepressants called selective serotonin reuptake inhibitors, or SSRIs. They state:

> One might speculate that variable results of trials of antidepressants are simply the consequence of modest effect sizes coupled with samples too small to overcome the inherent variability of the condition studied. Results, however, are consistent with effect sizes that vary greatly and unpredictably from study to study. With current knowledge, one cannot specify a particular study population, treatment protocol, or sample size that will regularly identify active [SSRI] agents.[25]

The problem with this argument is that Temple and Ellenberg are blaming the tools (the trial) when the carpenter (the drug's lack of clear effectiveness) is more likely to blame. If we can't specify which study population or trial protocol is appropriate to allow these antidepressants to show their effects, why do they think that the drugs work in real life (where populations and conditions vary even more widely than they do in trials)? In fact, there is a logical error in the idea that treatments can have "difference-telling" problems. They start by saying that they know a treatment works. Then, if a trial doesn't show it works, they say there is some unknown problem with the trial, but the treatment must work. Therefore, Temple and Ellenberg are begging the question.

Just imagine what would happen if we applied the idea that treatments could have "difference-telling" more generally. Every form of snake oil and ineffective pharmaceutical drug that was roughly as effective as a placebo (so would outperform placebos in some trials but not others) would be touted by their proponents as having "difference-telling" problems. Their proponents would say things like, "I know this new expensive treatment didn't prove superior to placebo in many trials. And I can't tell you what is wrong with the trials. But my wonderful treatment has 'difference-telling' problems that make it difficult to prove itself superior to placebos in many trials. Yet, I just know it works." As crazy as it sounds, this is just what Temple and Ellenberg do when they say, "In each case, however, the problem is not identifiable a priori by examining the study; it is recognized only by the observed failure of the trial to distinguish the drug and placebo treatments."[25]

Rather than making the illogical claim that treatments have "difference-telling" problems, the idea that the treatments are not effective in many cases needs to be taken more seriously. Temple and Ellenberg list only 11 treatments that have supposed "difference-telling" problems, they provide evidence for four (SSRIs, some painkillers, beta-blockers, and anti-vomiting drugs), and they go into detail about just one (SSRIs). The evidence they provide for the others is shoddy. They cite a single 1994 paper to support the claim that painkillers have difference-telling problems,[26] but it's well known that painkillers are not all effective for all types of pain.[27] So, the variable results of placebo-controlled trials of painkillers are probably due to the fact that some analgesics are effective for some types of pain, while others are not. They cite a single 1985 paper to support the claim that beta-blockers have difference-telling problems.[28] But the authors of the paper they cite encourage using of larger trials and systematic reviews to detect the intervention effect. This suggests that the explanation for the variable results of beta-blockers is that the effect size is small and could be solved by larger trials. They cite another single paper as evidence that anti-vomiting drugs have difference-telling problems,[29] but again the problem was likely that the trial was small.

When it comes to their prized example of SSRIs, Temple and Ellenberg pretend to be oblivious to the controversy about whether the small benefits of these drugs outweigh the risks. The very idea that serotonin levels are linked to depression is contested,[30] and the antidepressant effects of SSRIs are not definitive. The most recent megastudy concludes that there are small differences between active placebo and SSRIs,[31] while other systematic reviews barely detected benefits of SSRIs over placebo controls.[32,33] Worse, SSRIs seem to increase the risk of suicide by a small amount.[34,35]

There is also evidence that SSRIs are little more than active place-bos for depression. It seems that if you replace SSRIs with different drugs that are not antidepressants, they have the same antidepressant effect as SSRIs. Some trials comparing drugs that are *not* considered to be antidepressants (amylobarbitone, lithium, liothyronine, and adin-azolam) find the same antidepressant effects as SSRIs when compared with placebo.[32] But how could these drugs, which are not antidepres-sants, have antidepressant effects? One hypothesis is that the other drugs do *something*, leading to patients believing they are getting a great new treatment. The beliefs generate positive expectations about recovery, and lower depression compared with placebo (see chapter 8). Finally, Temple and Ellenberg ignore the widely cited potential prob-lems of publication bias (whereby negative results are less likely to be published) [36,37] and bias inherent in industry-sponsored trials,[38-40] both of which are known to exaggerate apparent treatment benefits.

To recap, placebo-controlled trials are no better than active controlled trials at detecting differences. It is a logical mistake to claim that treatments have "difference-telling problems." This pulls the rug out from under Temple and Ellenberg's argument. But there's more misinformation in their arguments that needs to be exposed.

Trials Comparing a New Treatment with Established Treatment *Can* Tell the Difference between Two Treatments

In addition to claiming that only placebo-controlled trials can tell the difference between an active treatment and a placebo, Temple and Ellenberg also claim that only placebo-controlled trials can tell the difference between any two treatments. This is also a mistake. The statistical tests used to detect whether new treatments are superior to established treatments are identical to the tests used to detect dif-ferences between new treatments and placebos. The statistical tests don't know whether the control treatment is a placebo or a proven treatment. It is therefore simply untrue that placebo-controlled trials are better at detecting differences than trials comparing a new treatment with a proven one. Temple and Ellenberg know this, so they switch the goal posts. Instead of talking about trials comparing a new treatment with a proven one where we're looking to see whether the new one is *better*, they switch to a subtype of active controlled trial where we look to see whether the new treatment is *as good as* the old one.

However, instead of saying "as good as" (which everyone gets) they use the obtuse statistical term "noninferior." A trial designed to tell whether a new treatment is as good as the old one is (they say) not good at detecting a difference because that's not the point of looking for "as good as." They are wrong about that too, but it gets technical, so I've left it in appendix 8.

The final reason Temple, Ellenberg, and the authors of the International Conference on Harmonisation provide to support the methodological superiority of placebo-controlled trials is the mistaken idea that placebo-controlled trials provide a measure of absolute effect size.

Placebo-Controlled Trials Do Not Provide Absolute Effect Sizes

Temple and Ellenberg claim that placebo-controlled trials provide a measure of absolute effect size. They implicitly define absolute effect size as the effect size compared with placebo control, and the word "absolute" implies that it is unchanging or definite. According to this view, if a new treatment outperforms a placebo by 10%, then that treatment has a 10% effect size. Whereas if a new treatment is better than a proven treatment by 10%, we don't know how big the effect is compared to a placebo control. It might be 15%, 20%, 25% (or some other amount) better than a placebo. We would have to indirectly infer how much better the proven control was compared with a placebo in that trial. This is why Temple and Ellenberg say that trials comparing a new drug with a proven one provide a measure of *relative* effect size.

But the idea that placebo-controlled trials provide a measure of absolute effect size is based on the mistaken assumption of additivity (see chapter 7). As I described in detail in numerous places in the book, placebo effects vary widely and can interact with active treatment effects. For example, in 1983 Daniel Moerman did a megastudy of an ulcer drug called cimetidine. The effect of the drug was quite constant, but the placebo effect was not. The placebo effect ranged from 10% to 90% of the drug effect. An update of his study yielded more dramatic results, with the placebo effect ranging from between 0% and 100% of the (again, roughly constant) drug effect.[41] A similar study of treatments for irritable bowel syndrome (IBS) found that the placebo response ranged from 16.0% to 71.4% of the (roughly constant) experimental treatment.[42] Moerman looked for reasons that could logically explain why the placebos had such different responses. He didn't find any difference based on the age or gender of those who took the drugs. But he did find national differences. The "placebo" response rate was less than half the average in Brazil and twice the average in Germany. Moerman infers that "Placebo effects seem to be highly variable regardless of the axis on which you examine them."[41]

Because placebo effects vary so much, placebo-controlled trials do not provide a measure of absolute effect size. Instead, they provide a measure of *relative* effect size, with the effect size being relative to the effectiveness of the placebo in that trial and context. You could say that the effect size in a trial comparing the new treatment with a proven one is somehow doubly relative: relative to the effect of the proven treatment in that trial and relative to how much better the proven treatment would have been against a placebo. This is true, but it is still untrue that placebo-controlled trials provide a measure of absolute effect size.

There is also another factor to consider. If a new treatment is compared with a placebo instead of a proven treatment, we are still left with the question of deciding which treatment—the new treatment or the proven one—is best. This important question needs to be answered with educated yet inaccurate guesses whereas a trial comparing the two treatments would have provided a more accurate answer that allows patients and doctors to make the right treatment choice.

Not the Best of Both Worlds: Three-Armed Trials

Some people might be tempted to propose trials that include both a placebo and an established treatment as controls. That way we get to compare the new treatment with the placebo and the established treatment. Three-armed trials are slightly better than standard placebo-controlled trials because patients will at least have a chance to get the established treatment. They also solve the supposed assay sensitivity problems noted by Temple and Ellenberg. However, they do not solve the ethical problem that doctors may be violating their ethical codes of conduct by facilitating the allocation of some patients to receiving a placebo when they could be getting a proven treatment. Also, they are only justified if adding a placebo adds some advantage in cases where there is a proven therapy, which it doesn't.

Other Mistaken Arguments Promoting Placebo-Controlled Trials

Several other arguments are sometimes offered in favor of placebo-controlled trials that I will review here.

Smaller Sample Sizes

Placebo-controlled trials supposedly require fewer participants for their statistical tests. If this were true, then it would save money, which is usually a good thing, especially if public tax dollars are used to fund the trials. But this only applies to noninferiority trials not to superiority trials, and even then, it only applies where the size of the acceptable difference in the noninferiority trial is small (see appendix 8).

Developing Nations

I've often heard colleagues say that even if there is a proven therapy, we can still use placebo-controlled trials in developing nations. This is because, they say, placebos are cheaper than the established treatments. After all, the poor people in the developing nations would not be able to afford the established therapy. Letting them enroll in a placebo-controlled trial is giving these poor people at least a chance of getting the great new drug.

In a way, what they are saying is that while there might be a proven treatment for wealthy people, the proven treatment is not available in the developing country. In that sense, they might say that there is not really a proven treatment in the developing country. This position is cruel and mistaken. First, the new treatment could turn out to be harmful. In 2006, a drug called TGN1412 was tested on six healthy volunteers, who were paid £2,000 (about $2,500) each to participate in the trial. Within minutes of being given these very low doses, the white blood cells in the human volunteers disappeared.[43] This led to catastrophic organ failure with the victims fighting for their lives, over a month of hospitalization, and likely permanent damage to their immune systems that will leave them vulnerable to disease for the rest of their lives. One of the victims lost all his toes and the tips of all his fingers. Not only did the drug operate differently in animals than in humans (which is obvious to many people), but the extremely serious organ failure was not predicted by scientists who had studied how the drug activated various body parts for many years. In addition to activating the system they thought it would activate, the drug acted on other parts with disastrous consequences.

Second, sometimes placebos (for trials) are more expensive than the established therapy. This surprised me when I did my first placebo-controlled trial, but it's true. The reason is that the companies that make the placebos for the trials must make very small batches, and they have to look exactly like the new drug. There are no economies of scale. Third, if the drug turns out to work, the company stands to make billions of dollars. And if it turns out not to work, they'll stop wasting money on it. Given the massive profits or savings of the companies, they should give patients in developing countries the chance of getting something that will help them rather than exposing then to potential harm.

Allowing placebo-controlled trials in developing nations even when there is a proven therapy is also a perversion of what the World Medical Association says. In a clarification of the updated Declaration of Helsinki, Delon Human (the World Medical Association's Secretary General) stated that the nonavailability of drugs should not be used as a justification to conduct placebo-controlled trials as it "would lead to poor countries of the world being used as the laboratory of research institutions of the developed world."[44]

Avoiding Nocebo Effects in Clinical Trials: The Need to Make Ethics Committees More Ethical

Whereas there is a debate about the use of placebo controls in clinical trials, there is no reason to not take great care to avoid nocebo effects in clinical trials. As mentioned in part I, my previous research showed that half of the people in clinical trials who take placebos report at least one negative side effect, and one in 20 have such bad side effects that they drop out of the trial. Not all of these are nocebo effects, but many are. My other background research found that the way information about potential trial intervention harms is presented is very unbalanced. Sometimes, several pages are dedicated to describing all the bad things that might happen to patients, and no space is devoted to describing the potential benefits. There is a wide variety in the way ethics committees believe in the need to describe potential harms, and the way some of them insist on doing it causes unnecessary harm.

The reason for the undue focus on the need to share information about harms is that ethicists are eager to avoid the horribly unethical trials conducted by the Nazis and others. Patients need to be informed of and agree to participate in trials in which they might be harmed. I agree with this requirement. The problem is that the way we share information about harms can cause harm. In many trials, professional (often self-proclaimed) ethicists sometimes insist on forcing information about potential harms upon patients without thinking of ways to share this information in a less scary way. I have witnessed this myself in some of the trials I have been involved with. Together with actual patients who might end up enrolled in the trial, we initially develop a patient information leaflet that describes the potential benefits and harms in a clear, understandable, and balanced way. Then we send it to the ethics committee, which usually gets back to us and insists that we reformulate the leaflet to deemphasize the potential benefits and spend more time discussing the harms. The committees also often insist that we use legalistic language to describe the harms, which patients don't understand. Presumably, they are thinking about protecting themselves against possible lawsuits from patients who might be harmed then say they didn't know about the potential harm.

I think it is good to protect against legal action of this kind, but the need to respect autonomy is a double-edged sword. If patients do not want to be forced to learn about all the harms, however rare, this violates their autonomy. On top of this, the ethics committee standards are inconsistent. A different ethics committee could make a completely different decision. And if you disagree with them, there is nothing you can do because appealing is often more difficult than simply obeying. All you can do is squirm and take time to change your protocol to meet the ethics committee's demands. This can waste public resources if the research is state funded. Sadly, it might take legal action to change this. For example, researchers who have had what they take to be an unfair decision from an ethics committee might sue the institution at which the committee is based. Or patients might be scared away from a trial in which they could have benefited because of Dr. Vetigan–type behavior. These patients might sue the institution for failing to disclose adequate information about the potential benefits of a trial treatment. These kinds of lawsuits may force ethics committees to behave in a more balanced way.

There is no easy solution to the problem of how to be honest about potential trial treatment harms without scaring people unnecessarily.

However, the fact that it is difficult is no reason to shy away from it. I'm leading a Medical Research Council–funded trial with a great team at Cardiff University to start to try to solve the problem. We've discovered that there are some easy ways to reduce unnecessary harms— for example, by balancing information about potential harms of a new treatment with information about potential benefits (if there were no potential benefits, they wouldn't be doing the trial!).[45]

Reassessing the Methodological Quality of Placebo-Controlled Trials

It's not sound science to have a trial that compares the new treatment with a placebo if a proven treatment could be used instead. Comparing the new treatment (which could turn out to be harmful) with a placebo puts patients at risk of harm that could be reduced by comparing the new treatment with what we know works. Because doctors are required to help patients and avoid harms, it is unethical for them to enroll patients in placebo-controlled trials when there is an established treatment. This makes common sense and it's why the World Medical Association's Declaration of Helsinki initially stated that placebo-controlled trials are unethical if we have an established therapy. The so-called scientific reasons why we need placebo-controlled trials to show that new treatments work can be easily debunked. One reason they may have survived this long is that they are shrouded in complex, confusing, and confounded jargon.

The World Medical Association moved away from the commonsense position and claimed that placebo-controlled trials are sometimes acceptable even when we have an established treatment. They state that there are "scientific" reasons for the new position. When unveiled in plain English, they are plainly false. At best, they apply to some noninferiority trials, which are rarely justified. There are no methodological advantages of placebo-controlled trials over trials that compare a new treatment with an established one. The revised declaration puts doctors in a compromised ethical position because they are not offering patients the best available options. It also lacks common sense: we need to compare available options when we buy dishwashers, so why should good comparative information be withheld when it comes to our health and clinical trials?

Yet, because of the World Medical Association's unethical position, unethical placebo-controlled trials persist.[46] With that in mind, the World Medical Association should revert to their initial position. In the meantime, ethics committees should refuse to approve placebo-controlled trials when we have an established treatment. They should also investigate requests to approve noninferiority trials very carefully as they are rarely justified.

There is no justification for the way in which nocebo effects seem to be increased in trials due to unbalanced information about potential trial treatment harms.

CHAPTER 11

Public Health, Surgery, and Alternative Medicine

Special Topics

Special Topic 1: Nocebo and Placebo Public Health Messages
Negative Nocebo Public Health Messages

In 2010, anti-windfarm campaigners in Australia spread news about a "wind turbine syndrome." The alleged syndrome was supposedly caused by subaudible infrasound generated by wind turbines. The symptoms of the supposed syndrome included heart palpitations, headaches, and nausea. Coinciding with the scary news about the alleged syndrome, health authorities noticed a growing number of complaints reporting the purported symptoms. Yet researchers quickly found that complaints were concentrated in regions where anti-windfarm campaigners were actively spreading news about the supposed syndrome.[1] In an experiment, people who were randomly allocated to watch scary news about the harms of windfarms reported an increase of symptoms.[1] Researchers concluded that wind turbine syndrome was caused by misinformation rather than by wind turbines. Something similar seems to have happened with side effects of statin therapy. In 2018, a study found that people living in countries with more Google search results about statin adverse events were more likely to report statin intolerance. Authors of the study concluded that exposure to online information contributed to these adverse effects.[2]

The COVID-19 era was fertile ground for the proliferation of harmful nocebo public health messages. A positive test for COVID-19, combined ith some initial symptoms and alarming mass-media health news, could aggravate coughs, fever, pains, and breathlessness.[3] While I'm not aware of any reports of this happening, the evidence presented earlier in this book suggests that shock caused by negative information might even precipitate death in severely ill patients by aggravating heart disorders or affecting the respiratory system already attacked by the virus. The social isolation imposed in many countries, well known to be linked to illness and death, could have exacerbated these effects.[4]

The anti–wind turbine messages, the messages about statin side effects, and the public health messages about COVID-19 are not medical treatments, but they all produced negative health effects. The mechanisms by which these negative effects are produced are probably the same as the way nocebo effects of medical treatments are produced.

Positive Placebo Public Health Messages

Perhaps the most common form of positive public health placebos is drug marketing where people are led to have very positive expectations about new treatments. Somewhat paradoxically (yet understandably), a kind of negative nocebo message often precedes the positive message. For example, as part of the marketing for Prozac, its manufacturer educated the public about depression. Their message was that millions of people were depressed but just didn't know it. Academic researchers, often well paid by the company,[5] presented data about the epidemic of undiagnosed depression. The education about the condition included promotion of the idea that feeling down sometimes wasn't really normal, and that people could be happy all the time. The education also included claims that the depressive feelings were not a result of life circumstances but rather they were caused by a chemical imbalance in the brain.[6,7] Because the cause was a chemical imbalance in the brain, the cure was a convenient pill. (Note: after I drafted this chapter, a major study found no evidence that depression was related to serotonin levels.)[8] In one of their infomercials, Freda Lewis-Hall (an Eli Lilly psychiatrist) said "Public education about depression, including a significant campaign by national advocacy groups to reduce stigma, has helped raise awareness around the seriousness of depression and appropriate treatments."[9] Raising social consciousness is a wonderful thing, but some have argued that the company went further than that by making people who were not depressed believe they were depressed.[5]

Television ads promoting Prozac often started with background images of gray skies and people looking sad. One of them had a voiceover of a teary voice saying, "I remember being happy, graduating from college . . . becoming a mother . . . following my dreams. . . . Then one day the colors just didn't seem as bright."[10] This is misleading because almost everyone felt amazing the day they graduated from college or had their first child. The world *does* look bright to most people when they graduate from college because we're full of potential then. We're in our early twenties, the day of graduation is usually part of a graduation week when we attend lots of parties and are not worried about exams. A college graduation party on Saturday night and seeing a newborn for the first time are *inherently* more exciting than lots of the stuff that happens later in life such as being woken up at 3 a.m. by a crying toddler, paying taxes, or failing to get an anticipated promotion.

After the negative phase, people are led to have very positive expectations about recovery. In the ads for Prozac, people take the drug, the music becomes happier, the sun comes out, and people with perfect white teeth start smiling. Prozac was marketed to consumers in the United States in this way before it was formally approved for marketing (a practice illegal outside the United States and New Zealand). Even the name was carefully chosen to sound positive and powerful (see chapter 3). The result of this ingenious campaign is that the number of people diagnosed with depression increased thirtyfold after Prozac was approved for marketing, and many of the newly depressed people demanded prescriptions. Sales of Prozac skyrocketed to levels unheard of (for antidepressant drugs) in the past.[6,11]

The campaigns to promote the benefits of Prozac were amazing for generating positive expectations in people about its benefits. As I've explained in previous chapters, the expectations can produce a benefit. Similar stories can be found in relation to other drugs, including drugs to treat a new condition called prediabetes (which can supposedly affect young slim people who will almost certainly not get diabetes),[12-14] and those at a low risk of heart disease (most of whom will never have a heart attack).[15-17]

Evidence for the Effects of Public Health Messages

One giant review of 36 reviews found that mass-media interventions for reducing smoking and illicit drug use, improving sexual health, and improving physical activity were cost-effective.[18] The successful campaigns included positive messages (eliciting happiness, satisfaction, or hope) and negative messages (eliciting fear, sadness, guilt, anger, or disgust), and that both of these were effective, with positive messages being slightly more effective.

Other evidence about the effects of public health messages comes from studies showing that placebo effects in pain trials have increased over time in the United States (these were described in chapter 7 as well).[17] A reason for this could be that drug companies are allowed to advertise directly to consumers in the United States, and their marketing tactics could have become more successful.

Improving Public Health Messages with the Science of Placebos

Imagine what would happen if the genius and money spent on public health campaigns for education about the need for pills to treat conditions people were not previously aware they had were applied to something like exercise. Exercise, after all, reduces depression and heart disease while increasing libido. I imagine the campaign for promoting exercise going something like this: First, there would be a scene in the hospital for diseases that can be at least partly prevented by healthy lifestyle choices—ailments like type 2 diabetes, cardiovascular disease, and obesity. Then they could show how much happier, stronger, healthier, and virile exercise makes us. With the money saved on treating people with these (to some degree) preventable diseases, we could build, fun outdoor spaces or outdoor gyms, and enjoy engaging activities. That would do away with the need for most of the pills for most people with mild depression or low risk of heart disease or diabetes. I'll discuss how something like that might be done in chapter 12.

Paradoxically, it probably helps for background public health messages to avoid promoting expectations that are too high. In a 1994 paper, D. Mark Chaput de Saintonge and Andrew Herxheimer found it is easier to deliver effective positive messages if expectations are not unreasonably high. I have quoted them at length below.

> Do not promote perfect health as a realistic goal. Aside from economic considerations, 70–80% of people have a complaint on any one day, which suggests that perfect health is unattainable. The best way to increase a nation's health is to increase the expectation of disease. This would at least allow the pessimism of the half-empty to be transformed to into the satisfaction of the half-full. A more realistic goal than perfect health is to aim for . . . 70% benefit. . . . Anything more is a bonus.[20]

The Ethics of Public Health Placebos

By and large, public health placebo and nocebo ethics are like medical ethics. Just as doctors must avoid harm and do their best to benefit patients, it is unethical for public health interventions to cause unnecessary harm and avoid helping. Some negative messages are helpful for preventing people from starting to smoke and can therefore be justified. On the other hand, the daily tsunami of doomsday news about the coronavirus pandemic, often based on questionable statistical predictions that have turned out to be exaggerated, is probably causing harm that could be avoided with more tempered and rational language.

Against this, one could argue that inducing fear is required to get people to follow the rules and stay home. This is true. But when fear is used to change behavior, people get tired of the message and start to ignore it altogether.[21]

Special Topic 2: Sham Surgery

Sham surgery usually involves cutting the skin then stitching it back up without doing the other "essential" parts of the surgery. The first report of sham surgery I'm aware of was published in 1953. In that report, Kenneth Livingston describes giving four patients with psychosis a skin incision and removing a fragment of the skull bone, but nothing was done to the brain itself.[22] The sham procedure did not work, and all the patients subsequently underwent the real surgery, in which the brain was operated upon. The real surgery probably didn't work and was also harmful, but that's another subject.

In a 1961 paper, the great pioneer of placebo research Henry Knowles Beecher describes a surgical treatment for chest pain that was widely used from the 1930s until the late 1960s. The surgical procedure involved tying up one of the arteries, which was supposed to increase blood flow to other areas and reduce chest pain. The initial results of the procedure were astonishing, with the surgeons reporting large increases of between 5 and 10 cubic centimeters per minute of blood flow and reduced pain following the procedure.[23] Beecher hypothesized that the apparent benefits of the procedure could be placebo effects. In the late 1950s, two landmark placebo-controlled trials of sham surgery were done to evaluate the procedure.[24,25] The sham surgery involved giving patients local anaesthesia, cutting into the skin, then sewing it up but not doing anything to the artery. The real surgery and the placebo surgery both worked equally well.

Sham surgery was made famous a few decades later by Bruce Moseley, who was the team surgeon for the Houston Rockets basketball team. Dr. Moseley performs a lot of knee surgeries called arthroscopies. To perform these surgeries, Dr. Moseley inserts a small metal tube called an arthroscope into the knee and then uses it to repair damaged cartilage and remove loose bone fragments that cause pain. A million knee arthroscopies are performed each year in the United States at a cost of $5,000 each, making a total annual bill of $5 billion. By observing that players with positive attitudes seemed to recover more quickly, Dr. Moseley got the idea that *placebo* arthroscopy for osteoarthritis might be almost as good as the real thing. He found 180 patients who had such bad knee pain that even the strongest drugs had failed to work for more than six months. Many were in so much pain that they had trouble getting out of their chairs. Moseley enrolled them in a trial of real compared with placebo arthroscopic surgery.

Moseley gave two-thirds of the patients real arthroscopy and a third placebo arthroscopy. Patients in the placebo arthroscopy group were given anaesthetics and doctors made a small incision on their knees, but there was no arthroscope, no repairing of damaged cartilage, and no cleaning out of loose fragments of bone. To keep the patients blinded, the doctors and nurses talked through a real procedure and mimicked the sounds of real surgery even when they were performing the placebo procedure.

Moseley and his team then monitored the patients for two years, asking them how much pain they felt and measuring how far they could walk and how many stairs they could climb before their pain got in the way. After two years, even Moseley was surprised. The placebo was not almost as good as the real surgery—it was equally good. Both those in the placebo and real surgery group had an average of 10% less pain and 10% better function.

Eutenio Perez was one of the patients in Moseley's trial. Before the surgery, he had such bad knee pain that he could barely walk. A scan revealed damage to his cartilage and bones. When interviewed, a teary-eyed Eutenio reported that before the surgery the pain "could not be any worse," and that it stopped him from doing pastimes that he enjoyed such as fishing, playing basketball, and dancing. He was very pleased to enroll in Moseley's trial because he was a big Houston Rockets fan. Within a few weeks he was dancing and playing basketball again (according to his wife, he could dance all night). But Eutenio had received the sham surgery.

Moseley's trial is dramatic because it was a large-scale, high-quality trial with interesting results. It received a lot of press and seemed to kick off a lot of placebo-controlled trials of surgery interventions. For example, in 2009, researchers from Australia took 78 patients with spinal fractures of the kind that are often treated by vertebroplasty.[26] Vertebroplasty involves making a small incision in someone's back then injecting bone glue into a damaged vertebra. Half the patients got real vertebroplasty, and the other half got placebo vertebroplasty. In the placebo vertebroplasty, surgeons cut the skin and touched the bone to simulate the glue injection but did not inject any cement. The sham procedure performed as well as the real thing. A similar trial in the United States also revealed that sham surgery was as good as genuine vertebroplasty.[27] Worse, the cement glue used can leak,[28] possibly causing more fractures.[29]

In 2014 my colleagues published a review of all placebo-controlled surgery trials. They found 53 trials, and sham surgery was as good as the real thing in over half. Besides knee, back, and shoulder surgery whose aim is to reduce pain (skeptics will always complain that pain is subjective and that the trials don't mean much), pretending to insert brain implants works as well as real implants for reducing migraine attacks, fake laser surgery works as well as real laser surgery to stop gastrointestinal bleeding, and fake surgery works as well as real surgery for improving sphincter function. What makes this even more striking is that the real surgery is associated with greater harm, which shouldn't surprise us because the more invasive the procedure, the more harm that can be done.

Placebos on Steroids: How So-Called Placebo Surgery Works

So-called placebo surgery does several things all at once. First, it generates very high expectations. Surgeons are usually the most eminent clinicians in the hospital and they are usually a last resort. Their powerful techniques are used only if less invasive options, such as drugs or rehabilitation, fail. Then, during the surgery itself, patients are lying down in prone, submissive positions giving someone the power to cut them. This requires an enormous amount of trust in the surgeon's authority, knowledge, and skill. When eminent surgeons say they are going to perform an operation, it is believable and leads to high expectations about recovery. The high expectations can then contribute to the recovery.

In addition, surgery is very meaningful—perhaps the most meaningful of medical interventions. Operations take place in the surgical theater, where the surgeon is the star of the show, surrounded by a supporting cast of assistants and nurses. Crucially, surgery involves cutting the skin and the letting of blood. We all know about sacrifice by letting blood (of innocent lambs or even people), usually for redemption. Even atheists can't escape having imbibed powerful memes of bloodletting through literature, art, film, and just talking (who doesn't know what a "sacrificial lamb" is?). Surgery therefore invokes much of the latent cultural meaning that we ascribe to bloodletting. Moreover, the way surgical procedures work is also easy to understand: cutting away a bad tumour, gluing the bone together, clearing out the pieces of cartilage, making the sphincter smaller. Being able to understand what's happening can also contribute to high expectations about recovery, because it all makes sense at an understandable, mechanical level. By contrast, what happens to our bodies after ingesting drugs can be obscure. Trust in the authority of a clinician, understanding *how* something is going to get better, and the deep meaning surrounding the letting of blood—all of these create extremely fertile ground for patients to develop powerful and effective expectations about their postsurgical recovery.[30] If taking a pill in a doctor's office has meaning (and it does), then an eminent surgeon cutting your skin in a hospital has meaning on steroids. And if meaning has an effect, surgery has a bigger effect. Hence it is unsurprising that authors have argued that historical bloodletting and modern surgery are super-placebos.[31]

Surgery and the Wound-Healing Cascade

Surgery isn't just meaning. At a very concrete, physical level, placebo surgery activates the body's power of regeneration, known as the *wound-healing cascade*.[32] All living organisms are very good at regenerating themselves when they get cut or injured. If you cut a planarian flatworm's head off, it completely grows back. You can't grow a human head back if it gets chopped off, but many parts of your body can repair and regenerate themselves. Whether a cut is from a thorn that scrapes you on a walk in the woods, or a friendly surgeon's scalpel, the wound-healing cascade begins. It starts immediately with blood clotting in the injured region to stop the bleeding. Then the area swells up, and white blood cells phagocytose damaged cells and potentially harmful bacteria. (Phagocytose is a fancy name for saying that the white blood cells devour and destroy the unwanted cells.) Next, the body gets back to work making new tissue and blood vessels to feed the tissue and closing up the wound. Finally, the wound is healed when new scar tissue and skin cover it.

The wound-healing cascade is activated in patients who received sham surgery, and this could generate a physiological change to the problematic area. For example, sham surgery could fire up a process that heals vertebrae and even clear away some of the debris that causes knee pain. Eutenio, who had a strong response to the placebo surgery, may have had an unusually effective wound healing cascade. That might have changed the mechanics of his knee in ways that made it less painful and more functional.

Placebo surgery that includes painkillers—which it usually does before the incision—has an additional mechanism. Whether you get the real or placebo surgery, you are often given a hefty dose of local painkiller. This can cause back pain to subside even if a fracture isn't healed. With less pain, people feel freer to move around, and the moving around might have a benefit. In fact, exercise reduces back pain.[33]

Ethics of Placebo Surgery

Many people initially reacted to the stories of placebo-controlled surgery trials by saying it was unethical. How can you give potentially harmful fake surgery to people? For example, Ruth Macklin states: "Sham surgery is ethically unacceptable as a placebo control. . . . Sham surgery, with accompanying anesthesia, poses the risks of any surgical intervention that would not be used alone for therapeutic purposes."[34]

Sam Horng and Franklin Miller do not condemn placebo surgery trials outright. Instead, they say that those promoting placebo surgery trials need to jump over an additional hurdle: "Use of an invasive procedure as a placebo control poses risks to research subjects assigned to the control group, without the prospect of a benefit from their participation, and the burden of proof is therefore on those who argue that placebo surgery is warranted as a means of evaluating the efficacy of surgical procedures."[35]

Unfortunately, as is too often the case,[36] professional ethicists make strong untested claims about procedures for which we need strong evidence. They assume—without any investigation—that the risks of placebo surgery outweigh the benefits. When it was investigated (though placebo-controlled surgery trials!) it has proved to be false. Not only does sham surgery often have a great benefit, but the more invasive real surgery causes more harm. If the more invasive and more harmful real procedure does not outperform sham surgery, then the placebo surgery is more ethical than the real surgery not less ethical.

In ethics-speak, since sham surgery helps, and since the more invasive real surgery might cause harm, placebo-controlled trials of surgery are no more or less ethical than placebo-controlled trials of any other intervention. Of course, the devil is in the details: it depends on whether we have good reason to know that the surgical technique works without doing a trial.[37] For example, we know that appendectomy for confirmed acute appendicitis has a dramatic effect. We know this because many people with acute appendicitis get extremely ill or die without appendectomy, and most of those who get appendectomy do not get very ill and die. Therefore, it would not be ethical to test appendectomy for confirmed acute appendicitis against a placebo. We would not be in *equipoise* (roughly, most people would not have equal faith in the placebo surgery and the real appendectomy) in a trial of appendectomy for acute appendicitis. On the other hand, Bruce Moseley had good reason to believe that placebo effects played a strong role in the recovery after knee arthroscopy. Moseley was therefore not acting unethically when he did his sham surgery trial.

In practice it isn't always easy to determine whether a surgical technique or any other treatment is effective without doing a placebo-controlled trial. This is because surgeons and other practitioners—not to mention those with financial conflicts of interest—believe that their treatments work and that there is no need for a trial.[37,38] For example, some people suggested that it would be unethical to perform placebo-controlled trials of antiarrhythmic drugs, because the drugs–in their eyes—obviously worked.[4] Yet, a placebo-controlled trial subsequently revealed the drugs to be deadly (see chapter 10). Led by Jane Blazeby and David Beard, scientists have recently done a great deal of research on the methods and ethics of placebo-controlled surgery trials.[39,40] They urge researchers to ensure that there is a strong methodological and ethical rationale for a placebo-controlled surgery trials before performing them which is more sensible than blanket condemnation.

The Paradox of So-Called Placebo Surgery

After a placebo-controlled trial of antiarrhythmic drugs showed that the drugs were no better than placebos (and even harmful), their use stopped overnight. Not so after trials of placebo surgery. Take knee arthroscopy as an example (the same thing happened for many surgical techniques that have failed to outperform their sham versions). Besides Moseley's high-profile trial, three systematic reviews all concluded no benefit of knee arthroscopy for osteoarthritis compared with sham.[41-43] Nobody can avoid the conclusion that *on average*, "real" knee arthroscopy for osteoarthritis is no better than "placebo" knee arthroscopy. Based on these facts, we would expect that the knee arthroscopy business was dire. Yet, over a million arthroscopies are still performed in the United States each year,[44] and about 40,000 of these are done in the United Kingdom.[45] At a cost of about £1,681 in the UK and $5,000 in the US, this means that £67,000,000 in the UK and $5 billion in the US are spent each year on knee arthroscopies. That doesn't include the costs of treating side effects.

How can we explain the fact that the knee arthroscopy for osteoarthritis business (and other surgical procedures that have failed to outperform sham surgery) continues to thrive? Sure, financial conflicts of interest play a role because many surgeons and companies that make the relevant equipment profit from them. But there's more to it. Remember that, to be eligible for the trial, Eutenio and the others in Moseley's trial failed to respond to maximum drug doses for at least six months. For them, the placebo surgery *worked*. And it worked well— almost certainly better than a pill or injection placebo would have. This leaves surgeons in a bit of a bind. Either they carry on performing knee arthroscopies despite the cost and evidence that the procedures don't outperform sham versions. Or they stop doing them and allow patients like Eutenio to carry on suffering. The way out from between this rock and a hard place is to look more closely at whether sham surgery is actually a placebo.

Placebo Surgery Is Not a Placebo

A placebo is something that has no effect on the target disorder by itself, but whose meaningful features and the context in which it is delivered combine to generate an effect. Tiny amounts of sugar have no effect on pain, but when it is given in pill form by a trusted doctor, when the patient believes it is very expensive, and so on, it can reduce pain. This doesn't apply to placebo surgery. Whether the patient believes the procedure is very expensive, or the surgeon inspires confidence, the cut (which is an essential part of placebo surgery)[46] activates the wound-healing cascade. The wound-healing cascade, in turn, can have a direct effect on the problems that the surgical procedure is designed to rectify. When painkillers are used as part of the placebo surgery in advance of the incision (and they usually are), these can also have a direct effect. In short, the sham surgery does not fit the definition of a placebo.

So-called sham surgery is therefore more accurately described as minimally invasive surgery. Because the surgery allows surgeons to have a look, it is also what is called scoping surgery. A better name for so-called placebo surgery is therefore "minimally invasive scoping surgery." Patients suffering from conditions where the placebo surgery has performed as well as the more invasive, expensive, and risky surgery could be offered the option of minimally invasive scoping surgery. They could be given honest instructions about what the procedure involved. They could be told something like this:

> Hello, I'm Dr. Osler. I understand that you've had shoulder pain for several months and that painkillers aren't helping. We've seen a scan of your shoulder and found some bone spurs (which are pieces of bone that have grown in a way that can cause irritation) and other soft tissue we believe are causing the pain. There are two options. First, we could go ahead with a more invasive option and remove the bone spurs to repair the damage. This procedure is called arthroscopic subacromial decompression. It often relieves pain, but also comes with some risks including infection and minor nerve damage. Another option is to do minimally invasive scoping surgery. For the second option, we open the shoulder surgically, and have a look to confirm the extent of the damage, then sew it back up. We don't repair the damage ourselves. However, the act of cutting the skin near the damage can cause the body to do things that make the pain go away. Just as your body forms scar tissue when you get a cut, it can do similar things to the shoulder. Of course, if we find that the damage to your shoulder is very severe during the scoping procedure, we can do the regular arthroscopic subacromial decompression. Feel free to ask me any questions you have, and you can take your time to decide which option you prefer.

Replacing the false concept of placebo or sham surgery with a more accurate description (minimally invasive scoping surgery) solves the current conundrum about how to implement the evidence that real surgery doesn't work better than the so-called sham options, but that they both work.

Alternative Medicine and the Placebo

I don't believe the term "alternative medicine" is useful and don't want to give it too much airtime. Not only is the term vague, but it is a red herring: Either medical interventions are based on evidence or they are not. Some treatments that are considered to be conventional, even in the recent past, are not based on evidence.[47] And some interventions that are considered to be alternative have pretty good evidence to support their effects.[48]

I'm going to ignore all these problems with the term "alternative medicine" and make a generalization that is not completely true: alternative practitioners are better at eliciting placebo effects than conventional practitioners. Conventional medicine has benefited from great advances in pharmaceutical and surgical (and other) science. Since doctors in the past had very little in their toolkits that wasn't a placebo, they had to rely on excellent bedside manner and placebos. The advent of modern scientific, powerful medicine meant that this bedside manner didn't matter as much. It doesn't matter how nice the doctor who gives you an adrenaline injection for anaphylactic shock: adrenaline works. Because they have powerful treatments in their toolboxes, and because of the insane amount of paperwork they have to do,[49] many conventional doctors have lost their skills and have less time for good bedside manner and eliciting strong placebo effects.

Meanwhile, the holistic theories supporting many alternative practices require their practitioners to take time with patients to speak about their physical problems, emotions, and other aspects of their lives. Their worldview often forces them to do many of the things that the science of placebos says we should do if we want to enhance placebo

effects. Things like warm, compassionate communication, takin.
to set up a healing environment, and taking time to get to know
tients in a more holistic way.

Of course, newspapers sometimes report cases of weird alternative treatments like homeopathy for stage 4 cancer, which doesn't work, drinking urine, or coffee enemas. However, it is important to keep in mind that the reason these stories make headlines is that they are exceptions. Numerous surveys conclude that between a third and half of people in the US and UK use "complementary or alternative medicine."[50,51] If this was all harmful there would be a much higher rate of adverse events or even death. In fact, most people take "alternative" medicine because they are treating something that is not life-threatening and because their conventional doctors are not communicating with as much empathy and hope as they would like in environments that are not as healing as they would like. There is no reason why all health care practitioners cannot leverage placebo effects and minimize nocebo effects, and I'll suggest just how this can be done in chapter 12.

CHAPTER 12

The Next Placebo Revolution

Helping Dad

So many gods, so many creeds,
So many paths that wind and wind,
While just the art of being kind
Is all the sad world needs.

—ELLA WHEELER WILCOX, *The Voice of the Voiceless*

Putting the Research from This Book into Practice: Helping David

David is 61 years old and delivers groceries full-time for a major supermarket in Minnesota. He developed back and knee pain about 10 years ago (he forgets exactly when), and it started getting really bad about seven years ago. He eventually told his doctor, who told him to take iboprofen three times a day. The doctor emphasized that he shouldn't take ibuprofen on an empty stomach. He was already overweight, and to follow the doctors' instructions, he filled his stomach with food he liked to eat before taking the pills: cakes, chocolate bars, and whole milk. Within a few months, his weight reached 264 pounds (120 kilograms). At just under six feet tall, this made him obese. His pain also got worse; sometimes, it was so bad that he couldn't sleep properly, and the only way he could get himself in the mood to go to work was to eat junk food.

After about a year of this, he went back to his doctor. The doctor asked David a few questions, but David is a man of few words who was brought up to grin and bear it. He didn't really explain why he was gaining weight or convey how much pain he was suffering. The doctor was too busy to try to get David to talk more and wasn't sure whether, like many other people he sees, David was faking it to get off work. The doctor said that his pain was due to normal wear and tear for people who had done manual labor their whole lives; there wasn't much he could do other than prescribe co-codamol, which he did. (Co-codamol pills contain acetaminophen and codeine, which is a kind of morphine.)

David left the office feeling down. He had hoped that the doctor could make things better, but it seemed that his problem was unavoidable wear and tear. If the doctor had bothered to question him a bit more, and if David was more inclined to share his feelings, he almost certainly would have diagnosed him with mild depression. Despite feeling down, David took the co-codamol regularly and his decline slowed but didn't stop. It got to the point where he could barely stand up straight and shuffled when he walked. He couldn't afford to quit his job because he had to build up his pension before retiring.

His wife and children told him repeatedly to go see the doctor again, but he just wanted to rest when he wasn't working. He had a bad hernia too, but didn't mention it to the doctor.

David's wife was frustrated that he wouldn't get off the sofa and call the doctor, so she called their eldest son, Melvyn, to help. Melvyn is a charming building contractor who runs his own company, and he convinced his Dad to make an appointment and urged him to tell the doctor the truth about how much pain he was in. David complied and called the doctor's office to book an appointment. It was during the pandemic, so there were no face-to-face appointments, and he missed the first call. The doctor's office said they would call back later that afternoon, but by the time they did, David was at work. They didn't make any plans to set up a new appointment. This cat-and-mouse game went on until the doctor finally reached David on the phone. The doctor listened for a few minutes, then gave him a prescription for a higher dose of co-codamol.

In the meantime, Melvyn was getting frustrated. He had been looking up the side effects of co-codamol and learned some scary facts. Some people get hooked, and some of those who get hooked overdose and die. Apparently, it happens to more 136 people in the United States every day. Melvyn went to see David and watched over him as he called the doctor several times and insisted on a face-to-face appointment.

The next day, he drove David to the doctor's office. When they arrived, they went to the receptionist who sat behind what looked like bullet-proof glass that had a sign saying, "Abuse will not be tolerated." It took a while to get the receptionist's attention, and when they did, she told them to have a seat.

"Do you know how long it will be?" Melvyn asked.

"We can't tell, sir; please sit down," the receptionist answered, without looking at him.

They went to sit down in a crowded waiting room. Something didn't smell quite right. The waiting room was dirty and had marks on the floor. The walls were plastered with posters with scary pictures of germs warning people about the flu and what happens if you don't wash your hands. A sign on the wall read, "Only one problem discussed per visit." Melvyn was hoping to ask about his father's back pain as well as the knees, but he decided not to because of the sign. Eventually they were ushered by a nurse into an office. They sat down and eventually a doctor came in. The doctor sat down and had a friendly face but was visibly preoccupied, probably because he had too many patients to see. Melvyn asked David to walk across the room. Seeing David shuffle, the doctor immediately ordered a back, hip, and knee scan. Exceptionally, because someone had dropped out, they were able to do the scan later on the same day.

The next day, David agreed to hand over power of attorney to Melvyn so that Melvyn could follow up. Melvyn called to get the scan results. Things were worse than the doctor expected. Not only had three vertebrae in David's spine degenerated so badly that he needed back surgery, but his hips and knees were worn out to the point where they needed replacing too. The most urgent concern was the back, so the doctor urged him to call an orthopedic surgeon. The surgeon confirmed that David needed the surgery. The problem was that he was overweight and that they couldn't do the surgery until he lost at least thirty pounds. David couldn't even be put on the waiting list (which, because of the surgeon's backlog, was currently at least 18 months long) until he lost the weight.

Melvyn tried to get David to eat less and do more exercise, and David tried. He stopped eating chocolate at night and tried to walk a bit more, but it hurt too much. David managed to lose about a pound every two weeks, but then Christmas came, and he gained it all back. His pain got worse, and it looked like he was never going to get the back surgery. Melvyn was worried that David would die of opioid dependence or injure himself badly at work.

Then something lucky happened. Melvyn was watching a football game on TV one Saturday night. At half-time the channel played a clip from a documentary about the quarterback for the Minnesota Vikings and his father. The quarterback's dad seemed to be a carbon copy of David: about the same age, didn't talk much, and was in excruciating back pain. The quarterback was so eager to help his father that he had set up a charity called "Helping Dad." It included a clinic where people like David could go to get proper care. They showed some clips of the clinic; it looked a bit too New Age for Melvyn. He didn't think David would go for it. But they said they were looking for volunteers to try the clinic as part of a pilot program to test whether the care they gave was cost-effective. The program was sponsored by an insurance company and promoted by the Vikings' quarterback. Melvyn looked up the website immediately and applied on David's behalf. As part of the application, they needed to send a picture, so Melvyn looked through his photographs of David, and found a recent one that showed him out of shape. He also accidentally came across a fifty-year-old picture of David at a Vikings game. David was a Vikings fan and went to games whenever he could afford a ticket. Melvyn included both pictures in the application, hoping that it would catch their attention.

It worked. A few days later, a representative called Melvyn to say that David had won a place at the new clinic. Melvyn was elated and called David. As Melvyn suspected, it all sounded a bit too New Age for David. But Melvyn insisted and drove him to the first appointment.

The first thing Melvyn noted at Helping Dad was parking. He had been to clinics and hospitals for the birth of his three children, and parking always seemed to be a drama. The parking lots were always full, or you had to park far away, and you never knew if you needed coins, a card, or an app to pay; more often than not, the machine turned out to be broken.

This parking lot was convenient and free. Melvyn and David went in and were greeted by a very friendly receptionist at a desk with no bullet-proof glass. She smiled and politely asked them to take a seat in the waiting room. The waiting room was clean, smelled nice, and there was even some pleasant classical music in the background playing at just the right volume. A minute after they sat down, an elderly woman approached them. She didn't have a uniform but wore a large official-looking name tag with her name (Mary) on it. She asked them whether they would like a cup of tea, coffee, or some water, and a cookie or some fruit. They said thank you and asked Mary for coffee, which she brought a few minutes later.

Melvyn and David both felt relaxed and started talking about the fishing trips they used to take when Melvyn was a kid. They were pleasantly interrupted by a friendly nurse who came into the room to say that the surgeon was waiting for them. On the way to the office, they passed a cleaner who smiled and said hello. They went to the office, and the surgeon greeted them with a beaming smile.

"Hi, I'm Michael," he said, shaking their hands firmly. He looked at David and said, "You're a brave man sticking it out at work while being in all that pain."

David looked down. "Yeah, it's been tough," he said.

"Well, you've got a complex case that's hard to fix. I won't promise miracles, but we are going to do our best to make things better."

Michael then looked at Melvyn.

"You're David's son?"

"Yes," Melvyn answered.

Michael looked at David. "You must be proud to have such a caring son."

David smiled. In truth, one of the reasons his body was in such bad shape is that he had spent more than three decades doing manual labor, usually seven days a week, in order to be able to give Melvyn and his other two children what they needed. He didn't expect anything in return, but it felt good to have it noticed.

Then, somehow, Michael got David to talk about his pain and suffering. About how much he would like to run after his grandchildren again. Melvyn couldn't remember the last time he had heard his dad speak that much. The surgeon was obviously trained in communication skills as well as fixing backs. Then the surgeon raised the tough topic of David's obesity.

"David, we're going to have to discuss your weight now. If it was easy, nobody would be overweight. I'm going to give you some advice and even support. But I can't actually lose the weight for you. You'll have to do that yourself. You need to be the quarterback here. It's no good me blocking and setting passing lanes for you if you don't throw the ball. I don't need you to be perfect, but we're not going anywhere if you don't take charge. How does that sound?"

David nodded, "Understood," he said.

The surgeon then set him up with a health coach who they went to see right away. The health coach spoke with David to find out how much he knew and what kind of things would help. He recommended eating more fruits and vegetables, and not eating for a few hours before bedtime, and smaller portions. He also recommended a multivitamin. The health coach was open about the fact that there was only weak evidence that multivitamins worked. He said, "The science suggests that the vitamin D in these multivitamins might have a beneficial effect. Even though I'm not 100% sure. I still want you to take them because they can act as a kind of reminder. Whenever you take them, I want you to think of the other things I've said. So when you're taking the pill, you're reminding yourself of the benefits of this program we're setting up for you."

Finally, the health coach recommended aqua aerobics. He even gave David a *prescription* for aqua aerobics. The prescription was signed by

Michael and included the words "I'll see you there," which seemed a bit odd to David and Melvyn. They weren't sure whether to take it literally. The coach then arranged a subsidized membership to the fitness club. This was easy because it was owned by the insurance company that partnered with Helping Dad.

To David's surprise, when David showed up to the aqua aerobics, the surgeon was there too!

David started losing two pounds per week and took less co-codamol. He followed most of the health coach's other small tips as well—making sure that he didn't eat right before going to bed. That helped him sleep better. When he slept better, he felt more energized to do a bit more exercise and had more willpower to avoid chocolate. He started losing two and a half pounds per week and was feeling better than he had in years. Within three months, his weight was low enough to have the back surgery.

They made an appointment for the back surgery, and scheduled it for the next month. Two weeks before the surgery, the surgeon and coach met with David for a talk. They asked him what he hoped to be able to do after the surgery, and they told him what he could optimistically expect. They made a specific plan that David agreed to follow after the surgery in order to speed up the recovery. The plan included developing realistic yet positive expectations, as well as exercises to follow. Eventually, the plan was to get him off co-codamol altogether. To help with this, they recommended enrolling him in a trial that would involve replacing some of the co-codamol with placebo tablets from time to time without him knowing which pills were the real co-codamol and which were the placebos. David knew what placebos were but didn't understand how they could work. "If I get in that trial and don't like it, can I get off the placebos and on to real co-codamol?" He asked.

"Of course," they replied.

"Okay, why not; sign me up," David said.

Then they explained the risks of surgery, including serious ones, as well as the benefits, to make sure David still wanted to go ahead with it. They also offered David the option of minimally invasive scoping surgery, which they explained in great detail. They took time to answer his questions. David opted for minimally invasive scoping surgery.

The surgery went well, and David followed the post-surgical follow-up program. Within four weeks he was back at work part-time. Within six weeks he was completely off co-codamol. He continued exercising and maintained his lower weight. He looked and felt 10 years younger. More importantly to him, he was able to chase after his grandkids and even teach them to throw a football. Whereas he had loathed going to work for a few years, he now remembered the things he liked about it, especially the contact with his colleagues. He was even considering staying on after his official retirement date to make a bit of extra cash so that he could take his wife on a nice holiday. This was a dramatic shift. Before the experience with Helping Dad, working beyond retirement would have been unthinkable.

Melvyn was happy about David's progress. He was also curious about something. His experience with business made him certain that Helping Dad was losing money. It must be expensive to have clean waiting rooms, pay the people serving tea and coffee, so much time with the surgeon, the health coach, the subsidized gym memberships, and so on. He took advantage of the fact that David was part of a trial and that he had power of attorney to make an appointment with one of the Helping Dad senior administrators to ask some questions.

"Lose money?" asked the administrator, smiling. "No! Sure, some of those things cost money. But look at what is saved. Just losing the weight and exercising means that your dad is less likely to need a hip replacement. Even better, economic models suggest that people going through the Helping Dad program keep working longer. That means paying more taxes. Compared with similar people who don't go through our program, ours are less likely to need follow-up care, and are more likely to get back to work and pay taxes. So the government actually saves money, and based on this they've given us an incentive called a social impact bond. If we can show that we have good outcomes—if the people we care for get better—they keep paying us, and they say it saves them money."

"That seems a bit like communism to me, with the government paying," said Melvyn.

"I hear people say that, but it's the other way around. The government spends *less* money on health care because the side effects of the Helping Dad program are positive. Our patients have fewer mental health problems, fewer hospital admissions, and they stay working (and paying taxes) longer. Also, as you saw with your own dad, our system gets people to take individual responsibility for their health. Sure, we support them to take responsibility, but we don't do it for them. In fact, we have as much support from those on the political right as we do from those on the left. Those on the left see it as taking care of people, and those on the right see that we are encouraging personal responsibility and saving the state money.

"There are two other benefits that those on the right love. The first is that we are very thin on management. We don't believe in micromanaging, especially smart doctors who have spent 10 years studying. They're smart and they know that the success of Helping Dad depends on positive outcomes, so they are intrinsically motivated. Because we can't afford the complex and often crippling bureaucracy, we make sure that our systems are the most efficient. When we looked into this initially, we found that some systems for managing data take ten times longer than ours.

"The second is that we do our own research to find out which treatments are the best. Apparently, a lot of other health care providers make decisions based on whether a new treatment is better than a placebo. That doesn't tell most of our patients what they want to know. Most of our patients and doctors want to know what the best treatment is, from among all the available alternatives. People on the right love this because there is sometimes a winner, and the losing treatment doesn't get prescribed. To them, it's more like a capitalist market."

Melvyn was still curious. "Okay, but what about the people serving tea and coffee in the waiting room?" Melvyn asked. "I know from my own business that staff costs are huge."

"You mean Mary and her friends?" The administrator laughed, "They're volunteers. Most of them live alone, so their work here can be the highlight of their week. Volunteer work and helping others has a proven health benefit to the volunteer, all while helping others. It's the ultimate win-win."

Melvyn was still skeptical about one thing that he was sure the administrator wouldn't be able answer adequately. "But you are so nice to people and take so much time with them. You must have some lonely people who just come here to talk to you guys. They might even pretend they are sick just to get the cup of tea from Mary and have a short chat with the surgeon."

The administrator's answer surprised him. "Yes, we get that kind of patient from time to time, and we do our best to get them integrated into other social networks through volunteering—sometimes volunteering here. I admit that it doesn't always work, and we do have some patients who come here to socialize. The funny thing is that our economic modeling showed that it still saves money. If they didn't come to us for a friendly chat from time to time, many of them might deteriorate to the point where they need to be admitted to a mental health institution or the hospital for something more serious.

"One more thing that you haven't mentioned," the administrator added, "our rates of malpractice lawsuits and complaints are much lower, and our staff is much less likely to fall ill or burn out. It seems that patients are less eager to sue if they see that we are doing our very best and that we truly care about them. This saves us even more money. I'm not saying that we don't make mistakes, but the fact that our doctors are happy reduces the chances they make mistakes. Unsurprisingly, burnout and stress increase the chances of making mistakes."

Putting the Research from This Book into Practice: A Concise Blueprint

With the exception of the Helping Dad program (which is fictional), most of David's story is true, with details changed to preserve the patient's anonymity. The Helping Dad system is much (not all) of the research described in this book put into practice. It focuses on back pain because the condition is common and costly (more on that below). However, the same principles can be adapted for all but the rarest of health care consultations.

The components of the Helping Dad system are included in the book. They include enhanced communication training and improved health care space design (chapter 3), ethical placebos (chapter 9), avoiding negative communication (chapters 3 and 6), avoiding placebo-controlled trials to find the best treatments (chapters 4 and 10), and leveraging the power of placebo in surgery (chapter 11). The evidence-based need to design health-enhancing spaces has been established. To put the latter into context, hospitals are being built each year often at a cost exceeding $100 million each in the United States. Failure to build them in a way that promotes healing seems nonsensical.

The first impression of the Helping Dad program is that it is utopian. Some will be prepared to admit that it would be great, but object that we simply can't afford it. This is a mistake for two reasons. First of all, nobody has shown directly that the additional cost of the system exceeds its benefits. Moreover, there is a great deal of *indirect* evidence to show that it is highly cost-effective. Our recent overview of the cost-effectiveness of empathic care suggests that programs like Helping Dad could be highly cost-effective.[1] To see how this can be, look at back pain, which is the main problem in Helping Dad (although the principles here apply to many other ailments as well). Back pain affects over 10% of the world's population,[2] and back pain alone is the seventh greatest cause of reduction in disability adjusted life years worldwide.[3-5] In the United States, treating back pain costs an estimated $300 billion annually, with the cost rising to over $500 billion if we include loss of productivity.[6] This is 30% higher than the combined cost of treating cancer and diabetes. In the United Kingdom, treating back pain costs the National Health Services (NHS) over a billion pounds per year, and if lost productivity is taken into account, the amount increases to between £5 and 10 billion.[7] Other European countries show a similar trend,[6, 8-10] and the global prevalence and cost of low back pain is on the rise. Worldwide, back pain rose from the twelfth to the seventh most prevalent cause of morbidity between 1990 and 2010.[4] In about 15% of cases the cause of back pain is a fracture or an infection. In the remaining (85%-95%) of cases the cause of back pain is not clear,[11,12] and could be helped by the Helping Dad system. If we could reduce the cost of treating low back pain by just 10% in the US, it would save $30 billion, which is enough to pay half a million health coaches $60,000 per year to treat 300 million people twice per month. Even a 1% cost reduction would save $3 billion per year. Then, all the evidence suggests that programs like Helping Dad have additional benefits that I have listed below.

For patients, it reduces

- anxiety
- morphine use
- risk of opioid dependence
- length of stay in hospital
- function following surgery (and ability to return to work)

For practitioners, it reduces

- burnout
- stress
- risk of leaving profession

The clear benefits and likelihood that it's cost-effective raise the question: why isn't it done? At least part of the answer is that the way most doctors are paid prevents systems from being implemented that would help patients like David while saving money.

Ethics and Justice: Aligning Interests of Doctors and Payers

Doctors in ancient China, according to some accounts, were paid a monthly fee. But the fee would be withheld if the patient fell ill.[13] This system made it directly in the doctors' financial interest to keep the patients healthy. The practice recalls Hammurabi's four-thousand-year-old code "an eye for an eye, a tooth for a tooth," which has gained prominence recently through the work of Nassim Taleb, who calls it "skin in the game."[14]

While it is an overgeneralization, most doctors' pay is not linked directly to patient outcomes. Instead, doctors get paid for *processes* (how many tests and treatments they give). For the most part, the more patients they treat and the more tests and treatments they give, the more they get paid. This is called the "fee for service" model. Even in countries with nationalized health care like the United Kingdom and Australia, doctors are usually paid more for seeing more patients, and are given targets for prescribing certain tests and treatments.[15] The processes and targets are designed to improve patient outcomes, and they often do. Yet, they remain one step removed from actual *outcomes*. Also, because they incentivize quantity, they disincentivize spending more time with patients (the way they do in Helping Dad). This means that if most doctors spent more time with patients (which can help) they risk earning less and even bankrupcy. Very few people will volunteer to earn less money and risk bankruptcy. I doubt I would. Because of this, the system described in Helping Dad is blocked by the fee-for-service model. Squeezing more and more patients into the schedule also adds stress and paperwork for doctors, and contributes to the astronomical levels of burnout in the profession.

Fortunately, systems related to the ancient Chinese system are reemerging now as "value-based health care" whereby "providers are rewarded for helping patients improve their health, reduce the effects and incidence of chronic disease, and live healthier lives in an evidence-based way."[16] The problem is that the term "value-based health care" has too many meanings, so I prefer the term "skin-in-the-game health care." Below I will describe the emerging system in brief.

As in the Helping Dad example, achieving skin-in-the-game health care requires coordination between doctors, surgeons, health coaches, research units, and other staff. Health care practitioners are already supposed to do this in the form of what is called interprofessionalism. The problem (according to its proponents) is that interprofessionalism is not taught or implemented as much as it should be.[17] Skin-in-the-game health care would energize existing interprofessionalism and give the idea more real power to coordinate the different parts of the health care system for the good of patients. Another barrier to skin-in-the-game health care is that it involves spending money upfront and waiting for the good patient outcomes to emerge. This requires moving beyond short-term thinking, which can be challenging.[16] Despite the obstacles, skin-in-the-game health care is making inroads in the United States through accountable care organizations,[18] and in the United Kingdom and Europe with social-impact bonds.[19]

The challenges and short-term costs of skin-in-the-game health care need to be weighed with the costs of the fee-for-service model. With skin in the game, everyone in the system has an intrinsic motivation to get the patient better. With fee for service, the insurance company or government that pays the doctors needs to follow up to make sure that the doctors aren't giving unnecessary tests and treatments, and that they are giving the tests and treatments they are supposed to. This involves using bureaucratic managers to police doctors.

The problem is that managers get paid a great deal of money no matter what happens to patients. As I was writing this chapter, the NHS advertised to hire 42 new chief executives to be paid an average of £233,000 each ($322,000) per year. And that is just a drop in the ocean. There are so many managers in the NHS that a recent attempt to estimate just how many there were concluded that it was "extremely difficult to find an accurate figure for the number of managers in the NHS."[20,21] Worse, according to polls done in 2012 and 2013, between a quarter to a half of UK doctors' time is spent filling out paperwork.[22,23] If we take that into account, a major portion of the budget for paying doctors is being used for highly paid managers and doctors to do paperwork. This takes time away from treating patients. The problem seems to be worse in the United States. Data published in 2020 suggest that $812 billion, or about 34.2% of national health expenditure, is devoted to administration.[24]

The skin-in-the-game health care model could also be used to remunerate companies that make drugs, devices, and tests. Currently, these companies aren't paid based on outcomes but based on whether they follow certain processes related to getting their product approved. The processes are not bad, but once they follow the process, they get paid whether or not their product makes a difference. In some ways, they are disincentivized to make patients better because the sicker people are (or believe they are), the more they get paid. To demonstrate this, think of how much money many pharmaceutical companies would lose if people were just 10% happier, 10% slimmer, did 10% more exercise, and ate 10% more vegetables. If medical professionals were paid based on outcomes, it would incentivize them to align their profits more directly with patient health, and this includes incentivizing them to elicit placebo effects.

Medicine without Magic

The first revolution in placebo studies took placebo research from fringe into normal science. That revolution was a success and led to hundreds of studies that demonstrate placebo and nocebo effects, describe how the effects arise, and unshroud mysteries about what placebo and nocebo effects are. When considered in light of these arguments, placebo treatments are not just ethical; they are ethically required, and failure to reduce unnecessary nocebo effects is equally unethical. In parallel, the reasons for allowing placebo-controlled trials even if there is a proven therapy are bunk: we should only use placebo-controlled trials if there is no proven therapy.

What we've learned since that first revolution is that we don't need doctors to actually become shamans for patients to experience the benefits of placebo effects. We also don't need to believe in voodoo to know that nocebo effects are real. The first revolution provided incontrovertible evidence that communication, beliefs, environment, and setting, all make tangible differences to hard outcomes. The next revolution must catapult the knowledge we have about the effects of placebos and nocebos from within the walls of academia into the real world so that all patients and doctors can benefit.

The details of Adolf Grünbaum's model are best explained with the aid of figure 4.2 from the body of the chapter (see p. 75, recreated here in more detail as figure A.1.1). Beginning with the left-hand box in the diagram, we see that the therapeutic theory, ψ, differentiates between characteristic (C) and incidental (I) features. Even pill treatments that are often considered simple have several components. For example, a therapeutic theory may state that the therapy t is the administration of Prozac according to some given regime, the target disorder D being major depressive disorder. The therapeutic theory might also specify that the chemical fluoxetine hydrochloride is the "characteristic feature," C, of this therapy. The incidental features, I, of the therapy might include pill bulking agents, the potential disruption to the patient's life (they must take time every day to consume the pills), ingredients in the pill casing, the liquid with which the pills are swallowed, and perhaps most importantly expectations about the potential effects of fluoxetine hydrochloride and the patient/doctor interaction.

The four arrows in figure 4.2 represent *possible* effects. The top horizontal arrow represents the possible effect of the characteristic factors C on the target disorder D. The arrow that runs from the upper left to the lower right represents the possible side effects of the characteristic factors. The lower horizontal arrow represents potential effects of the incidental factors I on other things (not the target disorder), while the arrow from the bottom left to the upper right represents possible effects of the incidental factors I on the target disorder D. The four arrows of possible causal influences can be positive, negative, or, in some cases "empty": that is, they represent no effects at all. Henceforth when speaking about effects of features (both incidental and characteristic), I am referring to *possible* effects unless otherwise specified.

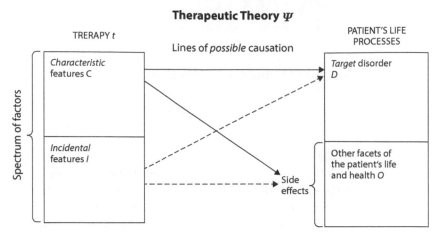

Therapeutic Theory ψ

TRERAPY *t*

Lines of *possible* causation

PATIENT'S LIFE PROCESSES

Spectrum of factors

Characteristic features C

Incidental features I

Target disorder D

Side effects

Other facets of the patient's life and health O

FIG. A1.1. Illustration of therapeutic theory ψ, used in clarifying the definition of "placebo" Based on Grünbaum A. The placebo concept in medicine and psychiatry. *Psychol Med.* Feb 1986;16(1):22. https://doi.org/10.1017/s0033291700002506.

Grünbaum appeals to the ideas in the figure to define placebos and related terms.

> *Nonplacebo.* A treatment process t is a nonplacebo for target disease D "if (and only if) one or more of the characteristic factors do have a positive therapeutic effect on the target disease D."[1]

The key feature of a nonplacebo is that its characteristic features must have a *positive* therapeutic effect on the target disorder *D*. The administration of Prozac therapy would thus be characterized as a nonplacebo for depression if and only if fluoxetine hydrochloride had some *positive* therapeutic effect for depression. Grünbaum then proceeds on this basis to characterize the notion of placebos and related terms:

> *Generic placebo.* A treatment process t is a generic placebo if none of the characteristic treatment factors C are remedial for D. Generic placebos come in two types: intentional and inadvertent.
>
> *Intentional placebo.* A treatment process t is an *intentional placebo* if and only if it satisfies the following four conditions—the fourth normally holding but, strictly speaking, being optional:
> - t is a generic placebo
> - the practitioner believes that the characteristic factors C all fail to be remedial for D (the practitioner believes that t is a generic placebo)

- the practitioner believes that some patients will benefit from the treatment due to one or more of its incidental features
- [optional] the practitioner "abets," or at least acquiesces in, [the patient's] belief that *t* has remedial efficacy for *D* by virtue of some constituents that belong to the set of characteristic factors [*C*]

Inadvertent placebo. A treatment process *t* is an *inadvertent* placebo if and only if it satisfies the first two of the following three conditions—the third normally holding but, strictly speaking, being optional:
- *t* is a generic placebo
- the practitioner believes that some of the characteristic features *C* are remedial for *D*
- [optional] the patient believes that the remedial effects on *D* are due to some characteristic feature of the treatment *t*.

Placebo effect. A placebo effect is either (a) one produced by the incidental features of some treatment (even when the treatment as a whole is a nonplacebo), or (b) any effect of a generic placebo. In Grünbaum's words: "a placebo control is an intentional generic placebo that is generally harmless."

Grünbaum's outline solves many of the problems with previous attempts at defining the placebo. His model allows for placebos to be active and have specific effects, provided that characteristic features do not cause these effects. It also allows for psychological factors to be both placebic and nonplacebic (depending on the therapeutic theory). However, Grünbaum solves the previous problems only to introduce a number of problems in his own model, some of which have been noted by critics such as John Greenwood[2] and Duff Waring.[5]

Failure to Define Therapeutic Theories

Grünbaum then makes a more murky claim that what counts as a placebo control is relative to a therapeutic theory. As others have noticed,[2–4] he fails to specify what a therapeutic theory is. Insofar as he does specify it, he does not put any restrictions on it, which takes us back to Asbjørn Hróbjartsson and Peter Gøtzsche's "anything goes" problem (more on this below). Reading between the lines charitably, a therapeutic theory has two features: First, it explains how an intervention works. Second, it tells us which features of a treatment are "characteristic" and which are "incidental." According to Grünbaum, a placebo *effect* is the effect of a placebo treatment process or the effect of an incidental feature.

To be sure, sometimes it is so obvious that it might seem artificial to talk about a theory at all. To take an example that Grünbaum cites, the "theory" underwriting accepted treatment for gallstones will make the surgical removal of the gallstones the characteristic feature. Other features such as the surgical consultation, the analgesia, and so on, would be classified as incidental. But in the psychotherapeutic and other fields, the dependence on theory is often crucial. There, which aspects of a particular interaction with a patient are characteristic will clearly be theory-dependent so that one and the same feature of a given interaction may be judged characteristic by one theory and incidental by another. For instance, according to Sigmund Freud, the characteristic features of his talking therapies included lifting a patient's presumed repressions, while the incidental features included the patient's faith in the analyst, emotional support from an authority figure, and the payment of a hefty fee.[1] Yet more pragmatic forms of talking therapies, such as cognitive behavioral therapy (CBT), do not regard these as characteristic.

The philosopher of science John Greenwood argues that because Grünbaum does not define therapeutic theories, his model has the absurd consequence of allowing pharmacologically active substances to be regarded as placebic.[2] It's hard to decipher what Greenwood means by this because he doesn't provide a real example to illustrate the apparently unhappy consequences of Grünbaum's model. (Aside: the failure of many philosophers of science to provide credible examples contributes to making them generally irrelevant to actual science.) Charitably, he might have in mind a case such as the following. Imagine that some treatment for bacterial pneumonia had the following treatment features:

a. the pill casing
b. a bulking agent
c. water with which the pills are swallowed
d. patient/doctor expectations
e. antibiotics

Imagine further that the therapeutic theory classified d and e as incidental while a, b, and c were classified as characteristic. Grünbaum's model would refer to this treatment as a "placebo" for treating pneumonia, and this would be a misuse of language.

But Greenwood's objection doesn't hold water. Classifying antibiotics as incidental would be a mistake that, if made, would subsequently be corrected. The fact that we have to revise our classification of features as incidental or characteristic is not a problem with Grünbaum's model but a consequence of the fact that *all* scientific theories are tentative and revisable in light of (hopefully reliable) new insights and evidence. Grünbaum explicitly acknowledged this: "if some of the incidental constituents of *t* are remedial but presently elude the grasp of ψ, the current inability of ψ to pick them out from the treatment process hardly lessens the objective specificity of their identity, mode of action, or efficacy."[1] In short, Greenwood's objection seems nitpicky and fails to take into account what Grünbaum actually said.

Failure to Provide Defining Features of Characteristic and Incidental Features

Related to the problem of failing to define therapeutic theories, Grünbaum does not tell us what the defining features of characteristic or incidental features are. To illustrate why this is a cause for concern, reconsider an example Grünbaum cites about surgery for the removal of gallstones. Recall that the "theory" underwriting accepted treatment for gallstones will define the surgical removal of the gallstones as characteristic. Other features, such as the surgical consultation, the analgesia, and so on, would be classified as incidental. But calling analgesia placebic does not reflect any etymological or current usage. It is not used to please the patient (except in a roundabout way), and it has an independent effect (albeit not always on the target disorder).

There are two ways to respond to this problem. The first is to say that analgesia is a characteristic feature. The problem with this solution is that analgesia does not have an effect on the target disorder, and indeed surgery was performed before the invention of modern analgesia. A defender of Grünbaum might insist that analgesia was placebic *relative* to surgery. However, that leads to a tangled way of thinking whereby placebos can be fatal (the "placebo" analgesia carries a small but statistically predictable risk of death). The second is to divide incidental features into placebic and nonplacebic. If a control treatment contains both placebic and nonplacebic incidental features, then one should not call it a placebo control. Instead, it is an intervention that (aims to) control for all but certain characteristic features such as surgical removal of gallstones. Such a control treatment simply needs to contain everything but the other elements of the experimental intervention. Placebo controls are a subset of these control treatments, namely, those whereby the incidental features are placebic. The third option—the one I prefer and that I defend in more detail in chapter 11—is that so-called placebo surgery is not really a placebo. Rather, it is a treatment that controls for some but not all aspects of (active) surgery.

It is also quite easy to provide a definition of characteristic features: they are features, such as lactose for the common cold, that would not have an independent effect on the target disorder if given alone.

Allowing Harmful Interventions to Count as Placebos

According to some critics (including myself in my previous writing on this topic), Grünbaum allows harmful interventions to be classified as placebos. The only distinguishing feature of placebos, according to Grünbaum's formal definition, is that they do not contain any characteristic features that have *positive* effects on the target disorder. This makes treatments whose characteristic features have *negative* effects on the target disorder generic placebos. This is at odds with ordinary usage. Imagine a therapeutic theory that classified deep scratching of the skin as the only characteristic feature in a treatment for hemophilia. This treatment would be classified as a placebo for treating hemophilia according to Grünbaum's model. Similarly, treatments whose characteristic features have no effects on the target disorder but that have negative effects on other life processes are classified as placebos. This implies that, for example, therapy aimed at treating pain that did not do so but that caused blindness would be classified as a placebo. I think this is an unfair, nitpicky criticism of Grünbaum because in other places he is clear that placebos are generally harmless. Also, the problem is easily solved by introducing a new category of treatments—namely, "harmful intervention"—to refer to treatments whose characteristic features have harmful effects on a target disorder or other life processes. Similarly, we use the term "nocebo" (which is Latin for "I shall harm") and "nocebo effects" to refer to the negative effects of certain incidental features. To be clear, some of the negative effects of the incidental features are nocebo effects, but not all of them are. If someone has a bad tummy reaction because of the bulking agent in the pill, it is not a nocebo effect, but rather a toxic effect of the noncharacteristic features.

Failure to Relativize to Individuals

Waring accuses Grünbaum of not relativizing placebos to individuals.[5] He uses the example of drugs that elicit "paradoxical responses" to argue that Grünbaum's model can classify the very same treatment both as a placebo and as a nonplacebo. A paradoxical response is an exacerbating response on the target disorder produced by a drug that is normally remedial.[5] A paradoxical effect is more than a negative side effect. It is a negative effect on the same disorder that the treatment sometimes cures. To use a "toy," but illustrative, example: swimming might be a wonderful treatment for rehabilitation or general well-being *but only for those patients who know how to swim.* Swimming could lead to death by drowning, a clear exacerbation of well-being, for non-swimmers. Whether Prozac is an antidepressant, whether swimming improves health, and (more generally) whether a treatment is a placebo is relative to the patient. Paradoxical responses, he argues, highlight an apparent contradiction in Grünbaum's model. Waring contends that calling paradoxical effects "placebic" is a "misuse of language."[5]

Waring's critique betrays a superficial reading. The existence of paradoxical responses does not point to a contradiction in Grünbaum's model any more than it points to a contradiction in saying that swimming is good for rehabilitation, even though it leads to drowning for those who cannot swim. In fact, Waring's point is well known in pharmacology, with Manfred Hauben and Jeffrey Aronson having identified at least 60 drugs with paradoxical effects.[6] A careful reading of Grünbaum indicates that he presumed what counts as a placebo should be relativized to patients. When describing intentional placebos, he makes explicit reference to particular "victims": "Both explications are *relativized to disease victims of a specifiable sort*, as well as to therapists (practitioners) of certain kinds" (emphasis added).[1] I also believe that Grünbaum's explicit relativization to a target disorder implies relativization to individuals, since individuals have the disorder. In short, Waring's objection is another nitpicky one that doesn't hold water in the context of Grünbaum's entire paper.

Waring and Greenwood's Insistence on Expectancy and Therapeutic Relationships as Placebo Controls

Both Waring and Greenwood propose that the definition of placebo controls be tied more closely to expectancy and the patient/doctor relationship. For example, Waring states: "psychological factors such as a patient's expectations of benefit seem closer to what we intend by the placebo concept rather than remedial failure."[5] Greenwood states: "we [might] have an instance of a placebo effect, according to Grünbaum's definition, *even though no part of the effect is produced by psychological factors such as therapist/doctor commitment or client/patient expectancy.*"[2]

Waring and Greenwood are correct that expectancy and client/patient relationships are important as part of the context (see chapter 2). However, we must interpret their proposal very charitably for it to be acceptable. If their objection is interpreted as an argument that all psychological factors are placebos, this implies classifying all psychological therapy as placebic a priori which is a mistake. Their objection also presupposes an unfortunate and mistaken distinction between psychological and physiological. The charitable interpretation is that placebos must include features such as doctor commitment or patient expectancy, which is acceptable.

The idea is that expectations and practitioner commitment capture the intuition that many people have about placebos. It is also arguably justified etymologically. Grünbaum himself accepted this view: "Turning now to placebo controls, we must bear in mind that to assess the remedial merits of a given therapy t* for some [disorder] D, it is imperative to disentangle . . . improvements produced by the expectations aroused in both the doctor and the patient by their belief in the therapeutic efficacy of t*." Still, Grünbaum does not mention this explicitly in his definitional model.

Yet controlling for expectancy is neither necessary nor sufficient for an intervention to count as a placebo control. For example, it is not necessary for treating unconscious patients who are given injections. An unconscious patient has no (conscious) expectations by definition, so expectations do not need to be controlled for. (Note that it is nonetheless important to use a control treatment [placebo or not] in trials of unconscious patients to control for [unconscious] conditioning or learning effects, and the effects of unblinded practitioner enthusiasm; more on this in chapter 5).

Here's why controlling for expectations is not sufficient: One might control for expectations in a trial of invasive versus sham surgery, but unless one also controls for the effects of analgesia, it will not be an adequate control for the characteristic feature of the surgery.

Also—and this point helps answer the objection that all forms of talking therapy are placebos—not all expectancy is placebic, which means that controlling for expectancy is not necessary. To see why, consider the example of "positive psychology." The theory behind positive psychology is that patients should focus on the positive aspects of their lives. This encourages them to have more positive expectations. Positive psychology therapists provide patients with cognitive tools that help them change negative thoughts and expectations into positive ones. For purposes of this argument, assume that positive psychology's therapeutic theory classifies positive expectations about recovery arising as a result of a positive psychology consultation as the only characteristic feature and all other treatment features as incidental. Now imagine that positive psychology became very popular, with beautiful Hollywood stars using and endorsing it. Positive psychology's popularity could (again, at least in principle) lead to patients having positive expectations about the effectiveness of positive psychology before even having a positive psychology session. These positive expectations could lead to some benefit independent of the positive psychology session itself. On the other hand, a qualified positive psychology therapist might induce a further benefit for the patient by providing a strategy that helps them modify their thought pattern. That is, there are two potential sources of expectations that could be responsible for effectiveness of a positive psychology session: (1) expectations that positive psychology is effective (arising from, for example, Hollywood hype), and (2) expectations generated in the patient by the positive psychology therapy (arising from the remarks of a qualified positive psychology therapist).

A real example from my experience will help clarify the difference between the two types of expectation. When I was an athlete, I lost a hard-fought race and I wanted to win the next one. To achieve my goal, I had to improve my ability to focus. I called my first coach, whose name is Scott. Now Scott is a great coach, and I had positive expectations that my focus would improve after talking to him. These positive expectations arose before I spoke to him and were therefore independent of anything he actually said. They were analogous to the Hollywood hype in the positive psychology example. These expectations could, at least in principle, have led to an improved focus regardless of what he said and would legitimately be classified as placebo expectations. However, in addition to the positive expectations that arose at the mere thought of speaking to Scott, he gave me some cognitive tools that helped me develop positive expectations about potentially negative situations. The one I remember most is that whenever something negative happened, he would remind me to tell myself that "adversity is an opportunity." He then gave me examples of great athletes who used setbacks to regroup and come back stronger than ever. I used these cognitive strategies (telling myself that adversity is an opportunity and recalling real cases of great athletes who had been through hard times and succeeded) to turn my negative expectations about the future into positive ones. These latter expectations that were induced by a specific cognitive tool—perhaps similar to those used by positive psychology therapists—were independent, at least in principle, from expectations I had about the benefits of interacting with him.

Since the expectations generated by Hollywood hype surrounding positive psychology are placebic, they need to be controlled for. If the expectations induced by the positive psychology therapist during a positive psychology therapy session do not have any incremental benefits over and above the expectations that positive psychology is an effective method (Hollywood hype), then any benefits of positive psychology are not due to "characteristic features" of positive psychology, but due to the expectations patients have about the effectiveness of positive psychology, and positive psychology can safely be classified as a placebo.

If positive psychology effects were only due to Hollywood hype, one could replace an actual positive psychology session with a "sham" positive psychology session and have the same results. In fact, this is not the case. In one study, five positive psychology interventions designed to induce positive expectations (showing gratitude, listing three good things in life, identifying a time when the patient did their best, identifying strengths, and using strengths in a new way) were compared with a "placebo" control that involved writing about early memories.[7] The patients were blinded to the treatment condition, so expectations *that* positive psychology therapy was effective were the same in both groups. A systematic review including this and 38 additional randomized trials of positive psychology found that positive psychology outperformed the sham positive psychology. [8] The systematic review reported that positive psychology had a statistically significant overall effect for subjective well-being (standardized mean difference = 0.34) as well as depression (standardized mean difference = 0.23). This suggests that positive psychology therapy has an incremental benefit over and above Hollywood hype expectations and thus that it seems to contain a feature that counts as characteristic according to the criteria laid out above.

There are two ways to react to the examples illustrating that there are different types of expectations that have different sources, different effects, and possibly slightly different mechanisms. The first is to say that they are all placebos but that they all differ. In the same way that drugs come in different doses, strengths and modalities, the same might apply to placebos. On this view, expectations that a treatment is effective might be a milder placebo, while positive psychology might be a more powerful or more complex "super"-placebo. However, unlike different doses of the same drug, the two types of expectations I have described above are different in kind. To see this, consider the simple positive psychology technique of writing a letter of gratitude. A person might do so in different contexts.

They might visit a positive psychologist who ends up prescribing it as part of a treatment process. Or, a spontaneous thought might arise for them to write a letter to a family member in which they say thank you for something. In the latter case, where the idea and act of writing a letter of gratitude arises independently of its administration or prescription by a therapist, we might still expect the person to feel better. [9] When combined with administration by a positive psychologist, the technique might generate greater benefits. But it is reasonable to anticipate an improvement in mood independent of the treatment process. As such, positive psychology techniques like writing letters of gratitude involve characteristic features. Therefore, they are neither incidental nor placebic.

The arguments I have made about expectations also partly apply to therapist/doctor commitment, which was the other feature of Waring and Greenwood's proposal. There are different ways to cash out therapist/doctor commitment, including empathic care. Empathic care and other features of therapist/doctor commitment are not placebos, as I argued in chapter 2.

To recap this discussion of the philosophy of placebo controls, Grünbaum's model has advantages (its emphasis that placebos are complex treatments, and relativization), but fails because it does not define therapeutic theories or characteristic features. Waring and Greenwood's proposal to include expectancy and patient/doctor relationship as part of the placebo control is logical in a loose sense but needs to be spelled out in order to avoid pitfalls, including that it leads to classifying all forms of talking therapies as placebos. My proposal will take the advantages of Grünbaum, Waring, and Greenwood, while avoiding their pitfalls.

In short, the criticisms of Grünbaum's model generally arise from nitpicking philosophers' objections that fail to take into account the body of Grünbaum's work. At the same time, Grünbaum could have been more explicit on a number of points. I have therefore revised his model.

The Modified Version of Grünbaum's Model
The revision takes into account the problems with Grünbaum's model discussed above. It adds four lines of possible causation to the original (fig. A1.2), and introduces a definition of placebo controls that reflects Grünbaum's intentions.

Nonplacebo. A treatment process *t* is a nonplacebo for target disease *D*, therapeutic theory ψ, and patients *X* if (and only if) one or more of the characteristic factors *do have a positive therapeutic effect on the target disease D.*

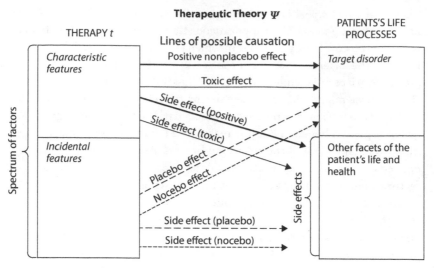

FIG. A1.2. A revised version of Grünbaum's model

Harmful Intervention. A treatment process *t* is a harmful intervention relative to a target disorder *D*, therapeutic theory ψ, and patients *X* if and only if (a) the characteristic features *C* do not have remedial effects on *D* and the characteristic features *C* have negative effects on the target disorder *D* or other life processes *O*.

Generic Placebo (revised). A treatment process *t* is a placebo when none of the characteristic treatment factors *C* are effective (remedial or harmful) in patients *X* for *D*.

Generic Nocebo. A treatment process *t* is a generic nocebo if it is a generic placebo whose incidental effects exacerbate the target disorder *D* in patients *X* or other life processes *O*.

Intentional Placebo. A treatment process *t* is an *intentional placebo* if and only if it satisfies the following conditions:
    (a) *t* is a (revised) generic placebo (b) to (d): (unchanged from original definition)

Inadvertent Placebo (unchanged)

Placebo Effect. A placebo effect is either (a) a remedial effect produced by the incidental features of some treatment (even when the treatment as a whole is a nonplacebo), or (b) any effect of a (revised) generic placebo.

Nocebo Effect. A nocebo effect is either (a) a negative effect produced by the incidental features of some treatment (even when the treatment as a whole is a nonplacebo), or (b) any negative effect of a generic nocebo.

Placebo Control (revised). A treatment functions as an adequate placebo control when it controls for *all* the effects of the experimental treatment *other than* the remedial effects of the characteristic features of the experimental treatment on the target disorder. Under conditions of informed consent, the placebo control must also mimic the sensory appearance of the experimental treatment in order to control for the effects of expectation *that* the treatment being given is (or in the case of a double blind trial) could be the experimental treatment.* This implies that the placebo control cannot contain any characteristic features that produce effects on the target disorder.

Characteristic Feature. A characteristic feature is a feature that:
1. Is not expectation *that* a treatment is effective, and
2. Has an incremental benefit on the target disorder over a legitimate placebo control in a well-controlled trial.

Concluding Reflections on Grünbaum's Model
Mistaken definitions of placebos have led to questionable estimates of placebo effects, unjustified "placebo" control treatments, and confused debates about the ethics of placebos. Hróbjartsson and Gøtzsche's suggestion to accept any treatment labeled as a "placebo" has unwanted consequences, and Nunn and Turner's suggestion to drop the term "placebo" is only warranted if we can't define the placebo, which I argued here is not the case. My modified version of Grünbaum's model captures what we mean by placebo controls and sheds light on complex cases such as that of acupuncture "placebos" whereas other proposals leave us in the dark. Grünbaum's main insights are: (1) all treatments are complex and the features of interventions can be classified into "characteristic" and "incidental"; and (2) what counts as a placebo is *relative* to a therapeutic theory, target disorder, and patient. The main problems with Grünbaum's model are his failure to specify what he means by a therapeutic theory and his failure to specify that expectation effects are placebo effects. With four modifications, Grünbaum's definition provides a defensible

---

*Controlling for expectations is not sufficient, and in some exceptional cases—those in which the expectations in question arise from, for example, cognitive strategies taught by a therapist or coach—they are not necessary.

account of placebos for the purpose of constructing placebo controls within clinical trials. The modifications I introduce are: (1) adding a special role for expectations, (2) insisting that placebo controls control for all and only the effects of the incidental treatment features, (3) relativizing the definition of placebos to patients, and (4) introducing harmful interventions and nocebos to the definitional model. I also provide guidance for classifying treatment features as characteristic or incidental.

APPENDIX 2
Binary Outcomes May Underestimate Placebo Effects

Binary outcomes give a yes-or-no answer to whether the treatment is believed to be effective. They usually involve a certain cutoff point that separates success from failure of a treatment. Penelope Greene and colleagues (2001) describe an imaginary scenario in which binary outcomes mask real effects:

> Imagine, hypothetically, smokers randomized to two groups—placebo (perhaps a placebo nicotine patch, or a "counselling" session unrelated to conventional smoking-cessation programs) and no-treatment—so that each group has a reasonably similar distribution of "numbers of cigarettes smoked." At the conclusion of the trial, the placebo group might have a significantly lower mean number of cigarettes smoked than at baseline (perhaps as dramatically as a 50+% average reduction). However, suppose not a single person in this "im-proved" placebo group stopped smoking entirely. Assume further that the number of cigarettes smoked by the no-treatment group remained the same. Drawing conclusions using the binary outcome, comparing proportions of smokers and nonsmokers, both groups began with 100% smokers and both ended with 100% smokers. "Therefore" the placebo was no different than no-treatment at all. *Q.E.D.* However, using the continuous outcome (the mean), the placebo group was, indeed, significantly "better" than no treatment at all. *Q.E.D.* (again!).[1, p. 302]

Real trials within Asbjørn Hróbjartsson and Peter Gøtzsche's review do the same. For example, Hanns-Peter Scharf and colleagues' 2006 trial compared acupuncture with sham acupuncture and no acupuncture (but 10 physician visits).[2] They defined the success rate as at least 36% improve-ment according to the Western Ontario and McMaster Universities Osteoarthritis Index (WOMAC) score at 26 weeks. WOMAC measures pain, stiffness, and physical functioning of the joints.[3] The choice of 36% was justified by citing a 1993 study that surveyed consultants and other professionals (but not patients) and arrived at the 36%.[4] However, there is a range of definition of clinically relevant differences, with a systematic review finding studies reporting between 8% and 40% as the correct threshold for minimally important differences.[5] According to the binary outcome, there was almost no difference between sham acupuncture and (so-called) no-treatment. (For the statistics nerds, the relative risk for sham acupuncture compared with conservative therapy was 1.73, with a 95% confidence interval of 1.42 to 2.11.) In spite of existing, the effect shows up as not significant in Hróbjartsson and Gøtzsche's review.

Had they reported continuous outcomes (which are not dichotomous but can take on a range of values), the results would be easier to understand and more impressive. Fifty-one percent of those in the sham acupuncture group reported a clinically relevant benefit, compared with 29% in the "untreated" group. This is an absolute difference of 22%, which is quite large, in medical terms. Yet, the very same effect gets almost completely obscured when it is measured in dichotomous terms.

Additivity versus Interaction

A Formalization

Say we have a treatment with both placebo and treatment features, whereby $p_1, p_2, p_3, \ldots p_n$ are the placebo treatment features (empathic body language, positive language, environment, etc.). The effects of these features are $f_1(p_1) + f_2(p_2) + f_3(p_3) + \ldots f_n(p_n)$.

Placebo treatment features as a whole are P, and their effects are $F(P)$.

$t_1, t_2, t_3, \ldots t_n$ are the treatment features

$g_1(t_1) + g_2(t_2) + g_3(t_3) + \ldots g_n(t_n)$ are their effects

Treatment features as a whole are T, and their effects are $G(T)$

Interactions will be synergistic (whole greater than sum of parts) when

$$F[(p_1, p_2, p_3, \ldots p_n), (t_1, t_2, t_3, \ldots t_n)] > [[f_1(p_1) + f_2(p_2) + f_3(p_3) + \ldots f_n(p_n)] + [g_1(t_1) + g_2(t_2) + g_3(t_3) + \ldots g_n(t_n)]]$$

and when

$$H(P,T) > F(P) + G(T)$$

Interactions will be antagonistic (whole less than sum of parts) when

$$F[(p_1, p_2, p_3, \ldots p_n), (t_1, t_2, t_3, \ldots t_n)] > [[f_1(p_1) + f_2(p_2) + f_3(p_3) + \ldots f_n(p_n)] + [g_1(t_1) + g_2(t_2) + g_3(t_3) + \ldots g_n(t_n)]]$$

and when

$$H(P,T) < F(P) + G(T)$$

Table A3.1. Additivity versus interaction

	Additivity	Interaction*
Of placebo treatment features	$p_1 + p_2 + p_3 + \ldots p_n =$ $f_1(p_1) + f_2(p_2) +$ $f_3(p_3) + \ldots f_n(p_n)$	$p_1 + p_2 + p_3 + \ldots p_n =$ $F(p_1, p_2, p_3, t) \ldots p_n)$
Of placebo treatment features (as a whole) and "active" treatment features (as a whole)	$P + T = F(P) + G(T)$	$P + T = H(P,T)$

*With interactions, almost anything goes. Two inert substances can create a flammable one, and placebo treatment factors can make the overall effect larger or smaller or negate it altogether.

The balanced placebo design uses four groups (table A4.1). Both groups in the top row (A and B) are told that they are receiving the experimental treatment, but only group A receives it. Group B is told that they are receiving the active treatment but do not. Both groups in the bottom row (C and D) are told they are *not* getting the experimental treatment, but one of them (group C) gets it. In the balanced placebo design, some patients are told the truth (that they are or are not getting the experimental treatment: groups A and D) and others are deceived (group B is told that they are getting the treatment but do not get it, and group C is told they are not getting the treatment but get it).

The balanced placebo design allows us to test for interactions in three ways:

1. The placebo effect can be measured in two ways: We can subtract the outcomes in group D from the outcomes in group B (B–D), and we can subtract the effect in group C from the effect in group A (A–C). If additivity held, then B–D should be the same* as C–A. If not, then additivity does not hold.

2. The effect of actually receiving the treatment can be calculated in two ways: We can subtract B from A (A–B), and we can subtract D from C (C–D). If additivity held, then the two values, A–B and C–D, should be the same. If not, then additivity does not hold.

3. The effect in group A (of receiving the treatment and being told the treatment is received) should be the same as adding up the effect of baseline (group D) to the effect of the placebo (measured in one of the two ways listed above) and the effect of the treatment (measured in one of the two ways listed above). If not, then additivity does not hold.

*Of course, the values need not be identical for additivity to hold; they need to be similar within appropriate statistical boundaries.[1]

Table A4.1. The Balanced Placebo Design

| | RECEIVED | |
	Treatment	Placebo
TOLD — *Treatment*	A	B
TOLD — *Placebo*	C	D

Table A4.2. The Expanded Balanced Placebo Design

| | | RECEIVED | | |
		Treatment	*Placebo*	*No Treatment*
	Treatment	A	B	C
TOLD	*Treatment or placebo (blind)*	D	E	F
	Placebo	G	H	I
	No treatment	J	K	L

The groups in the balanced placebo design are unlike those in a conventional clinical trial, in which patients are usually told that they *might* get the active treatment and they might not. The balanced placebo design can be expanded to have a third row, comprising people who are told that they might be getting the active treatment or that they might not. This third row would mimic the conditions of an actual clinical trial. One might also add a row in which patients were told they were not receiving any treatment at all. Similarly, we could also add a third column comprising people who were told they were receiving no treatment (table A4.2). A large trial using this expanded design could provide definitive evidence of additivity or interactions.

The balanced placebo design can also be truncated. In Fabrizio Benedetti and colleagues' studies of overt versus covert treatment groups, both groups receive the treatment, yet only one group is aware that they are receiving the treatment; they correspond to groups A and J in table A4.2. One problem with all these studies is that the so-called untreated groups are rarely untreated (see chapter 5). To deal with this, it is important to minimize the contact that the so-called untreated groups have with health care professionals and to ensure that any contact is mirrored in all other groups.

The Nocebo Effect as a Smokescreen in the Great Statin Debate

Blinded clinical trials of statin versus placebo show little difference in adverse events between both groups. Yet in actual clinical practice, about half of statin takers discontinue the medication within the first year.[1] Muscle pain is often the reported cause of discontinuation,[2] and studies suggest that statin discontinuation rates increase after periods of increased media coverage highlighting these effects.[3]

Ajay Gupta and colleagues report a trial of a statin versus placebo with more than 10,000 patients.[4] The trial had two periods: blinded statin versus placebo, followed by unblinded statin versus no treatment. In the blinded period, when patients didn't know whether they were receiving the statin or the placebo, there was barely a difference between the rates of reported muscle-related adverse events (2.00% versus 2.03%, not statistically significant). In the unblinded period, they report a small difference (1.26% versus 1.00%) that is statistically significant. They use this as evidence that muscle-related adverse events arise due to the nocebo effect. Some n-of-1 trials have used a related method to draw the same conclusions by investigating the extent to which statin side effects are nocebo effects.[5] One of these trials randomized 60 patients who had discontinued statin use to alternating periods of statin, placebo, or no treatment, switching every month for one year.[5] Then they recorded adverse events. They found that patients reported similar rates of side effects whether they were taking the statins or not. Again, they blamed the nocebo.

There are problems with these trials, however. I'll mention what I think are the main ones here. The way in which the Gupta and colleagues' trial collected adverse events may have prevented them from detecting the adverse events. The main report states:

> Reports of AEs by study participants were initially recorded verbatim and subsequently classified with use of the Medical Dictionary for Regulatory Activities into 26 separate system organ class (SOC) groups, 2288 unique

preferred terms, and 5109 separate low-level terms. For this report, two physicians (AW and DT) adjudicated the four AEOIs: muscle-related, erectile dysfunction, sleep disturbance, and cognitive impairment. Each of the adjudicators reviewed (blinded to baseline characteristics, randomised treatment, non-study statin use, and trial phase) all reported AEs for the presence of any of the four AEOIs and, on the basis of the description in the case report form, classified their degree of certainty (definite, probable, or possible) according to prespecified definitions. . . . Any disagreements between the two adjudicators were independently resolved by a third physician (AG), who was similarly blinded.[4, pp. 2475–2476.]

In the supplementary appendix, they noted the following exclusions from adverse events: chest pain, non-cardiac chest pain, "musculoskeletal chest pain," thoracic pain, abdominal pain, headache, lower back pain, neck pain, hand and foot pain, claudication and claudication-equivalent descriptions. However, unless blood flow is measured, it is hard to see how "claudication" (defined as muscle pain typically caused by restricted blood flow) can be disambiguated in an unbiased way from standard muscle cramps. Hence, the methods they used to detect adverse events may lead to an underestimate of all adverse events, leading to an underpowered trial.

The n-of-1 trial was too small and too short to detect statin adverse events. In fact, adverse events of statins (including muscle pain, diabetes, and strokes) that are too small to detect, often only arise in fewer than a handful out of 100 patients, and they often take more than a year to arise.[7] Pointing the finger at the nocebo effect is a scapegoat that veils the potential of these other harms.

Another potential problem with the trials claiming that statin side effects are nocebo effects is that they presuppose that the real side effects and nocebo effects add rather than interact. This may be a mistake, and to see why, consider the possibility that they interact in a certain way. It could be that both statin drugs and the expectation of a negative side effect both produce the adverse event. If that were the case, then:

- if an adverse event arose because of a negative expectation, then there is no room for statin-caused muscle-related adverse events; and
- if an adverse event arose because of the statin, then there is (less) room for a nocebo-induced adverse event.

Table A5.1. The Modified Balanced Placebo Design for Testing the Extent to Which Muscle-Related Adverse Effects after Taking Statins Are Nocebo Effects

	Receives statin	Receives no treatment
Told statin (low expectations about statin-related adverse effects)	A	B
Told no-treatment (high expectations about statin-related adverse effects)	C	D

That is, the simple trials conducted to test whether some statin side effects are misattributions, nocebo effects, or drug adverse events do not rule out interactions. To distinguish between the different possibilities, a balanced placebo design could be used (table A5.1).

If the side effects were reported in people who did not know they were receiving statins (group C), then they could not be nocebo effects. The side effects in this group could be compared with reported side effects in groups that were told they received statins (group A). Then the hypothesis of interactions could be calculated by comparing nocebo effect rates in two different ways: A–C and B–D. If those two values differed by a statistically significant amount, then it would offer support for interactions, calling into question the method used in the Gupta and n-of-1 trial. On the face of it, it may seem that such a trial would face insurmountable ethical and regulatory challenges.[8] However, it may not be the case. People could give their informed consent to receive or not receive statins without their knowledge. Then, because most people on statins are already taking other medications, the statins could be added to or not added to those other medications.

The Many Faces of Blinding: Clarifying the Terminology

Sometimes people use the word "mask" instead of "blind." "Mask" is preferred by some because it reflects what was done historically in the Mesmer trials. People can see through masks, and attempts to blind trials are rarely successful: people often manage to figure out what they're getting, much like what would have happened if the young man in Mesmer's experiment had had a faulty mask. However, because the word "blind" is more common, I'll use it.

Another problem is that "blinding" is used in dozens of ways to describe hiding knowledge of who got what. Here are the six groups from which we can hide knowledge of who got what:

1. Patients (participants): these are the people, usually patients, who receive the active treatment or control interventions
2. Doctors and nurses, psychiatrists, and exercise trainers: anyone giving the treatment
3. Data collectors who take the patients' blood pressure, ask how much pain patients are in, or take an X-ray
4. Outcome evaluators who decide whether the participant has suffered (or enjoyed) the outcome
5. Statisticians (data analysts) who make decisions about the type of statistical tests to perform and then perform the tests
6. People writing the paper

Often the same people can perform multiple roles (for example, the doctor might also collect the data and evaluate the outcomes), but in larger trials it is often different people. Unfortunately, most trials don't tell us which of the groups were blinded. One study found that the term "double blind" was used in over a dozen ways.[1] About a third defined "double masking" as masking of the participants and doctors (or nurses or others who administer the treatment). Definitions are getting better, and people are starting to be more explicit about which groups were blinded.[2]

How to Measure Blinding Success and More about Why We Need to Measure It

One way to measure the success of blinding uses chi-squared tests of independence, in which successful blinding is indicated by a null finding (patient guesses are not related to their intervention allocation).[3,4] However, this does not provide any directional information about the pattern of participant guesses.[5] Kenneth James's[6] and Heejung Bang's[5] blinding indexes address this concern by asking participants to guess their intervention assignment using three responses (active, placebo, or do not know). James's provides a single value that combines data from all arms ranging from 0 to 1, 0 being total lack of blinding, 1 being complete blinding, and 0.5 being completely random blinding. Bang's BI aims to provide a more sensitive measure of blinding within each experimental arm compared to James's by calculating a score from −1 to 1, 1 being complete lack of blinding, 0 being consistent with perfect blinding and −1 indicating opposite guessing, which may be related to unblinding.[5] As such, it can be used to detect where blinding may have failed while still assessing overall success. An even newer method is the use of video surveillance. This involves video-recording procedures in the trial and asking a professional familiar with the procedure to guess the intervention allocation.[7]

If blinding is perfect, then patients and doctors shouldn't be able to distinguish between the placebo control or the real treatment, but most trials don't test whether blinding has been a success. Even more disappointingly, the ones that have, found that only 2% of trials that test for blinding are successful.[8,9] The failure to keep patients and doctors blinded is no surprise. To succeed, the appearance, smell, taste, and side effects of the drug must be mirrored almost exactly by the placebo control. But that is almost impossible, because even in the simple case of drugs, they have distinctive smells and tastes that patients can identify. For interventions like surgery, diet, exercise, and acupuncture, it gets even harder. If most blinded trials are not successfully blinded, then they do not rule out the potential bias caused by expectations.

All but one megastudy investigating whether blinding makes a difference have found that on average, trials described as "double-blind" report at least 10% smaller treatment effects than similar trials that are not clearly double-blinded.[8,10–21] One study did not find a difference, but it had serious methodological limitations. The MetaBLIND study is the most recent systematic review of the effect of blinding and has results that disagree with a wealth of evidence from previous studies and systematic reviews.[20] Unfortunately, their conclusions are now being manipulated by researchers who do not critique the methods or results, yet insist that the paper is a "game changer" that questions the "dogma" that blinding or measuring its success are useful. I will list some problems with the review here. For my critique I've relied heavily on an extensive analysis by Michiel Tack,[22] as well as my own response published in the *BMJ*.[23]

1. They did not distinguish between successful and unsuccessful blinding. At best, the description of a trial, including descriptions from trial authors, refers to the report of whether a trial was blinded, not whether the trial actually was blinded. This distinction was blurred in the report. In fact, there is good reason to believe that the blinding was not successful. In most comparisons, there are significant differences in the intervention, the control arm, the length of treatment, the inclusion criteria, or the outcome measure used across trials. The differences between the intervention and control almost certainly led to unsuccessful blinding. And contrary to current evidence-based medicine standards, the success of blinding matters.[24]

2. The majority (68 of the 132 trials in their main analysis) came from two Cochrane reviews.[25,26] Neither tests the effectiveness of an intervention to treat a medical condition but rather tests the knowledge recall of participants who were given different types of information sheets. Testing recall of patient information sheets is not the same thing as testing for the success of blinding. The side effect of a treatment (say it makes my urine turn purple) could make it clear that I was not taking the placebo, yet I might not recall anything that was said on the information sheet. In fact, most patients don't read information sheets.[27] The authors of the only blinded trial from one of the reviews stated: "The 'standard' leaflet had been constructed without reference to this study, by consensus between a large number of specialist anaesthetists. In contrast, the knowledge questionnaires and the 'full' information sheet were designed by the investigators to address information thought important. It turned out that the information in the 'standard' leaflet (unlike the 'full' leaflet) did not actually cover all the issues addressed by the knowledge questionnaire."[28]

3. For some comparisons the data weren't relevant to clinical trials. Two analyses did not test the effectiveness of an intervention to treat a

medical condition; rather they tested knowledge recall of participants who were given different types of information sheets.

4. In the study of the treatment of pruritus, the two blinded trials compared rifampicin against placebo, while the one unblinded trial compared it against another treatment (phenobarbitone). For a fair comparison, the unblinded trial should compare it to placebo as well.

5. Perhaps the biggest problem was found in an analysis of "Strategies for Partner Notification for Sexually Transmitted Infections." Here the data extracted—the number of sexual partners notified—weren't relevant to the intervention: it wasn't an outcome measure.

In short, their conclusions were based on a small handful of trials, most of which seem to have had peculiarities that make comparisons between blinded and unblinded trials unfair which distorted the entire comparison. A new, better review needs to be published. When it is, I suspect it will reflect what the many anecdotes and previous large studies have shown, namely that successful blinding often improves the quality of trials.

An Open Letter to the World Medical Association

November 14, 2023
David O. Barbe
President, World Medical Association

Dear Dr. Barbe:

Earlier versions of the World Medical Association (WMA) Declaration of Helsinki forbade the use of placebo controls in cases where established effective therapy was available.[1] Yet the revised versions of the declaration (since 2004) allow for placebo-controlled trials even when there is established effective therapy: "Where for compelling and scientifically sound methodological reasons the use of any intervention less effective than the best proven one, the use of placebo, or no intervention is necessary to determine the efficacy or safety of an intervention."[2]

Comparing a new treatment (which could turn out to be harmful) with a placebo is putting the patient at risk of harm that could be avoided by comparing the new treatment with an established treatment. Because doctors are required to help patients and avoid harms, it is unethical for them to enroll patients in placebo-controlled trials when there is an established treatment, or indeed to treat patients in such trials. (An exception is placebo add-on trials, which are a separate class of placebo-controlled trials that are not ethically problematic; I am not referring to these here.) The earlier versions of the declaration reflected the professional requirements of medical practitioners to help and to avoid harm.

The revision to the declaration hinges on there being "compelling and scientifically sound methodological reasons" for overriding the strong case to avoid placebo-controlled trials when there is a proven therapy. Yet, the revised declaration did not provide detail regarding what these reasons might be. Investigations into these potential reasons have not withstood scrutiny and reveal a number of conceptual and statistical confusions.[3,4]

Opening the door to placebo-controlled trials even when there are established therapies has led to measurable harm. In one trial, a new antipsychotic was tested against placebos even though we know that other drugs reduce psychosis.[5] In another trial, a new drug for skin cancer was compared with placebos, even though we knew for more than five years before the trial that other treatments were also effective. Yet another compared steroid injections to a placebo (saline injection) for treating severe bruising in patients getting rhinoplasties in Brazil even though we already knew that other drugs were effective for treating severe bruising. The authors of these studies claimed that their trials complied with the World Medical Association's Declaration of Helsinki. You might say that these trials did not have "compelling and scientifically sound methodological reasons" for conducting placebo-controlled trials. Yet in the absence of clear guidance as to what these might be (and a robust scrutiny of the research which has questioned whether there are any valid ones), the door is left open for these kinds of trials to persist.

The World Medical Association has the power to stop or at least reduce the unethical use of placebo-controlled trials when there is an established therapy. We urge you to use this power to benefit patients and help doctors follow their professional duties untethered from unsound methodological considerations.

Faithfully yours,
Jeremy Howick

APPENDIX 8
More on Noninferiority Trials

Sometimes, being "as good as" (noninferior) is an improvement. For example, a very brave group of surgeons tested whether doing nothing was equivalent to (noninferior) doing surgery. The statistical test revealed that doing nothing was not worse (to within a margin of 3%) than surgery.[1] Here and in a few other cases,[2] noninferiority tests have led to the rejection of relatively risky, invasive, and expensive procedures.

More recently, and more often, noninferiority trials are used to promote drugs that are the same as what we already have but are often more expensive. The argument given is that the new more expensive treatment, while only "as good as" (and not better) than what we already have is that the new treatment might have fewer side effects. Or the new treatment might simply have different side effects that some people find easier to tolerate. Or it could be easier to take (for example, it might involve one daily dose rather than two).[3-6] But that is another way of saying that the new treatment is *better* than the existing one. And the best way to *prove* that one treatment is better than another is obviously to test whether it is superior. Testing whether it is "as good as" will not provide evidence of those claims. Moreover, comparing side effects of the new treatment with the old one is unfair. Existing treatments have been around for longer, so there will be more extensive data about their side effects. We don't know about the rare and long-term side effects of new treatments because fewer people have taken them. This makes comparing side effects in trials—which are usually short—unbalanced. More importantly, if the reason we are doing the noninferiority trial is to see whether the new treatment has a better side-effect profile, then we can test whether the side-effect profile is better (not whether it is as good as the established one).

Another reason why we might want more treatments that are as good as (but not better than) what we already have is in case people develop tolerance to the new drug, or the company making it goes bust, or whatever.

This justifies having more than one option, not dozens. Yet, the proliferation of roughly equivalent treatments is precisely what indiscriminate use of noninferiority trials encourages. For instance, at least six selective serotonin reuptake inhibitors (SSRIs) treat depression, as do numerous other pharmaceutical antidepressants ranging from the older tricyclic agents, monoamine oxidase inhibitors (MAOIs), serotonin norepinephrine reuptake inhibitors (SNRIs), noradrenergic and specific serotonergic antidepressants (NASSAs), norepinephrine (noradrenaline) reuptake inhibitors (NRIs), and norepinephrine and dopamine reuptake inhibitors (NDRIs). Many non-pharmaceutical therapies are used to treat depression, including St. John's wort, cognitive behavioral therapy (CBT), exercise, and self-help. None of these have demonstrated consistent superiority to others in trials, although some, such as exercise, are admittedly very different from others. Even if it were useful to have a few of these treatments available in case one of them suddenly turned out to be harmful or because patients somehow developed resistance, it is difficult to justify so many.

In reality, the real reason most noninferiority trials are done is to gain market share and improve drug company profits. You may suppose that having lots of imitation drugs creates competition that should drive prices down. But in reality, it seems that the opposite is the case. A study of the cost of medical treatment in British Columbia, Canada, showed that imitation drugs accounted for an 80% increase in drug expenditures between 1996 and 2003.[7] This is probably because the companies that market their imitation drugs spend a ton of money convincing us that the new "as good as" treatment's supposedly better side-effect profile is worth paying more money for.

An easy solution to overusing noninferiority trials is for governments to refuse to pay more for drugs that are merely as good as (but no better) than what we already have.

In sum, it's not true that trials comparing a new treatment with a proven one can't detect differences. At best, a specific type of trial comparing a new treatment with an existing one—namely, those that attempt to learn whether the new one is as good as the existing one (a noninferiority trial)—can't detect a difference. Yet even that is not true, as I will show below.

Statistical Tests of Noninferiority
To see where the word "noninferiority" comes from, it helps to look at its statistical roots. In a test of whether a new treatment is better than a

placebo or another treatment, we posit a null hypothesis that they are the same. Then, if the data allow us to *reject* the null hypothesis, we conclude that there is probably a difference.

One might be tempted to say that when the null hypothesis of equivalence is not rejected, we can conclude equivalence. But that's not how the logic of classical statistics works (it is different for Bayesian statistics). Unfortunately, many trials that claim equivalence (and hence can also claim noninferiority) are based on superiority trials in which the null hypothesis of equivalence was not rejected.[8]

To provide evidence that a new treatment is (roughly) equal to an established treatment, we have to reject two null hypotheses (in classical statistics):

> the null hypothesis that the new treatment is inferior to the established one (by more than some minimum amount Δ), and
> the null hypothesis that the new treatment is better than the established one (by at least some minimum 'equivalence margin' Δ).

If the first of the above hypotheses (that the new treatment is *inferior to* the existing one) is rejected, then the new treatment is *noninferior*.

Getting more technical, there three ways to test for equivalence: using confidence intervals, using a single null hypothesis in a two-sided test, or using two null hypotheses in separate one-sided tests. I will limit my discussion to significance tests. A number of textbooks explain the other ways.[9–11]

Let:

> T = (new) test treatment
> S = standard treatment control
> P = placebo control
> δ = the equivalence or noninferiority margin, which is the acceptable difference between T and S that is allowed in order to maintain equivalence

To be considered equivalent, two treatments don't need to be exactly equal (two things never are); rather, they need to be equal within the acceptable range ($-\delta, \delta$). The equivalence margin should generally be a fraction of the standard treatment control effect (over and above "placebo"), Δ. This is self-evident. If δ approaches or surpasses Δ, then a result of "equivalence" could mean that T is no more effective than "placebo." The

margin must be chosen at the design stage and not post hoc. The ICH E10 Guideline recommends that it be *at least* smaller than Δ,[12] but this may be too conservative.[10] The correct choice of Δ is usually chosen as "the smallest value that would be a clinically important effect."[6] Irving Hwang and Toshihiko Morikawa recommend that the margin be less than ½ Δ to be useful. At the same time, it cannot be too small, or the sample size will be impractically large.

For example, consider a trial of a new drug and a standard drug for hypertension. The primary endpoint will be supine diastolic blood pressure (SDBP, measured in mmHg). The minimum drug effect size Δ (standard drug–"placebo") in mean reduction from baseline in SDBP in many "placebo"-controlled trials was approximately 10 mmHg. A choice of $\delta = 3$ mmHg was considered reasonable based on clinical relevance and statistical judgment—it ensured that some clinically acceptable drug effect would be maintained without having an unrealistically large sample size.

In an equivalence trial, the null hypothesis, h_0, which investigators will try to reject, is that the difference is neither superior nor inferior to the upper and lower limits of the equivalence margin. The alternative hypothesis, h_a, is that the difference lies within the range of acceptable difference. That is:

$$h_0: T - S \leq -\delta \quad \text{or} \quad T - S \geq \delta$$
$$\text{vs. } h_a: -\delta < T - S < \delta$$

Alternatively, equivalence can be tested with a pair of one-sided null and alternative hypotheses:

$$h_0: T - S \leq -\delta \quad \text{vs.} \quad h_a: T - S > -\delta \text{ and}$$
$$h_0: T - S \geq \delta \quad \text{vs.} \quad h_a: T - S < \delta$$

Noninferiority trials can either use the first method in a one-sided test or the first pair of hypotheses in the second. Note that compared to placebo-controlled *superiority* trials, the null and alternative hypotheses in noninferiority trials are essentially reversed. In a placebo-controlled trial, the null and alternative hypotheses are:

$$h_0: T - S \leq 0 \quad \text{vs.} \quad h_a: T - S > 0$$

The relationship between the null and alternative hypotheses in "conventional," equivalence, superiority, and noninferiority trials is best explained pictorially (fig. A8.1).

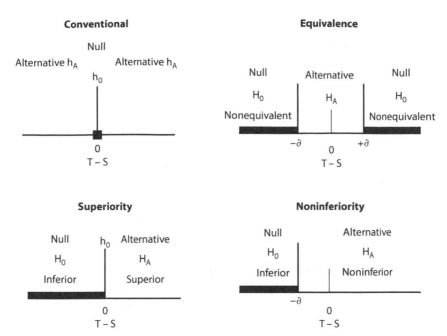

FIG. A8.1. Null and alternative hypotheses for equivalence, noninferiority, and superiority trials

The Second Assay Sensitivity Argument Fails

Recall from chapter 10 that the second assay sensitivity argument is that only placebo-controlled trials can detect differences. This is obviously false if the active-controlled trial is a superiority trial (the statistical tests for superiority don't know whether the control is a placebo or another treatment). So, the second assay sensitivity argument is not aimed at *superiority* active-controlled trials, but only *noninferiority* active-controlled trials. With the background about noninferiority trials out of the way, I will now show that noninferiority trials can also detect differences and therefore that the second assay sensitivity argument fails completely.

Both superiority and noninferiority can be tested using confidence intervals. A confidence interval represents a range within which the mean difference between experimental and control treatments is likely to lie. If the entire confidence interval lies to the right side of the line representing no difference, then we can conclude (in a probabilistic sense) that the experimental treatment is superior. If the entire confidence interval lies to the right of the lower bound of the equivalence margin ($-\partial$), then we can

conclude (again in a probabilistic sense) noninferiority. It is true that a positive result of a noninferiority trial does not provide evidence of a difference: a treatment could be noninferior and also roughly equal (the confidence interval could lie within the "equivalence margin" bound by $-\partial$ and $+\partial$). It is also true that the purpose of a noninferiority trial is not to detect a difference: we would be happy if the experimental treatment were roughly equal. It does not follow, however, that a noninferiority trial cannot detect a difference. Even if the purpose of the trial is to detect noninferiority, if we find that the confidence interval lies entirely to either side of the line representing no difference, then the trial will have provided evidence that a treatment difference exists.

One might object that the second assay sensitivity argument against active controlled trials is only apparent if we consider the null and alternative hypotheses used in superiority and noninferiority trials. Since I have used confidence intervals without referring to the null and alternative hypotheses, the objection proceeds, I have concealed the problem. Given that the confidence interval and hypothesis test methods are equivalent,[9] it would certainly be surprising if it turned out that consideration of the null and alternative hypotheses revealed that noninferiority trials are incapable of detecting differences. Thus, the second assay sensitivity argument, like the first, fails as a justification for the claim that placebo-controlled trials are methodologically superior to active controlled trials. I will now examine the argument that placebo-controlled trials (but not active controlled trials) provide a measure of absolute effect size.

Getting even more technical, we can look at the relationship between type I and type II errors in both superiority and noninferiority trials. A type I error, or a "false positive," is the error of rejecting a true null hypothesis (and instead "accepting" a false alternative hypothesis). A type II error, or "false negative," is the mistake of failing to reject a false null hypothesis (and "rejecting" a true alternative hypothesis). Both type I and type II errors can be controlled for and specified in advance of a trial. When the type I error rate, or "significance level" is sufficiently low, generally 1% or 5%, then rejection of the null hypothesis is said to be justified. Of note, it is often objected, notably by Bayesians, that the choice of a type I error rate (at which rejection becomes justified) is arbitrary, and that we should instead speak of hypotheses which are more or less probable.[13]

In a superiority trial, a type I error is the mistake of rejecting no difference (and "accepting" that the experimental treatment is superior) when there is a difference. If the type I error rate, or α, in a superiority trial is sufficiently low, then the trial will probably not assert a difference when there is none. To be sure, a low type I or type II error rate does not actually bear on the probability of a single trial, but applies only to the *long run*. That is, if the type I error rate is 1%, this means that if we ran the same trial a hundred times, we would expect one of the trials to give the wrong result. It says nothing about the probability of a particular trial being mistaken. I will ignore this problem with classical hypothesis testing for the purposes of my analysis.

However, nothing about type I errors tells us anything about the accuracy of the test where the null hypothesis is *not* rejected, which is achieved by lowering the type II error rate. A low type II error rate in a superiority trial means it is unlikely that failure to reject the null hypothesis is a mistake—that is, that some difference has not gone undetected. To speak loosely, a type I error in a superiority trial is the mistake of accepting that there is a difference when there is none; a type II error is the mistake of accepting no difference when there is one.

In a noninferiority trial, type I and type II errors, although defined in the same way, imply different things. In a noninferiority trial, a type I error would be the error of mistakenly rejecting the hypothesis of strict inferiority (negative difference) and accepting the hypothesis of equivalence or superiority. A type II error in a noninferiority trial, on the other hand, is the error of failing to reject inferiority when the experimental is either (roughly) equivalent or superior to the control treatment. To reduce the type II error rate in a noninferiority trial is therefore to make the trial very sensitive to differences: if the null is true and there is a difference (inferiority), then the trial will not reject it. Again, speaking loosely, a type I error in a noninferiority trial is the mistake of accepting equality or superiority (when there is inferiority), while a type II error is the mistake of accepting inferiority when there is equality or superiority.

The relationship between type I and type II error rates in superiority and noninferiority trials is clearly explained with the help of table A8.1.

Whether a trial is good at detecting differences depends on the degree of risk of type I and type II errors. A type I error, or "false positive," is the error of rejecting a true null hypothesis (and accepting a false alternative hypothesis). A type II error, or "false negative," is the mistake of failing to reject a false null hypothesis (and not accepting a true alternative hypothesis). In a superiority trial, a type I error is the mistake of accepting a positive difference when there is none, while a type II error is the mistake

Table A8.1. Classification of Possible Decisions Based on Hypothesis Tests (Adapted from Blackwelder)[11]

		TRUE HYPOTHESIS			
		Null	*Alternative*	*Null*	*Alternative*
DECISION	*Reject*	Type I error (α), i.e., mistake of "accepting" the alternative of *difference* (superiority)	correct	Type I error (α), i.e., mistake of "accepting" *no difference* (or superiority)	correct
	Don't reject	correct	Type II error (β), i.e., mistake of "accepting" the null alternative of *no difference* (or inferiority)	correct	Type II error (β), i.e., mistake of "accepting" *difference* (inferiority)

of accepting no difference or inferiority when the experimental treatment is superior.

Both type I and type II errors can be controlled for and specified in advance of a trial. To sensitize a superiority trial to differences, we reduce the type I error rate. To sensitize a noninferiority trial to differences, we must reduce the type II error rate.

With this in mind, it is straightforward to show that noninferiority trials are as good (or bad) at detecting differences as superiority trials. James Anderson postulates four conditions required to assume assay sensitivity.[14, p. 75] Using "D" to denote "difference between intervention and control group," and T to denote "trial," the conditions for asserting assay sensitivity (of the second kind) are:

D
T indicates D
D $\rightarrow$ (T indicates D)
not-D $\rightarrow$ not (T indicates D)

The first condition tells us that, ontologically speaking, there is a difference between the interventions being compared. The second tells us that the trial indicated a difference. The third tells us that the trial would indicate a difference if there were one. The fourth tells us that if there is no difference, then the trial will not indicate a difference. In the real world, of course, the modality of the conditionals in (3) and (4) is not necessity—actual trials deal in probability.

The four conditions for assay sensitivity will be satisfied in a superiority trial when:

> There is a difference (the experimental treatment is superior to placebo).
> The trial indicates a difference (there is a "positive" result).
> The type II error rate is sufficiently low (the trial did not wrongly suggest no difference).
> The type I error rate is sufficiently low (the trial did not wrongly indicate a difference).

In a noninferiority trial, the four conditions for affirming assay sensitivity will be satisfied when:

1. There is a difference (the experimental treatment is superior to placebo).
2. The trial indicates a difference (there is a "positive" result).
3. The type I error rate is sufficiently low.
4. The type II error rate is sufficiently low.

As long as we are able to reduce both the type I and type II error rates sufficiently, both superiority and noninferiority trials can be made equally assay sensitive. Anderson concludes, and he is surely correct, that "Contrary to the assay sensitivity argument, there is not an absolute difference between PCT [placebo-controlled trials] and ACT [active controlled trials] with respect to . . . the assay sensitivity assumption."[14]

There are two final notes about this assay sensitivity argument. First, since it is about classical hypothesis tests of the different trials, it would not apply to statistical tests using Bayesian methods. The other arguments against active controlled trials, on the other hand, could apply no matter which type of statistical tests one employs. Similarly, this assay sensitivity argument applies exclusively (and not merely more strongly) to noninferiority active controlled trials.

Chapter 1. A Manifesto for the Next Revolution in Nocebo and Placebo Studies

1. Plato. *Complete Works.* Cooper JM, Hutchinson DS, ed. and trans. Hackett; 1997.

2. Beecher HK. The powerful placebo. *J Am Med Assoc.* Dec 24 1955;159(17):1602–1606. https://doi.org/10.1001/jama.1955.02960340022006.

3. National Health Service. Diclofenac. Accessed June 8, 2022. https://www.nhs.uk/medicines/diclofenac/.

4. Hróbjartsson A. Clinical placebo interventions are unethical, unnecessary, and unprofessional. *J Clin Ethics.* Spring 2008;19(1):66–69.

5. Braillon A. Placebo is far from benign: It is disease-mongering. *Am J Bioeth.* 2009 Dec;9(12):36–38. https://doi.org/10.1080/15265160903234078.

6. Howick J. Unethical informed consent caused by overlooking poorly measured nocebo effects. *J Med Ethics.* 2021 Sep;47(9):590–594. https://doi.org/10.1136/medethics-2019-105903.

7. Howick J, Webster R, Kirby N, Hood K. Rapid overview of systematic reviews of nocebo effects reported by patients taking placebos in clinical trials. *Trials.* Dec 11 2018;19(1):674. https://doi.org/10.1186/s13063-018-3042-4.

8. Kirby N, Shepherd V, Howick J, Betteridge S, Hood K. Nocebo effects and participant information leaflets: Evaluating information provided on adverse effects in UK clinical trials. *Trials.* Jul 17 2020;21(1):658. https://doi.org/10.1186/s13063-020-04591-w.

9. Charlesworth JEG, Petkovic G, Kelley JM, et al. Effects of placebos without deception compared with no treatment: A systematic review and meta-analysis. *J Evid Based Med* 2017;10(2):97–107. https://doi.org/ 10.1111/jebm.12251.

10. Howick J. The relativity of placebos: Defending a modified version of Grünbaum's scheme. Synthese 2017;194(4):1363–96. https://doi.org/10.1007/s11229-015-1001-0.

11. Frank JD, Frank JB. *Persuasion and Healing: A Comparative Study of Psychotherapy.* 3d ed. Johns Hopkins University Press; 1991.

12. Kaptchuk TJ. Intentional ignorance: A history of blind assessment and placebo controls in medicine. *Bulletin of the History of Medicine* 1998;72.3:389–433. https://doi.org/10.1353/bhm.1998.0159.

13. Kaptchuk TJ. The placebo effect in alternative medicine: Can the performance of a healing ritual have clinical significance? *Ann Intern Med.* Jun 4 2002;136(11):817–825. https://doi.org/10.7326/0003-4819-136-11-200206040-00011.

14. Shapiro AK, Morris LA. The placebo effect in medical and psychological therapies. In: Garfield SL, Bergin AE, eds. *Handbook of Psychotherapy and Behavior Change: An Empirical Analysis.* 2d ed. Wiley; 1978:369–410.

15. Grünbaum A. The placebo concept in medicine and psychiatry. *Psychol Med.* Feb 1986;16(1):19–38. https://doi.org/10.1017/s0033291700002506.

16. Kirsch I. Response expectancy as a determinant of experience and behavior. *American Psychologist.* 1985;40(11):1189–1202. https://doi.org /10.1037/0003-066x.40.11.1189.

17. Bok S. The ethics of giving placebos. *Sci Am.* Nov 1974;231(5):17–23. http:// www.jstor.org/stable/24950213.

18. Brody H. The lie that heals: The ethics of giving placebos. *Ann Intern Med.* Jul 1982;97(1):112–118. https://doi.org/10.7326/0003-4819-97-1-112.

19. Freedman B, Glass KC, Weijer C. Placebo orthodoxy in clinical research. II: Ethical, legal, and regulatory myths. *J Law Med Ethics.* Fall 1996;24(3):252–259. https://doi.org/10.1111/j.1748-720x.1996.tb01860.x.

20. Freedman B, Weijer C, Glass KC. Placebo orthodoxy in clinical research. I: Empirical and methodological myths. *J Law Med Ethics.* Fall 1996;24(3):243–251. https://doi.org/10.1111/j.1748-720x.1996.tb01859.x.

21. Kuhn TS. *The Structure of Scientific Revolutions.* 2d ed. University of Chicago Press; 1970.

22. Gøtzsche P. Is there logic in the placebo? *Lancet* 1994;344(8927): 925–926. https://doi.org/10.1016/s0140-6736(94)92273-x

23. Commentary: Is the placebo powerless? *N Engl J Med. Catalyst.* 2001;345: 1276–1279. https://doi.org/10.1056/NEJM200110253451712.

24. Colquhoun D. Placebo effects are weak: Regression to the mean is the main reason ineffective treatments appear to work. *DC's Improbably Science* (blog). 2015. http://www.dcscience.net/2015/12/11/placebo-effects-are-weak-regression-to-the -mean-is-the-main-reason-ineffective-treatments-appear-to-work/.

25. Kleijnen J, de Craen AJ, van Everdingen J, Krol L. Placebo effect in double-blind clinical trials: A review of interactions with medications. *Lancet.* Nov 12 1994;344(8933):1347–1349. https://doi.org/10.1016/s0140-6736(94)90699-8.

26. Di Blasi Z, Harkness E, Ernst E, et al. Influence of context effects on health outcomes: A systematic review. *Lancet* 2001;357(9258):757–762. https://doi.org /10.1016/s0140-6736(00)04169-6.

27. Moerman DE. *Meaning, Medicine, and the "Placebo Effect."* Cambridge University Press; 2002.

28. Evans D. *Placebo: The Belief Effect.* HarperCollins; 2003.

29. Benedetti F. *Placebo Effects: Understanding the Mechanisms in Health and Disease.* 3d ed. Oxford University Press; 2020.

30. Kirsch I, Deacon BJ, Huedo-Medina TB, Scoboria A, Moore TJ, Johnson BT. Initial severity and antidepressant benefits: A meta-analysis of data submitted to the Food and Drug Administration. *PLoS Med.* Feb 2008;5(2):e45. http://doi.org/10.1371/journal.pmed.0050045.

31. Howick J, Friedemann C, Tsakok M, et al. Are treatments more effective than placebos? A systematic review and meta-analysis. *PLoS One* 2013;8(5):e62599. http://doi.org/10.1371/journal.pone.0062599.

32. Harris I. *Surgery, the Ultimate Placebo: A Surgeon Cuts through the Evidence.* NewSouth; 2016.

33. Louhiala P. *Placebo Effects: The Meaning of Care in Medicine.* Springer; 2020.

34. Kaptchuk TJ, Stason WB, Davis RB, et al. Sham device v inert pill: Randomised controlled trial of two placebo treatments. *BMJ.* Feb 18 2006;332(7538): 391–397. http://doi.org.10.1136/bmj.38726.603310.55.

35. Kaptchuk TJ, Kelley JM, Conboy LA, et al. Components of placebo effect: Randomised controlled trial in patients with irritable bowel syndrome. *BMJ.* May 3 2008;336(7651):999–1003. https://doi.org/10.1136/bmj.39524.439618.25.

36. Kaptchuk TJ, Friedlander E, Kelley JM, et al. Placebos without deception: A randomized controlled trial in irritable bowel syndrome. *PLoS One.* 2010;5(12):e15591. https://doi.org/10.1371/journal.pone.0015591.

37. Kelley JM, Kaptchuk T, Cusin C, Lipkin S, Fava M. Open-label placebo for major depressive disorder: A pilot randomized controlled trial. *Psychotherapy and Psychosomatics.* 2012;81:312–14. https://doi.org/10.1159/000337053.

38. Jonas WB, Crawford C, Colloca L, et al. To what extent are surgery and invasive procedures effective beyond a placebo response? A systematic review with meta-analysis of randomised, sham controlled trials. *BMJ Open.* Dec 11 2015;5(12):e009655. https://doi.org/10.1136/bmjopen-2015-009655.

39. Carvalho C, Caetano JM, Cunha L, Rebouta P, Kaptchuk TJ, Kirsch I. Open-label placebo treatment in chronic low back pain: A randomized controlled trial. *Pain.* Dec 2016;157(12):2766–2772. https://doi.org/10.1097/j.pain.0000000000000700.

40. Society for Interdisciplinary Placebo Studies. https://www.placebosociety.org.

41. Marchant J. *Cure: A Journey into the Science of Mind over Body.* Crown; 2016.

42. Dispenza J. *You Are the Placebo: Making Your Mind Matter.* Hay House; 2015.

43. Howick J. *Doctor You: Revealing the Science of Self-Healing.* Hodder & Stoughton; 2017.

44. Thomson J. *The Placebo Diet: Use Your Mind to Transform Your Body.* Hay House; 2016.

45. Saint Placebo. Accessed August 12, 2020. http://saintplacebo.com.

46. Meissner K. Placebo, nocebo: Believing in the field of medicine. *Front Pain Res (Lausanne)* 2022;3:972169. https://doi.org/10.3389/fpain.2022.972169.

47. Daston L, Galison P. *Objectivity.* Zone Books; 2007.

48. Harrington A. *The Placebo Effect: An Interdisciplinary Exploration*. Harvard University Press; 1997.

49. Raz A, Harris CS. *Placebo Talks: Modern Perspectives on Placebos in Society*. Oxford University Press; 2015.

50. Colloca L, ed. *Neurobiology of the Placebo Effect*. Elsevier; 2018.

51. Rotenstein LS, Torre M, Ramos MA, et al. Prevalence of Burnout Among Physicians: A Systematic Review. *JAMA* 2018;320(11):1131–1150. https://doi.org/10.1001/jama.2018.12777.

52. Dutheil F, Aubert C, Pereira B, et al. Suicide among physicians and healthcare workers: A systematic review and meta-analysis. *PLoS One* 2019;14(12):e0226361. https://doi.org/10.1371/journal.pone.0226361.

53. Rao SK, Kimball AB, Lehrhoff SR, et al. The Impact of Administrative Burden on Academic Physicians: Results of a Hospital-Wide Physician Survey. *Acad Med* 2017;92(2):237–43. https://doi.org/10.1097/ACM.0000000000001461.

54. Sinsky C, Colligan L, Li L, et al. Allocation of physician time in ambulatory practice: A time and motion study in 4 specialties. *Ann Intern Med* 2016;165(11):753–60. https://doi.org/10.7326/M16-0961.

55. General Medical Council. *The State of Medical Education and Practice in the UK*. 2019. https://www.gmc-uk.org/-/media/documents/somep-2019---full-report_pdf-81131156.pdf.

56. Sinsky CA, Dyrbye LN, West CP, et al. Professional Satisfaction and the Career Plans of US Physicians. *Mayo Clin Proc* 2017;92(11):1625–35. https://doi.org/10.1016/j.mayocp.2017.08.017.

57. OECD. Health Expenditure 2022 [Available from: https://www.oecd.org/els/health-systems/health-expenditure.htm; accessed November 28, 2022.

58. Mehta NK, Abrams LR, Myrskyla M. US life expectancy stalls due to cardiovascular disease, not drug deaths. *Proc Natl Acad Sci U S A* 2020;117(13):6998–7000. https://doi.org/10.1073/pnas.1920391117.

59. Minton J, Fletcher E, Ramsay J, et al. How bad are life expectancy trends across the UK, and what would it take to get back to previous trends? *J Epidemiol Community Health* 2020;74(9):741–46. https://doi.org/10.1136/jech-2020-213870.

60. Thirioux B, Birault F, Jaafari N. Empathy is a protective factor of burnout in physicians: New neuro-phenomenological hypotheses regarding empathy and sympathy in care relationship. *Frontiers in Psychology* 2016;7. https://doi.org/Artn 763.10.3389/Fpsyg.2016.00763.

61. Little P, White P, Kelly J, et al. Randomised controlled trial of a brief intervention targeting predominantly non-verbal communication in general practice consultations. *British Journal of General Practice* 2015;65(635):e351–356. https://doi.org/10.3399/bjgp15X685237.

62. Gagnon MA, Lexchin J. The cost of pushing pills: A new estimate of pharmaceutical promotion expenditures in the United States. *PLoS Med*. Jan 3 2008;5(1):e1. https://doi.org/ 10.1371/journal.pmed.0050001.

63. Bala A, Nguyen HMT, Hellstrom WJG. Post-SSRI sexual dysfunction: A literature review. *Sex Med Rev.* Jan 2018;6(1):29–34. https://doi.org/10.1016/j .sxmr.2017.07.002.

64. Chipidza FE, Wallwork RS, Stern TA. Impact of the doctor-patient relationship. *Prim Care Companion CNS Disord.* 2015;17(5). https://doi.org/10.4088/PCC.15f01840.

Part I. The Troubled Story of Placebos and Nocebos

1. Finniss DG, Kaptchuk TJ, Miller F, Benedetti F. Biological, clinical, and ethical advances of placebo effects. *Lancet.* Feb 20 2010;375(9715):686–695. https://doi.org/10.1016/S0140-6736(09)61706-2.

2. Nunn R. It's time to put the placebo out of our misery. *BMJ.* 2009;338:1015. https://doi.org/10.1136/bmj.b1568.

3. Turner A. "Placebos" and the logic of placebo comparison. *Biology & Philosophy.* May 2012;27(3):419–432. https://doi.org/10.1007/s10539-011-9289-8.

Chapter 2. Please Me, Please

1. Jefferson T. Letters of Thomas Jefferson. Ed. Irwin F. Sonbornton. Bridge Press; 1975.

2. Shapiro AK, Shapiro E. *The Powerful Placebo: From Ancient Priest to Modern Physician.* Johns Hopkins University Press; 1997.

3. Grünbaum A. The placebo concept in medicine and psychiatry. *Psychol Med.* 1986 Feb;16(1):19–38. https://doi.org/10.1017/s0033291700002506.

4. Bishop FL, Howick J, Heneghan C, Stevens S, Hobbs FD, Lewith G. Placebo use in the UK: A qualitative study exploring GPs' views on placebo effects in clinical practice. *Fam Pract.* Apr 15 2014. https://doi.org/10.1093/fampra/cmu016.

5. Hardman DI, Geraghty AW, Howick J, Roberts N, Bishop FL. A discursive exploration of public perspectives on placebos and their effects. *Health Psychol Open.* Jan–Jun 2019;6(1):2055102919832313. https://doi.org/10.1177 /2055102919832313.

6. Bishop FL, Aizlewood L, Adams AE. When and why placebo-prescribing is acceptable and unacceptable: A focus group study of patients' views. *PLoS One.* 2014;9(7):e101822. https://doi.org/10.1371/journal.pone.0101822.

7. Aronson J. Please, please me. *BMJ.* Mar 13 1999;318(7185):716. https://doi.org /10.1136/bmj.318.7185.716.

8. Chaucer G. *The Canterbury Tales,* ed. N Coghill. Penguin; 1978.

9. Chaucer G. *The Canterbury Tales.* http://eleusinianm.co.uk/author.html.

10. Sutherland A. *Attempts to Revive Antient Medical Doctrines, etc.* 1763.

11. Leibniz GWF, Papin D. *Leibnizens und Huygens' Briefwechsel mit Papin.* Ed. Gerland E. Martin Sändig oHG; 1966.

12. Smellie W. *A Treatise on the Theory and Practice of Midwifery.* D. Wilson; 1752.

13. Motherby G. *A New Medical Dictionary: or, General Repository of Physic.* 3d ed. J. Johnson, 1791.

14. Beecher HK. The powerful placebo. *JAMA*. Dec 24 1955;159(17):1602–1606. https://doi.org/10.1001/jama.1955.02960340022006.

15. Grünbaum A. The placebo concept in medicine and psychiatry. *Psychol Med*. Feb 1986;16(1):19–38. https://doi.org/10.1017/s0033291700002506.

16. Shapiro AK, Morris LA. The placebo effect in medical and psychological therapies. In: Garfield SL, Bergin AE, eds. *Handbook of Psychotherapy and Behavior Change: An Empirical Analysis*. 2d ed. Wiley; 1978:369–410.

17. Grencavage LM, Norcross JC. Where are the commonalities among the therapeutic common factors? *Professional Psychology: Research and Practice*. 1990;21(5):372–378.

18. Benedetti F. *Placebo Effects: Understanding the Mechanisms in Health and Disease*. 3d ed. Oxford University Press; 2020.

19. Howick J, Friedemann C, Tsakok M, et al. Are treatments more effective than placebos? A systematic review and meta-analysis. *PLoS One*. 2013;8(5):e62599. https://doi.org/10.1371/journal.pone.0062599.

20. Hróbjartsson A, Gøtzsche PC. Placebo interventions for all clinical conditions. *Cochrane Database Syst Rev*. Jan 20 2010;(1):CD003974. https://doi.org /10.1002/14651858.CD003974.pub3.

21. American Medical Association. *Code of Medical Ethics*. October 30, 2019. https://www.ama-assn.org/about/publications-newsletters/ama-principles-medical -ethics.

22. Gøtzsche P. Is there logic in the placebo? *Lancet*. Oct 1 1994;344(8927):925– 926. https://doi.org/10.1016/s0140-6736(94)92273-x.

23. Hróbjartsson A, Gøtzsche P. Is the placebo powerless? An analysis of clinical trials comparing placebo with no treatment. *N Engl J Med*. May 24 2001;344(21): 1594–602. https://doi.org/10.1056/NEJM200105243442106.

24. Nunn R. It's time to put the placebo out of its misery. *BMJ*. 2009;338:1015. https://doi.org/10.1136/bmj.b1568.

25. Charlesworth JEG, Petkovic G, Kelley JM, et al. Effects of placebos without deception compared with no treatment: A systematic review and meta-analysis. *J Evid Based Med*. May 2017;10(2):97–107. https://doi.org/10.1111 /jebm.12251.

26. Blease CR. Psychotherapy and placebos: Manifesto for conceptual clarity. *Front Psychiatry*. 2018;9:379. https://doi.org/10.3389/fpsyt.2018.00379.

27. Babel P. The effect of question wording in questionnaire surveys on placebo use in clinical practice. *Eval Health Prof*. Dec 2012;35(4):447–461. https://doi.org /10.1177/0163278711420285.

28. Fassler M, Meissner K, Schneider A, Linde K. Frequency and circumstances of placebo use in clinical practice—a systematic review of empirical studies. Review. *BMC Medicine*. 2010;8:15. https://doi.org/10.1186/1741-7015-8-15.

29. Woff HG, Dubois EF, Gold H. Cornell conferences on therapy: Use of placebos in therapy. *New York Journal of Medicine*. 1946; 46:1718.

30. Howick J, Bishop FL, Heneghan C, Wolstenholme J, Stevens S, Hobbs FD, Lewith G. Placebo use in the United Kingdom: Results from a national survey of primary care practitioners. *PLoS One.* 2013;8(3):e58247. https://doi.org/10.1371/journal.pone.0058247.

31. Coelho P. *The Zahir: A Novel of Obsession.* HarperCollins; 2006.

32. Miller FG, Colloca L. Semiotics and the placebo effect. *Perspectives in Biology and Medicine.* Autumn 2010;53(4):509–516. https://doi.org/10.1353/pbm.2010.0004

33. Dossey L. *Be Careful What You Pray For—You Just Might Get It: What We Can Do about the Unintentional Effects of Our Thoughts, Prayers, and Wishes.* HarperSan-Francisco; 1997.

34. Cannon WB. *Bodily Changes in Pain, Hunger, Fear and Rage: An Account of Recent Researches into the Function of Emotional Excitement.* 2d ed. College Park; 1929.

35. Cavendish R. *A History of Magic.* Sphere; 1978.

36. Cannon, WB. "'Voodoo' Death." *American Anthropologist.* 1942; 44(2): 169–81.

37. Adapted from Reeves RR, Ladner ME, Hart RH, Burke RS. Nocebo effects with antidepressant clinical drug trial placebos. *Gen Hosp Psychiatry.* May–June 2007;29(3):275–277. https://doi.org/10.1016/j.genhosppsych.2007.01.010.

38. Kennedy WP. The nocebo reaction. *Med World.* Sep 1961;95:203–205.

39. Kirby N, Shepherd V, Howick J, Betteridge S, Hood K. Nocebo effects and participant information leaflets: Evaluating information provided on adverse effects in UK clinical trials. Trials. Jul 17 2020;21(1):658. https://doi.org/10.1186/s13063-020-04591-w.

40. Amanzio M, Mitsikostas DD, Giovannelli F, Bartoli M, Cipriani GE, Brown WA. Adverse events of active and placebo groups in SARS-CoV-2 vaccine randomized trials: A systematic review. *Lancet Reg Health Eur.* 2022 Jan;12:100253. https://doi.org/10.1016/j.lanepe.2021.100253.

41. Fragoulis GE, Bournia VK, Mavrea E, Evangelatos G, Fragiadaki K, Karamanakos A, Kravariti E, Laskari K, Panopoulos S, Pappa M, Mitsikostas DD, Tektonidou MG, Vassilopoulos D, Sfikakis PP. COVID-19 vaccine safety and nocebo-prone associated hesitancy in patients with systemic rheumatic diseases: A cross-sectional study. *Rheumatol Int.* 2022 Jan;42(1):31–39. https://doi.org/10.1007/s00296-021-05039-3.

Chapter 3. Placebo Components and Meaningful Contexts

1. Dossey L. *Be Careful What You Pray For—You Just Might Get It.* Harper San Francisco; 1997.

2. O'Brian P. *Master and Commander.* Collins; 1970.

3. Engel G. The need for a new medical model: A challenge for biomedicine. *Science.* 1977;196:129–136.

4. Blackwell B, Bloomfield SS, Buncher CR. Demonstration to medical students of placebo responses and non-drug factors. *Lancet.* Jun 10 1972;1(7763):1279–1282. https://doi.org/ 10.1016/s0140-6736(72)90996-8.

5. De Craen AJ, Roos PJ, Leonard de Vries A, Kleijnen J. Effect of colour of drugs: Systematic review of perceived effect of drugs and of their effectiveness. *BMJ.* Dec 21–28 1996;313(7072):1624–1626. https://doi.org/ 10.1136/bmj.313 .7072.1624.

6. Moerman DE. *Meaning, Medicine, and the "Placebo Effect."* Cambridge University Press; 2002.

7. Branthwaite A, Cooper P. Analgesic effects of branding in treatment of headaches. *Br Med J (Clin Res Ed).* May 16 1981;282(6276):1576–1578.

8. Waber RL, Shiv B, Carmon Z, Ariely D. Commercial features of placebo and therapeutic efficacy. *JAMA.* Mar 5 2008;299(9):1016–1017. https://doi.org/10.1001 /jama.299.9.1016.

9. MacKrill K, Gamble GD, Bean DJ, Cundy T, Petrie KJ. Evidence of a media-induced nocebo response following a nationwide antidepressant drug switch. *Clinical Psychology in Europe.* 2019;1(1):1–12. https://doi.org/10.32872/cpe.v1i1.29642.

10. MacKrill K, Petrie KJ. What is associated with increased side effects and lower perceived efficacy following switching to a generic medicine? A New Zealand cross-sectional patient survey. *BMJ Open.* Oct 18 2018;8(10):e023667. https://doi .org/10.1136/bmjopen-2018-023667.

11. Colloca L, Panaccione R, Murphy TK. The clinical implications of nocebo effects for biosimilar therapy. *Front Pharmacol.* 2019;10:1372. https://doi.org /10.3389/fphar.2019.01372

12. Moore A. Eternal sunshine. *The Guardian.* May 13, 2007. https://www .theguardian.com/society/2007/may/13/socialcare.medicineandhealth.

13. Gasteiger C, Jones ASK, Kleinstauber M, et al. Effects of message framing on patients' perceptions and willingness to change to a biosimilar in a hypothetical drug switch. *Arthritis Care Res.* Sep 2020;72(9):1323–1330. https://doi.org/10.1002 /acr.24012.

14. Sims R, Michaleff ZA, Glasziou P, Thomas R. Consequences of a diagnostic label: A systematic scoping review and thematic framework. *Front Public Health,* 2021 Dec 22;9:725877. https://doi.org/10.3389/fpubh.2021.725877.

15. Buckalew LW, Coffield KE. An investigation of drug expectancy as a function of capsule color and size and preparation form. *J Clin Psychopharmacol.* Aug 1982;2(4):245–248.

16. Blackwell B, Bloomfield SS, Buncher CR. Demonstration to medical students of placebo responses and non-drug factors. *Lancet.* Jun 10 1972;1(7763):1279–1282. https://doi.org/ 10.1016/s0140-6736(72)90996-8.

17. De Craen AJ, Moerman DE, Heisterkamp SH, Tytgat GN, Tijssen JG, Kleijnen J. Placebo effect in the treatment of duodenal ulcer. *Br J Clin Pharmacol.* Dec 1999;48(6):853–860. https://doi.org/10.1046/j.1365-2125.1999.00094.x.

18. De Craen AJ, Tijssen JG, de Gans J, Kleijnen J. Placebo effect in the acute treatment of migraine: Subcutaneous placebos are better than oral placebos. *J Neurol.* Mar 2000;247(3):183–188. https://doi.org/10.1007/s004150050560.

19. Zhang W, Robertson J, Jones AC, Dieppe PA, Doherty M. The placebo effect and its determinants in osteoarthritis: Meta-analysis of randomised controlled trials. *Ann Rheum Dis.* Dec 2008;67(12):1716–1723. https://doi.org/10.1136/ard.2008.092015.

20. Grenfell RF, Briggs AH, Holland WC. A double-blind study of the treatment of hypertension. *JAMA.* Apr 15 1961;176:124–128. https://doi.org/10.1001/jama .1961.03040150040010.

21. Kaptchuk TJ, Stason WB, Davis RB, et al. Sham device v inert pill: Randomised controlled trial of two placebo treatments. *BMJ.* Feb 18 2006;332(7538): 391–397. https://doi.org/10.1136/bmj.38726.603310.55

22. Meissner K, Fassler M, Rucker G, et al. Differential effectiveness of placebo treatments: A systematic review of migraine prophylaxis. *JAMA Intern Med.* Nov 25 2013;173(21):1941–1951. https://doi.org/10.1001/jamainternmed.2013.10391.

23. Harris I. *Surgery, the Ultimate Placebo: A Surgeon Cuts through the Evidence.* NewSouth; 2016.

24. Lidgett CD. Improving the patient experience through a commit to sit service excellence initiative. *Patient Experience Journal.* 2016;3(2):67–72. https:// pxjournal.org/cgi/viewcontent.cgi?article=1148&context=journal.

25. Benedetti F. *Placebo Effects: Understanding the Mechanisms in Health and Disease.* 3d ed. Oxford University Press; 2020.

26. Lintz KC, Penson RT, Chabner BA, Lynch TJ. Schwartz Center Rounds: A staff dialogue on caring for an intensely spiritual patient: Psychosocial issues faced by patients, their families, and caregivers. *Oncologist.* 1998;3(6):439–445.

27. Balint M. *The Doctor, His Patient and the Illness.* Pitman Medical; 1960.

28. Sinclair S, Beamer K, Hack TF, et al. Sympathy, empathy, and compassion: A grounded theory study of palliative care patients' understandings, experiences, and preferences. *Palliat Med.* May 2017;31(5):437–447. https://doi.org/10.1177 /0269216316663499.

29. Perez-Bret E, Altisent R, Rocafort J. Definition of compassion in healthcare: A systematic literature review. *Int J Palliat Nurs.* Dec 2016;22(12):599–606. https:// doi.org/10.12968/ijpn.2016.22.12.599.

30. Howick J, Moscrop A, Mebius A, et al. Effects of empathic and positive communication in healthcare consultations: A systematic review and meta-analysis. *J R Soc Med.* Jan 1 2018:141076818769477. https://doi.org/10.1177 /0141076818769477.

31. *The Oxford English Dictionary,* online version. www.oed.com.

32. Mercer SW, Reynolds WJ. Empathy and quality of care. *Br J Gen Pract.* Oct 2002;52 Suppl:S9–S12.

33. Howick J, Bizzari V, Dambha-Miller H, Oxford Empathy P. Therapeutic empathy: What it is and what it isn't. *J R Soc Med.* Jul 2018;111(7):233–236. https:// doi.org/10.1177/0141076818781403.

34. Halpern J. *From Detached Concern to Empathy: Humanizing Medical Practice.* Oxford University Press; 2011.

35. Winter, R., et al., Assessing the effect of empathy-enhancing interventions in health education and training: A systematic review of randomised controlled trials. *BMJ Open,* 2020. 10(9): e036471. https://doi.org/10.1136/bmjopen-2019-036471.

36. Howick J, Moscrop A, Mebius A, et al. Effects of empathic and positive communication in healthcare consultations: A systematic review and meta-analysis. *J R Soc Med.* Jan 1 2018:141076818769477. https://doi.org/10.1177/0141076818769477.

37. Chassany O, Boureau F, Liard F, et al. Effects of training on general practitioners' management of pain in osteoarthritis: A randomized multicenter study. *J Rheumatol* 2006;33(9):1827–1834.

38. Lloyd SM, Cantell M, Pacaud D, Crawford S, Dewey D. Brief report: Hope, perceived maternal empathy, medical regimen adherence, and glycemic control in adolescents with type 1 diabetes. *J Pediatr Psychol.* Oct 2009;34(9):1025–1029. https://doi.org/10.1093/jpepsy/jsn141.

39. Boswell K, Cook C, Burch S, Eaddy M, Cantrell R. Associating medication adherence with improved outcomes: A systematic literature review. *Am J Pharm Benefits.* 2012;4(4):e97–e108.

40. Butler CC, Pill R, Stott NC. Qualitative study of patients' perceptions of doctors' advice to quit smoking: Implications for opportunistic health promotion. *BMJ.* Jun 20 1998;316(7148):1878–1881. https://doi.org/10.1136/bmj.316.7148.1878.

41. Choi SM, Lee J, Park YS, Lee CH, Lee SM, Yim JJ. Effect of verbal empathy and touch on anxiety relief in patients undergoing flexible bronchoscopy: Can empathy reduce patients' anxiety? *Respiration.* 2016;92(6):380–388. https://doi.org/10.1159/000450960.

42. Knight LK, Stoica T, Fogleman ND, Depue BE. Convergent neural correlates of empathy and anxiety during socioemotional processing. *Front Hum Neurosci.* 2019;13:94. https://doi.org/10.3389/fnhum.2019.00094.

43. Kroenke K, Outcalt S, Krebs E, et al. Association between anxiety, health-related quality of life and functional impairment in primary care patients with chronic pain. *Gen Hosp Psychiatry.* Jul–Aug 2013;35(4):359–65. https://doi.org/10.1016/j.genhosppsych.2013.03.020.

44. Pereira Gray DJ, Sidaway-Lee K, White E, Thorne A, Evans PH. Continuity of care with doctors—a matter of life and death? A systematic review of continuity of care and mortality. *BMJ Open.* Jun 28 2018;8(6):e021161. https://doi.org/10.1136/bmjopen-2017-021161.

45. Thomas KB. General practice consultations: Is there any point in being positive? *BMJ (Clin Res Ed).* 1987 May 9;294(6581):1200–1202. https://doi.org/10.1136/bmj.294.6581.1200.

46. Howick J, Lyness E, Albury C, et al. Anatomy of positive messages in healthcare consultations: Component analysis of messages within 22 randomised trials. *European Journal for Person-Centered Healthcare.* 2020;7(4).

47. Barnes K, Faasse K, Geers AL, et al. Can positive framing reduce nocebo side effects? Current evidence and recommendation for future research. *Front Pharmacol.* 2019;10:167. https://doi.org/10.3389/fphar.2019.00167.

48. Benedetti F, Maggi G, Lopiano L, et al. Open versus hidden medical treatments: The patient's knowledge about a therapy affects the therapy outcome. *Prevention and Treatment.* 2003;6(1). https://doi.org/10.1037/1522-3736.6.1.61a.

49. Colloca L, Barsky AJ. Placebo and nocebo effects. *N Engl J Med.* Feb 6 2020;382(6):554–561. https://doi.org/10.1056/NEJMra1907805.

50. Howe LC, Goyer JP, Crum AJ. Harnessing the placebo effect: Exploring the influence of physician characteristics on placebo response. *Health Psychology.* 2017;36(11):1074–1082. https://doi.org/10.1037/hea0000499.

51. Kaptchuk TJ, Kelley JM, Conboy LA, et al. Components of placebo effect: Randomised controlled trial in patients with irritable bowel syndrome. *BMJ.* May 3 2008;336(7651):999–1003. https://doi.org/10.1136/bmj.39524.439618.25.

52. Beckman HB, Frankel RM. The effect of physician behavior on the collection of data. *Ann Intern Med.* Nov 1984;101(5):692–696. https://doi.org/10.7326/0003-4819-101-5-692.

53. Langewitz W, Denz M, Keller A, Kiss A, Ruttimann S, Wossmer B. Spontaneous talking time at start of consultation in outpatient clinic: Cohort study. *BMJ.* Sep 28 2002;325(7366):682–683. https://doi.org/10.1136/bmj.325.7366.682.

54. Beecher HK. Relationship of significance of wound to pain experienced. *JAMA* Aug 25 1956;161(17):1609–1613. https://doi.org/10.1001/jama.1956.02970170005002.

55. Ulrich RS. View through a window may influence recovery from surgery. *Science.* Apr 27 1984;224(4647):420–421. https://doi.org/10.1126/science.6143402.

56. Ulrich RS, Cordoza M, Gardiner SK, et al. ICU patient family stress recovery during breaks in a hospital garden and indoor environments. *HERD.* Aug 7 2019:1937586719867157. https://doi.org/10.1177/1937586719867157.

57. Donovan GH, Gatziolis D, Douwes J. Relationship between exposure to the natural environment and recovery from hip or knee arthroplasty: A New Zealand retrospective cohort study. *BMJ Open.* Sep 20 2019;9(9):e029522. https://doi.org/10.1136/bmjopen-2019-029522.

58. Tse MM, Ng JK, Chung JW, Wong TK. The effect of visual stimuli on pain threshold and tolerance. *J Clin Nurs.* Jul 2002;11(4):462–469. https://doi.org/10.1046/j.1365-2702.2002.00608.x.

59. Diette GB, Lechtzin N, Haponik E, Devrotes A, Rubin HR. Distraction therapy with nature sights and sounds reduces pain during flexible bronchoscopy: A complementary approach to routine analgesia. *Chest.* Mar 2003;123(3):941–948. https://doi.org/10.1378/chest.123.3.941.

60. Sandal LF, Thorlund JB, Moore AJ, Ulrich RS, Dieppe PA, Roos EM. Room for improvement: A randomised controlled trial with nested qualitative interviews

on space, place and treatment delivery. *Br J Sports Med.* Mar 2019;53(6):359–367. https://doi.org/10.1136/bjsports-2016-097448.

61. Zhang Y, Tzortzopoulos P, Kagioglou M. Healing built-environment effects on health outcomes: Environment–occupant–health framework. *Building Research & Information.* 2018;47(6):747–766. https://doi.org/10.1080 /09613218.2017.1411130.

62. Eklund A, De Carvalho D, Page I, et al. Expectations influence treatment outcomes in patients with low back pain: A secondary analysis of data from a randomized clinical trial. *Eur J Pain.* Aug 2019;23(7):1378–1389. https://doi.org /10.1002/ejp.1407.

63. Rief W, Shedden-Mora MC, Laferton JA, et al. Preoperative optimization of patient expectations improves long-term outcome in heart surgery patients: Results of the randomized controlled PSY-HEART trial. *BMC Med.* Jan 10 2017;15(1):4. https://doi.org/10.1186/s12916-016-0767-3.

64. Rosenthal R, Jacobson LF. *Pygmalion in the Classroom: Teacher Expectation and Pupils' Intellectual Development.* Irvington Publishers; 1992.

65. Gracely RH, Dubner R, Deeter WR, Wolskee PJ. Clinicians' expectations influence placebo analgesia. *Lancet.* Jan 5 1985;1(8419):43. https://doi.org/10.1016 /s0140-6736(85)90984-5.

66. Chen PA, Cheong JH, Jolly E, Elhence H, Wager TD, Chang LJ. Socially transmitted placebo effects. *Nat Hum Behav.* Dec 2019;3(12):1295–1305. https://doi .org/10.1038/s41562-019-0749-5.

67. RxList. Morphine Tablets. WebMD. Accessed May 21, 2021. https://www .rxlist.com/morphine-tablets-drug.htm.

68. Thirioux B, Birault F, Jaafari N. Empathy is a protective factor of burnout in physicians: New neuro-phenomenological hypotheses regarding empathy and sympathy in care relationship. *Frontiers in Psychology.* May 26 2016;7. https://doi .org/Artn 76310.3389/Fpsyg.2016.00763.

69. Physician burnout: A global crisis. *Lancet.* Jul 13 2019;394(10193):93. https://doi.org/10.1016/S0140-6736(19)31573-9.

70. Rotenstein LS, Torre M, Ramos MA, et al. Prevalence of burnout among physicians: A systematic review. *JAMA.* Sep 18 2018;320(11):1131–1150. https://doi .org/10.1001/jama.2018.12777.

71. Fahrenkopf AM, Sectish TC, Barger LK, et al. Rates of medication errors among depressed and burnt-out residents: Prospective cohort study. *BMJ.* Mar 1 2008;336(7642):488–491. https://doi.org/10.1136/bmj.39469.763218.BE.

72. Kumar G, Mezoff A. Physician burnout at a children's hospital: Incidence, interventions, and impact. Pediatr Qual Saf. Sep–Oct 2020;5(5):e345. https://doi .org/10.1097/pq9.0000000000000345.

73. 66. Di Blasi Z, Harkness E, Ernst E, Georgiou A, Kleijnen J. Influence of context effects on health outcomes: A systematic review. *Lancet.* Mar 10 2001;357(9258):757–762. https://doi.org/10.1016/s0140-6736(00)04169-6.

74. Moerman DE. *Meaning, Medicine, and the "Placebo Effect."* Cambridge University Press; 2002.

75. Benedetti F. *Placebo Effects: Understanding the Mechanisms in Health and Disease.* 3d ed. Oxford University Press; 2020.

Chapter 4. It Depends

1. de Craen AJ, Kaptchuk TJ, Tijssen JG, Kleijnen J. Placebos and placebo effects in medicine: historical overview. *J R Soc Med.* 1999 Oct;92(10):511-5. doi: 10.1177/014107689909201005.

2. Howick J. Reviewing the unsubstantiated claims for the methodological superiority of 'placebo' over 'active' controlled trials: Reply to open peer commentaries. *Am J Bioeth.* 2009;9(9):W5–W7. https://doi.org/10.1080/15265160903149417.

3. Howick J. Questioning the methodologic superiority of 'placebo' over 'active' controlled trials. *Am J Bioeth.* Sep 2009;9(9):34–48. https://doi.org/10.1080/15265160903090041.

4. Flint A. A contribution toward the natural history of articular rheumatism: Consisting of a report of thirteen cases treated solely with palliative measures. *American Journal of Medical Science.* 1863;46:17–36.

5. Chalmers I, Tröhler U, Badenoch D, Glasziou P, Podolsky S. *The James Lind Library.* Accessed August 20. 2018. http://www.jameslindlibrary.org/

6. Haygarth J. *Of the Imagination, as a Cause and as a Cure of Disorders of the Body: Exemplified by Fictitious Tractors, and Epidemical Convulsions.* R. Crutwell; 1800.

7. Hermann D. Amtlicher Bericht des Herrn D. Herrmann über die homöopathische Behandlung im Militärhospitale zu Tulzyn in Podolien. *Annalen der homöopathischen Klinik* 1831;2:380–399.

8. Lichtenstädt J. Beschluss des Kaiserl. Russ. Menicinalraths [sic] in Beziehung auf die homöopathische Heilmethode. *Litterarische Annalen der gesammten Heilkunde* 1832;24:412–420 [German translation of: Ministry of Internal Affairs (Conclusion of the Medical Council regarding homeopathic treatment). *Zhurnal Ministerstva Vnutrennih del 1823.* 1823;3:49–63.

9. Stolberg M. Inventing the randomized double-blind trial: The Nuremberg salt test of 1835. *J R Soc Med.* Dec 2006;99(12):642–643. https://doi.org/10.1258/jrsm.99.12.642

10. Dean ME. An innocent "deception": Placebo controls in the St Petersburg homeopathy trial. *JLL Bulletin.* 2003:1829–1830. https://doi.org/10.1177/014107680609900726.

11. Golomb BA, Erickson LC, Koperski S, Sack D, Enkin M, Howick J. What's in placebos: who knows? Analysis of randomized, controlled trials. *Ann Intern Med.* 2010 Oct 19;153(8):532–535. http://doi.org/10.7326/0003-4819-153-8-201010190-00010.

12. Webster RK, Howick J, Hoffmann T, Macdonald H, Collins GS, Rees JL, et al. Inadequate description of placebo and sham controls in a systematic review of recent trials. *Eur J Clin Invest.* 2019;49(11):e13169. https://doi.org/10.1111/eci.13169.

13. Howick J. *The Philosophy of Evidence-Based Medicine.* Wiley-Blackwell; 2011.

14. Folegatti PM, Ewer KJ, Aley PK, et al. Safety and immunogenicity of the ChAdOx1 nCoV-19 vaccine against SARS-CoV-2: A preliminary report of a phase 1/2, single-blind, randomised controlled trial. *Lancet.* Aug 15 2020;396(10249):467–478. https://doi.org/10.1016/S0140<H>>6736(20)31604-4

15. Furukawa T, McGuire H, Barbui C. Low dosage tricyclic antidepressants for depression. *Cochrane Database Syst Rev.* 2003;(3):CD003197. https://doi.org/10.1002/14651858.CD003197.

16. Moncrieff J, Wessely S, Hardy R. Active placebos versus antidepressants for depression. *Cochrane Database Syst Rev.* 2004;(1):CD003012. https://doi.org/10.1002/14651858.CD003012.pub2.

17. Jefferson T, Jones M, Doshi P, Spencer EA, Onakpoya I, Heneghan CJ. Oseltamivir for influenza in adults and children: Systematic review of clinical study reports and summary of regulatory comments. *BMJ.* 2014;348:g2545. https://doi.org/10.1136/bmj.g2545.

18. Golomb B. Paradox of placebo effect. *Nature.* Jun 15 1995;375(6532):530.

19. Gyotoku T, Aurelian L, Neurath AR. Cellulose acetate phthalate (CAP): An "inactive" pharmaceutical excipient with antiviral activity in the mouse model of genital herpesvirus infection. *Antivir Chem Chemother.* Nov 1999;10(6):327–332. https://doi.org/10.1177/095632029901000604

20. BBC News. Pill coating "kills HIV." Accessed July 23, 2008. http://news.bbc.co.uk/1/hi/health/398041.stm.

21. Loprinzi CL, Ellison NM, Schaid DJ, et al. Controlled trial of megestrol acetate for the treatment of cancer anorexia and cachexia. *J Natl Cancer Inst.* Jul 4 1990;82(13):1127–1132. https://doi.org/10.1093/jnci/82.13.1127.

22. Osterlund P, Ruotsalainen T, Peuhkuri K, et al. Lactose intolerance associated with adjuvant 5-fluorouracil-based chemotherapy for colorectal cancer. *Clin Gastroenterol Hepatol.* Aug 2004;2(8):696–703. https://doi.org/10.1016/s1542-3565(04)00293-9

23. Almutairi R, Basson AR, Wearsh P, Cominelli F, Rodriguez-Palacios A. Validity of food additive maltodextrin as placebo and effects on human gut physiology: Systematic review of placebo-controlled clinical trials. *Eur J Nutr.* Mar 1 2022. https://doi.org/10.1007/s00394-022-02802-5.

24. Sihvonen R, Paavola M, Malmivaara A, et al. Arthroscopic partial meniscectomy versus sham surgery for a degenerative meniscal tear. *N Engl J Med.* Dec 26 2013;369(26):2515–2524. https://doi.org/10.1056/NEJMoa1305189.

25. Moseley JB, O'Malley K, Petersen NJ, et al. A controlled trial of arthroscopic surgery for osteoarthritis of the knee. *N Engl J Med.* Jul 11 2002;347(2):81–88.

26. Zeidan F, Johnson SK, Diamond BJ, David Z, Goolkasian P. Mindfulness meditation improves cognition: Evidence of brief mental training. *Consciousness and Cognition.* Jun 2010;19(2):597–605. https://doi.org/10.1016/j.concog.2010.03.014

27. Semple RJ. Does mindfulness meditation enhance attention? A randomized controlled trial. *Mindfulness.* June 1 2010;1(2):121–130. https://doi.org/10.1007 /s12671-010-0017-2.

28. Posadzki P, Pieper D, Bajpai R, et al. Exercise/physical activity and health outcomes: An overview of Cochrane systematic reviews. *BMC Public Health.* Nov 16 2020;20(1):1724. https://doi.org/10.1186/s12889-020-09855-3.

29. McCall MC, Heneghan C, Nunan D. Does physical exercise prevent or treat acute respiratory infection (ARI)? Oxford Centre for Evidence-Based Medicine. Accessed June 4, 2021. https://www.cebm.net/covid-19/does-physical-exercise -prevent-or-treat-acute-respiratory-infection-ari/.

30. Brown BS, Payne T, Kim C, Moore G, Krebs P, Martin W. Chronic response of rat brain norepinephrine and serotonin levels to endurance training. *Journal of Applied Physiology: Respiratory, Environmental and Exercise Physiology.* Jan 1979;46(1):19–23. https://doi.org/10.1152/jappl.1979.46.1.19.

31. Koch G, Johansson U, Arvidsson E. Radioenzymatic determination of epineph-rine, norepinephrine, and dopamine in 0.1 mL plasma samples: Plasma catecholamine response to submaximal and near maximal exercise. *Journal of Clinical Chemistry and Clinical Biochemistry.* 1980:367–372. https://doi.org/10.1515/cclm.1980.18.6.367.

32. McCann IL, Holmes DS. Influence of aerobic exercise on depression. *J Pers Soc Psychol.* May 1984;46(5):1142–1147. https://doi.org/10.1037//0022-3514.46 .5.1142.

33. Dunn AL, Trivedi MH, Kampert JB, Clark CG, Chambliss HO. The DOSE study: A clinical trial to examine efficacy and dose response of exercise as treat-ment for depression. *Control Clin Trials.* Oct 2002;23(5):584–603. https://doi.org /10.1016/s0197-2456(02)00226-x.

34. Benson H. *The Relaxation Response.* Morrow; 1975

35. Jorm AF, Morgan AJ, Hetrick SE. Relaxation for depression. *Cochrane Database Syst Rev.* Oct 8 2008;(4):CD007142. https://doi.org/10.1002/14651858.CD007142.pub2.

36. Brinsley J, Schuch F, Lederman O, et al. Effects of yoga on depressive symptoms in people with mental disorders: A systematic review and meta-analysis. *Br J Sports Med.* May 18 2020. https://doi.org/10.1136/bjsports-2019-101242.

37. Kaptchuk TJ. The placebo effect in alternative medicine: Can the performance of a healing ritual have clinical significance? *Ann Intern Med.* Jun 4 2002;136(11):817–825. https://doi.org/10.7326/0003-4819-136-11-200206040-00011.

38. Streitberger K, Kleinhenz J. Introducing a placebo needle into acupuncture research. *Lancet.* Aug 1 1998;352(9125):364–365. https://doi.org/10.1016/S0140 -6736(97)10471-8.

39. Linde K, Niemann K, Meissner K. Are sham acupuncture interventions more effective than (other) placebos? A re-analysis of data from the Cochrane review on placebo effects. *Forschende Komplementarmedizin.* Oct 2010;17(5):259–264. https:// doi.org/10.1159/000320374.

40. Furlan AD, van Tulder M, Cherkin D, et al. Acupuncture and dry-needling for low back pain: An updated systematic review within the framework of the Cochrane collaboration. *Spine*. Apr 15 2005;30(8):944–963. https://doi.org/10.1097/01.brs.0000158941.21571.01.

41. Ernst E. Acupuncture—a critical analysis. *Journal of Internal Medicine*. Feb 2006;259(2):125–137. https://doi.org/10.1111/j.1365-2796.2005.01584.x.

42. Kaptchuk TJ, Kelley JM, Conboy LA, Davis RB, Kerr CE, Jacobson EE, Kirsch I, Schyner RN, Nam BH, Nguyen LT, Park M, Rivers AL, McManus C, Kokkotou E, Drossman DA, Goldman P, Lembo AJ. Components of placebo effect: Randomised controlled trial in patients with irritable bowel syndrome. *BMJ*. 2008 May 3;336(7651):999–1003. https://doi.org/10.1136/bmj.39524.439618.25.

43. Chen YW, Wang HH. The effectiveness of acupressure on relieving pain: a systematic review. Pain Manag Nurs. 2014 Jun;15(2):539–50. https://doi.org/10.1016/j.pmn.2012.12.005.

44. Laudan L. A confutation of convergent realism. *Philosophy of Science*. 1981;48(Mar. 1981)(1):19–49.

45. Frank JD, Frank JB. *Persuasion and Healing: A Comparative Study of Psychotherapy*. 3d ed. Johns Hopkins University Press; 1991.

46. Kirsch, I. Placebo psychotherapy: Synonym or oxymoron? *J Clin Psychol*, 61(2005)(7), 791–803. https://doi.org/10.1002/jclp.20126.

47. Aycock DM, Hayat MJ, Helvig A, Dunbar SB, Clark PC. Essential considerations in developing attention control groups in behavioral research. *Res Nurs Health*. Jun 2018;41(3):320–328. https://doi.org/10.1002/nur.21870.

48. Barth J, Munder T, Gerger H, et al. Comparative efficacy of seven psychotherapeutic interventions for patients with depression: A network meta-analysis. *PLoS Med*. 2013;10(5):e1001454. https://doi.org/10.1371/journal.pmed.1001454.

49. Blease CR. Psychotherapy and placebos: Manifesto for conceptual clarity. *Front Psychiatry*. 2018;9:379. https://doi.org/10.3389/fpsyt.2018.00379.

50. Jakobsen JC, Lindschou Hansen J, Storebo OJ, Simonsen E, Gluud C. The effects of cognitive therapy versus 'treatment as usual' in patients with major depressive disorder. *PLoS One*. 2011;6(8):e22890. https://doi.org/10.1371/journal.pone.0022890.

51. Jakobsen JC, Hansen JL, Simonsen E, Gluud C. The effect of interpersonal psychotherapy and other psychodynamic therapies versus "treatment as usual" in patients with major depressive disorder. *PLoS One*. Apr 27 2011;6(4):e19044. https://doi.org/10.1371/journal.pone.0019044.

52. Aycock, D. M., Clark, P. C., & Hayat, M.(2016). Reducing stroke risk in young adult African Americans: A feasibility study. *Research in Nursing and Health, 40*, 153–164. https://doi.org/10.1002/nur.21776.

53. Pagoto SL, McDermott MM, Reed G, et al. Can attention control conditions have detrimental effects on behavioral medicine randomized trials? *Psychosom Med.* Feb 2013;75(2):137–143. https://doi.org/10.1097/PSY.0b013e3182765dd2.

54. Frank J. Expectation and therapeutic outcome: The placebo effect and the role induction interview. In Frank JD, Hoehn-Saric R, Imber S, Liberman BL, and Stone AR. Effective ingredients of successful psychotherapy, pp. 1–47. 1978: Burnner/Mazel.

55. Lipsey MW, Wilson DB. The efficacy of psychological, educational, and behavioral treatment: Confirmation from meta-analysis. *Am Psychol.* Dec 1993;48(12):1181–1209. https://doi.org/10.1037//0003-066x.48.12.1181

56. Golomb BA, Erickson LC, Koperski S, Sack D, Enkin M, Howick J. What's in placebos: who knows? Analysis of randomized, controlled trials. *Ann Intern Med.* Oct 19 2010;153(8):532–5. https://doi.org/10.7326/0003-4819-153-8-201010190-00010.

57. Webster RK, Howick J, Hoffmann T, et al. Inadequate description of placebo and sham controls in a systematic review of recent trials. *Eur J Clin Invest.* Nov 2019;49(11):e13169. https://doi.org/10.1111/eci.13169.

58. Bello S, Wei M, Hilden J, Hróbjartsson A. The matching quality of experimental and control interventions in blinded pharmacological randomised clinical trials: A methodological systematic review. *BMC Med Res Methodol.* 2016;16:18. https://doi.org/10.1186/s12874-016-0111-9.

54. Senn S, Chalmers I. Giving and taking: Ethical treatment assignment in controlled trials. *Journal of the Royal Society of Medicine.* 2021;114(11):525–530. https://doi.org/10.1177/01410768211049972.

55. Turner A. "Placebos" and the logic of placebo comparison. *Biology & Philosophy.* May 2012;27(3):419–432. https://doi.org/10.1007/s10539-011-9289-8.

56. Gøtzsche P. Is there logic in the placebo? *Lancet.* Oct 1 1994;344(8927):925–926. https://doi.org/10.1016/s0140-6736(94)92273-x

57. Grünbaum A. The placebo concept in medicine and psychiatry. *Psychol Med.* Feb 1986;16(1):19–38. https://doi.org/10.1017/s0033291700002506.

58. Dunn AL, Trivedi MH, Kampert JB, Clark CG, Chambliss HO. Exercise treatment for depression: Efficacy and dose response. *Am J Prev Med.* Jan 2005;28(1):1–8. https://doi.org/10.1016/j.amepre.2004.09.003

Part II. In Search of Placebo and Nocebo Effects

1. Moerman DE. *Meaning, Medicine, and the 'Placebo Effect.'* Cambridge University Press; 2002.

2. Klopfer B. Psychological variables in human cancer. *J Proj Tech.* Dec 1957;21(4):331–340. https://doi.org/10.1080/08853126.1957.10380794.

3. Moses J. Did a man cure his lymphoma with the power of belief? The case of Mr. Wright. *A Better Question.* Accessed September 16, 2021. https://www.youtube.com/watch?v=j7JtmTdlDqE.

Chapter 5. How (Not to) Measure Nocebo and Placebo Effects

1. Kirsch I, Sapirstein G. Listening to Prozac but hearing placebo: A meta-analysis of antidepressant medication. *Prevention & Treatment*. June 26 1998;1(2). https://doi.org/10.1037/1522-3736.1.1.12a.

2. Beecher HK. The powerful placebo. *J Am Med Assoc*. Dec 24 1955;159(17):1602–1606. https://doi.org/10.1001/jama.1955.0296034002200.

3. Howick J. *The Philosophy of Evidence-Based Medicine*. Wiley-Blackwell; 2011.

4. Symington B. When less is more; or, Acknowledging the value of tincture of time. *J Clin Oncol*. Jul 20 2020;38(21):2463–2465. https://doi.org/10.1200/JCO.20.00720.

5. Jessy T. Immunity over inability: The spontaneous regression of cancer. *J Nat Sci Biol Med*. Jan 2011;2(1):43–9. https://doi.org/10.4103/0976-9668.82318.

6. Cochrane JA. *Effectiveness and Efficiency: Random Reflections on Health Services*. Nuffield Provincial Hospitals Trust; 1972.

7. Kienle GS, Kiene H. The powerful placebo effect: fact or fiction? *J Clin Epidemiol*. Dec 1997;50(12):1311–1318. https://doi.org/10.1016/s0895-4356(97)00203-5.

8. Kirsch I, Sapirstein G. Listening to Prozac but hearing placebo: A meta-analysis of antidepressant medication. In Kirsch I, ed., *How Expectancies Shape Experience*. American Psychological Association (1999), 303–20. https://doi.org/10.1037/10332-012.

9. Hróbjartsson A, Gøtzsche P. Is the placebo powerless? An analysis of clinical trials comparing placebo with no treatment. *N Engl J Med*. May 24 2001;344(21):1594–1602. https://doi.org/10.1056/NEJM200105243442106.

10. Hróbjartsson A, Gøtzsche P. Placebo interventions for all clinical conditions. *Cochrane Database Syst Rev*. 2004b;(3):CD003974. https://doi.org/10.1002/14651858.CD003974.pub2.

11. Hróbjartsson A, Gøtzsche P. Placebo interventions for all clinical conditions. *Cochrane Database Syst Rev*. Jan 20 2010;(1):CD003974. https://doi.org/10.1002/14651858.CD003974.pub3.

12. Herbert JD, Gaudiano BA. Moving from empirically supported treatment lists to practice guidelines in psychotherapy: The role of the placebo concept. *J Clin Psychol*. Jul 2005;61(7):893–908. https://doi.org/10.1002/jclp.20133.

13. Kirsch I. Placebo psychotherapy: Synonym or oxymoron? *J Clin Psychol*. Jul 2005;61(7):791–803.https://doi.org/10.1002/jclp.20126.

14. Lambert MJ. Early response in psychotherapy: Further evidence for the importance of common factors rather than "placebo effects." *J Clin Psychol*. Jul 2005;61(7):855–69. https://doi.org/10.1002/jclp.20130.

15. Wampold BE, Minami T, Tierney SC, Baskin TW, Bhati KS. The placebo is powerful: Estimating placebo effects in medicine and psychotherapy from randomized clinical trials. *J Clin Psychol*. Jul 2005;61(7):835–54. https://doi.org/10.1002/jclp.20129.

16. Higgins JJ, Green S. *The Cochrane Handbook for Systematic Reviews of Interventions*. Version 5.1.0 [updated March 2011] The Cochrane Collaboration; 2011.

17. Kirsch I. Yes, there is a placebo effect, but is there a powerful antidepressant effect? *Prevention and Treatment* 2002;5(22).

18. Scharf HP, Mansmann U, Streitberger K, et al. Acupuncture and knee osteoarthritis: A three-armed randomized trial. *Ann Intern Med*. Jul 4 2006;145(1):12–20. https://doi.org/10.7326/0003-4819-145-1-200607040-00005.

19. Etter JF, Laszlo E, Zellweger JP, Perrot C, Perneger TV. Nicotine replacement to reduce cigarette consumption in smokers who are unwilling to quit: A randomized trial. *J Clin Psychopharmacol*. Oct 2002;22(5):487–95. https://doi.org/10.1097/00004714-200210000-00008.

20. Ditto B, France CR, Lavoie P, Roussos M, Adler PS. Reducing reactions to blood donation with applied muscle tension: A randomized controlled trial. *Transfusion*. Sep 2003;43(9):1269–75. https://doi.org/10.1046/j.1537-2995.2003.00488.x.

21. Krogsbøll LT, Hróbjartsson A, Gøtzsche PC. Spontaneous improvement in randomised clinical trials: Meta-analysis of three-armed trials comparing no treatment, placebo and active intervention. *BMC Med Res Methodol*. 2009 Jan 5;9:1. https://doi.org/10.1186/1471-2288-9-1.

22. Hróbjartsson A, Gøtzsche P. Is the placebo powerless? Update of a systematic review with 52 new randomized trials comparing placebo with no treatment. *J Intern Med*. Aug 2004;256(2):91–100. http://doi.org/10.1111/j.1365-2796.2004.01355.x.

23. Saretsky G. The OEO P.C. Experiment and the John Henry Effect. *Phi Delta Kappan*. 1972;53(9):578–581. https://www.jstor.org/stable/20373317.

24. Roethlisberger FJ, Dickson WJ. *Management and the Worker*. Harvard University Press; 1939.

25. Franke RH, Kaul JD. The Hawthorne Experiments: First statistical interpretation. *American Sociological Review*. 1978;43(5):623–643. https://www.jstor.org/stable/2094540.

26. McCambridge J, Witton J, Elbourne DR. Systematic review of the Hawthorne effect: New concepts are needed to study research participation effects. *J Clin Epidemiol*. Mar 2014;67(3):267–277. https://doi.org/10.1016/j.jclinepi.2013.08.015.

27. Mayo E. *The Human Problems of an Industrial Civilization*. Routledge; 2003.

28. Gøtzsche P. Blinding during data analysis and writing of manuscripts. *Control Clin Trials*. Aug 1996;17(4):285–290; discussion 290–293. https://doi.org/10.1016/0197-2456(95)00263-4.

29. Fisher JP, Hassan DT, O' CN. Minerva. *BMJ*. 1995;310(70). https://doi.org/10.1136/bmj.310.6971.70.

30. Meador CK. Hex death: Voodoo magic or persuasion? *South Med J*. Mar 1992;85(3):244–247.

31. Howick J, Webster R, Kirby N, Hood K. Rapid overview of systematic reviews of nocebo effects in clinical trials. *Trials*. 2018 Dec 11;19(1):674. https://doi.org/10.1186/s13063-018-3042-4.

32. Mitsikostas DD, Chalarakis NG, Mantonakis LI, Delicha EM, Sfikakis PP. Nocebo in fibromyalgia: Meta-analysis of placebo-controlled clinical trials and implications for practice. *Eur J Neurol*. May 2012;19(5):672–680. https://doi.org/10.1111/j.1468-1331.2011.03528.x.

33. Mitsikostas DD, Mantonakis L, Chalarakis N. Nocebo in clinical trials for depression: A meta-analysis. *Psychiatry Res*. Jan 30 2014;215(1):82–86. https://doi.org/10.1016/j.psychres.2013.10.019.

34. Mitsikostas DD, Mantonakis LI, Chalarakis NG. Nocebo is the enemy, not placebo: A meta-analysis of reported side effects after placebo treatment in headaches. *Cephalalgia*. Apr 2011;31(5):550–61. https://doi.org/10.1177/0333102410391485.

35. Chou R, Dana T, Blazina I, Daeges M, Jeanne TL. Statins for prevention of cardiovascular disease in adults: Evidence report and systematic review for the US Preventive Services Task Force. *JAMA*. Nov 15 2016;316(19):2008–2024. https://doi.org/10.1001/jama.2015.15629.

36. Finegold JA, Manisty CH, Goldacre B, Barron AJ, Francis DP. What proportion of symptomatic side effects in patients taking statins are genuinely caused by the drug? Systematic review of randomized placebo-controlled trials to aid individual patient choice. *Eur J Prev Cardiol*. Apr 2014;21(4):464–474. https://doi.org/10.1177/2047487314525531.

37. Howick J. *Doctor You: Revealing the Science of Self-Healing*. Hodder & Stoughton; 2017.

38. Vinogradova Y, Coupland C, Brindle P, Hippisley-Cox J. Discontinuation and restarting in patients on statin treatment: Prospective open cohort study using a primary care database. *BMJ*. Jun 28 2016;353:i3305. https://doi.org/10.1136/bmj.i3305.

39. Zhang H, Plutzky J, Skentzos S, et al. Discontinuation of statins in routine care settings: A cohort study. *Ann Intern Med*. Apr 2 2013;158(7):526–534. https://doi.org/10.7326/0003-4819-158-7-201304020-00004.

Chapter 6. Missing the Forest for the Trees

1. Caspi O, Bootzin RR. Evaluating how placebos produce change: Logical and causal traps and understanding cognitive explanatory mechanisms. *Evaluation & the Health Professions*. Dec 2002;25(4):436–464. https://doi.org/10.1177/0163278702238056.

2. Benedetti F. *Placebo Effects: Understanding the Mechanisms in Health and Disease*. 3d ed. Oxford University Press; 2020.

3. Colloca L, ed. *Neurobiology of the Placebo Effect*. Elsevier; 2018.

4. Colloca L, Barsky AJ. Placebo and nocebo effects. *N Engl J Med*. Feb 6 2020;382(6):554–561. https://doi.org/10.1056/NEJMra1907805.

5. Wolf S. Effects of suggestion and conditioning on the action of chemical agents in human subjects: The pharmacology of placebos. *J Clin Invest.* (1950) 29:100–109. https://doi.org/10.1172/JCI102225.

6. Lasagna L, Laties VG, Dohan JL. Further studies on the pharmacology of placebo administration. *J Clin Invest.* (1958) 37:533–537. https://doi.org/10.1172/JCI103635.

7. Benedetti, Fabrizio. Historical evolution of the scientific investigation of the placebo analgesic effect. *Frontiers in Pain Research.* 3 (2022): 961304. https://doi.org/10.3389/fpain.2022.961304.

8. Levine JD, Gordon NC, Fields HL. The mechanism of placebo analgesia. *Lancet.* 1978 Sep 23;2(8091):654–7. https://doi.org/10.1016/s0140-6736(78)92762-9.

9. Petrovic P, Kalso E, Petersson KM, Andersson J, Fransson P, Ingvar M. A prefrontal non-opioid mechanism in placebo analgesia. *Pain.* Jul 2010;150(1):59–65. https://doi.org/10.1016/j.pain.2010.03.011.

10. Zubieta JK, Bueller JA, Jackson LR, et al. Placebo effects mediated by endogenous opioid activity on mu-opioid receptors. *J Neurosci.* Aug 24 2005;25(34):7754–7762. https://doi.org/10.1523/JNEUROSCI.0439-05.2005.

11. Bingel U, Lorenz J, Schoell E, Weiller C, Buchel C. Mechanisms of placebo analgesia: rACC recruitment of a subcortical antinociceptive network. *Pain.* Jan 2006;120(1–2):8–15. https://doi.org/ 10.1016/j.pain.2005.08.027.

12. Wager TD, Scott DJ, Zubieta JK. Placebo effects on human mu-opioid activity during pain. *Proc Natl Acad Sci.* Jun 26 2007;104(26):11056–61. https://doi.org/10.1073/pnas.0702413104.

13. Benedetti F, Amanzio M, Casadio C, Oliaro A, Maggi G. Blockade of nocebo hyperalgesia by the cholecystokinin antagonist proglumide. *Pain.* Jun 1997;71(2):135–140. https://doi.org/10.1016/s0304-3959(97)03346-0.

14. Skvortsova A, Veldhuijzen DS, Pacheco-Lopez G, et al. Placebo effects in the neuroendocrine system: Conditioning of the oxytocin responses. *Psychosom Med.* Jan 2020;82(1):47–56. https://doi.org/10.1097/PSY.0000000000000759.

15. Benedetti F, Amanzio M, Rosato R, Blanchard C. Nonopioid placebo analgesia is mediated by CB1 cannabinoid receptors. *Nat Med.* Oct 2 2011;17(10):1228–1230. https://doi.org/10.1038/nm.2435.

16. Scott DJ, Stohler CS, Egnatuk CM, Wang H, Koeppe RA, Zubieta JK. Individual differences in reward responding explain placebo-induced expectations and effects. *Neuron.* Jul 19 2007;55(2):325–336. https://doi.org/10.1016/j.neuron.2007.06.028.

17. Elsenbruch S, Roderigo T, Enck P, Benson S. Can a brief relaxation exercise modulate placebo or nocebo effects in a visceral pain model? *Front Psychiatry.* 2019;10:144. https://doi.org/10.3389/fpsyt.2019.00144.

18. Eippert F, Finsterbusch J, Bingel U, Buchel C. Direct evidence for spinal cord involvement in placebo analgesia. *Science.* Oct 16 2009;326(5951):404. https://doi.org/10.1126/science.1180142.

19. Goffaux P, Redmond WJ, Rainville P, Marchand S. Descending analgesia: When the spine echoes what the brain expects. *Pain*. Jul 2007;130(1–2):137–143. https://doi.org/10.1016/j.pain.2006.11.011.

20. Petrovic P, Kalso E, Petersson KM, Ingvar M. Placebo and opioid analgesia: Imaging a shared neuronal network. *Science*. Mar 1 2002;295(5560):1737–40. https://doi.org/10.1126/science.1067176.

21. Wager TD, Rilling JK, Smith EE, et al. Placebo-induced changes in FMRI in the anticipation and experience of pain. *Science*. Feb 20 2004;303(5661):1162–1167. https://doi.org/10.1126/science.1093065.

22. Scott DJ, Stohler CS, Egnatuk CM, Wang H, Koeppe RA, Zubieta JK. Individual differences in reward responding explain placebo-induced expectations and effects. *Neuron*. Jul 19 2007;55(2):325–336. https://doi.org/10.1016/j.neuron .2007.06.028.

23. Hall KT, Loscalzo J, Kaptchuk TJ. Genetics and the placebo effect: The placebome. *Trends Mol Med*. May 2015;21(5):285–294. https://doi.org/10.1016/j .molmed.2015.02.009.

24. Colagiuri B, Schenk LA, Kessler MD, Dorsey SG, Colloca L. The placebo effect: From concepts to genes. *Neuroscience*. Oct 29 2015;307:171–190. https://doi .org/10.1016/j.neuroscience.2015.08.017.

25. Okusogu C, Wang Y, Akintola T, et al. Placebo hypoalgesia: racial differences. *Pain*. Mar 21 2020. https://doi.org/10.1097/j.pain.0000000000001876.

26. Wendt L, Albring A, Benson S, et al. Catechol-O-methyltransferase Val-158Met polymorphism is associated with somatosensory amplification and nocebo responses. *PLoS One*. 2014;9(9):e107665. https://doi.org/10.1371/journal. pone.0107665.

27. Petrovic P, Dietrich T, Fransson P, Andersson J, Carlsson K, Ingvar M. Placebo in emotional processing—induced expectations of anxiety relief activate a generalized modulatory network. Neuron. Jun 16 2005;46(6):957–969. https://doi .org/10.1016/j.neuron.2005.05.023.

28. Colloca L. Nocebo effects can make you feel pain. *Science*. Oct 6 2017; 358(6359):44. https://doi.org/10.1126/science.aap8488.

29. Lorenz J, Hauck M, Paur RC, et al. Cortical correlates of false expectations during pain intensity judgments—a possible manifestation of placebo/nocebo cognitions. *Brain Behav Immun*. Jul 2005;19(4):283–295. https://doi.org/10.1016/j .bbi.2005.03.010.

30. Vogtle E, Barke A, Kroner-Herwig B. Nocebo hyperalgesia induced by social observational learning. *Pain*. Aug 2013;154(8):1427–1433. https://doi.org/10.1016/j .pain.2013.04.041.

31. de la Fuente-Fernandez R, Ruth TJ, Sossi V, Schulzer M, Calne DB, Stoessl AJ. Expectation and dopamine release: Mechanism of the placebo effect in Parkinson's disease. *Science*. Aug 10 2001;293(5532):1164–1166. https://doi.org /10.1126/science.1060937.

32. Benedetti F, Colloca L, Lopiano L, Lanotte M. Overt versus covert treatment for pain, anxiety, and Parkinson's disease. *Lancet Neurology*. 2004;3(Nov 2004). https://doi.org/10.1016/S1474-4422(04)00908-1.

33. Howick J, Webster R, Kirby N, Hood K. Rapid overview of systematic reviews of nocebo effects in clinical trials. *Trials*. 2018 Dec 11;19(1):674. https://doi.org/10.1186/s13063-018-3042-4.

34. Luparello TJ, Leist N, Lourie CH, Sweet P. The interaction of psychologic stimuli and pharmacologic agents on airway reactivity in asthmatic subjects. *Psychosom Med*. Sep–Oct 1970;32(5):509–513. https://doi.org/10.1097/00006842-197009000-00009.

35. Luparello T, Lyons HA, Bleecker ER, McFadden ER, Jr. Influences of suggestion on airway reactivity in asthmatic subjects. *Psychosom Med*. Nov–Dec 1968;30(6):819–825. https://doi.org/10.1097/00006842-196811000-00002.

36. Schweiger A, Parducci A. Nocebo: The psychologic induction of pain. *Pavlov J Biol Sci*. Jul–Sep 1981;16(3):140–143. https://doi.org/10.1007/BF03003218.

37. Mondaini N, Gontero P, Giubilei G, et al. Finasteride 5 mg and sexual side effects: how many of these are related to a nocebo phenomenon? *J Sex Med*. Nov 2007;4(6):1708–1712. https://doi.org/10.1111/j.1743-6109.2007.00563.x.

38. Silvestri A, Galetta P, Cerquetani E, et al. Report of erectile dysfunction after therapy with beta-blockers is related to patient knowledge of side effects and is reversed by placebo. *Eur Heart J*. Nov 2003;24(21):1928–1932. https://doi.org/10.1016/j.ehj.2003.08.016.

39. Kaptchuk TJ, Friedlander E, Kelley JM, et al. Placebos without deception: A randomized controlled trial in irritable bowel syndrome. *PLoS One*. 2010;5(12):e15591. https://doi.org/10.1371/journal.pone.0015591.

40. McMillan FD. The placebo effect in animals. *J Am Vet Med Assoc*. Oct 1 1999;215(7):992–999.

41. Munana KR, Zhang D, Patterson EE. Placebo effect in canine epilepsy trials. *J Vet Intern Med*. Jan–Feb 2010;24(1):166–170. https://doi.org/10.1111/j.1939-1676.2009.0407.x.

42. Ongaro G, Kaptchuk TJ. Symptom perception, placebo effects, and the Bayesian brain. *Pain*. Jan 2019;160(1):1–4. https://doi.org/10.1097/j.pain.0000000000001367.

43. Peerdeman KJ, Geers AL, Della Porta D, Veldhuijzen DS, Kirsch I. Underpredicting pain: an experimental investigation into the benefits and risks. *Pain*. 2021 Jul 1;162(7):2024–2035. https://doi.org/10.1097/j.pain.0000000000002199.

44. Cranston-Cuebas MA, Barlow DH, Mitchell W, Athanasiou R. Differential effects of a misattribution manipulation on sexually functional and dysfunctional men. *J Abnorm Psychol*. Nov 1993;102(4):525–533. https://doi.org/10.1037//0021-843x.102.4.525.

45. Geers AL, Helfer SG, Kosbab K, Weiland PE, Landry SJ. Reconsidering the role of personality in placebo effects: Dispositional optimism, situational

expectations, and the placebo response. *J Psychosom Res.* Feb 2005;58(2):121–127. https://doi.org/10.1016/j.jpsychores.2004.08.011.

46. De Pascalis V, Chiaradia C, Carotenuto E. The contribution of suggestibility and expectation to placebo analgesia phenomenon in an experimental setting. *Pain.* Apr 2002;96(3):393–402. https://doi.org/10.1016/S0304-3959(01)00485-7.

47. Pecina M, Azhar H, Love TM, et al. Personality trait predictors of placebo analgesia and neurobiological correlates. *Neuropsychopharmacology.* Mar 2013;38(4):639–646. https://doi.org/10.1038/npp.2012.227.

48. Schweinhardt P, Seminowicz DA, Jaeger E, Duncan GH, Bushnell MC. The anatomy of the mesolimbic reward system: A link between personality and the placebo analgesic response. *J Neurosci.* Apr 15 2009;29(15):4882–4887. https://doi.org/10.1523/JNEUROSCI.5634-08.2009.

49. Beecher HK. Relationship of significance of wound to pain experienced. *J Am Med Assoc.* Aug 25 1956;161(17):1609–1613. https://doi.org/10.1001/jama.1956.02970170005002.

50. Engel G. The need for a new medical model: A challenge for biomedicine. *Science.* 1977;196:129–136. https://doi.org/10.1126/science.847460.

51. Howick J. *Doctor You: Revealing the Science of Self-healing.* Hodder & Stoughton; 2017.

52. Bradford A, Meston CM. Placebo response in the treatment of women's sexual dysfunctions: A review and commentary. *J Sex Marital Ther.* 2009;35(3):164–181. https://doi.org/10.1080/00926230802716302.

53. McGlashan TH, Evans FJ, Orne MT. The nature of hypnotic analgesia and placebo response to experimental pain. *Psychosom Med.* May–Jun 1969;31(3):227–246. https://doi.org/10.1097/00006842-196905000-00003.

54. Evans FJ. The placebo control of pain: A paradigm for investigating non-specific effects in psychotherapy. In: Brady JP, Mendels J, Reiger WR, T. OM, eds. *Psychiatry: Areas of Promise and Advancement.* Plenum Press; 1977:249–271.

55. Vase L, Robinson ME, Verne GN, Price DD. Increased placebo analgesia over time in irritable bowel syndrome (IBS) patients is associated with desire and expectation but not endogenous opioid mechanisms. *Pain.* Jun 2005;115(3):338–347. https://doi.org/10.1016/j.pain.2005.03.014.

56. Hadamitzky M, Sondermann W, Benson S, Schedlowski M. Placebo effects in the immune system. *Int Rev Neurobiol.* 2018;138:39–59. https://doi.org/10.1016/bs.irn.2018.01.001.

57. Ader R, Mercurio MG, Walton J, et al. Conditioned pharmacotherapeutic effects: A preliminary study. *Psychosom Med.* Feb 2010;72(2):192–197. https://doi.org/10.1097/PSY.0b013e3181cbd38b.

58. Goebel MU, Meykadeh N, Kou W, Schedlowski M, Hengge UR. Behavioral conditioning of antihistamine effects in patients with allergic rhinitis. *Psychother Psychosom.* 2008;77(4):227–234. https://doi.org/10.1159/000126074.

59. Olness K, Ader R. Conditioning as an adjunct in the pharmacotherapy of lupus erythematosus. *J Dev Behav Pediatr.* Apr 1992;13(2):124–125. https://doi.org/10.1097/00004703-199204000-00008.

60. Vits S, Cesko E, Enck P, Hillen U, Schadendorf D, Schedlowski M. Behavioural conditioning as the mediator of placebo responses in the immune system. *Philos Trans R Soc Lond B Biol Sci.* Jun 27 2011;366(1572):1799–1807. https://doi.org/10.1098/rstb.2010.0392.

61. Schenk LA, Krimmel SR, Colloca L. Observe to get pain relief: Current evidence and potential mechanisms of socially learned pain modulation. *Pain.* Nov 2017;158(11):2077–2081. https://doi.org/10.1097/j.pain.0000000000000943.

62. Goodman JE, McGrath PJ. Mothers' modeling influences children's pain during a cold pressor task. *Pain.* Aug 2003;104(3):559–565. https://doi.org/10.1016/s0304-3959(03)00090-3.

63. Colloca L, Benedetti F. Placebo analgesia induced by social observational learning. *Pain.* Jul 2009;144(1–2):28–34. https://doi.org/ 10.1016/j.pain.2009.01.033.

64. Hunter T, Siess F, Colloca L. Socially induced placebo analgesia: A comparison of a pre-recorded versus live face-to-face observation. *Eur J Pain.* Aug 2014;18(7):914–922. https://doi.org/10.1002/j.1532-2149.2013.00436.x.

65. Chen PA, Cheong JH, Jolly E, Elhence H, Wager TD, Chang LJ. Socially transmitted placebo effects. *Nat Hum Behav.* Dec 2019;3(12):1295–1305. https://doi.org/10.1038/s41562-019-0749-5.

66. Crick F. *The Astonishing Hypothesis: The Scientific Search for the Soul.* Simon & Schuster; 1994.

67. Rao M, Gershon MD. The bowel and beyond: The enteric nervous system in neurological disorders. *Nat Rev Gastroenterol Hepatol.* Sep 2016;13(9):517–528. https://doi.org/10.1038/nrgastro.2016.107.

68. Eryomin AL. Biophysics of evolution of intellectual systems. *Biophysics* (Oxford). 2022;67(2):320–326. https://doi.org/10.1134/S0006350922020051.

69. Sheldrake R. The sense of being stared at, 2: Its implications for theories of vision. *Journal of Consciousness Studies.* 2005;12:10–31. https://www.sheldrake.org/files/pdfs/papers/The-Sense-of-Being-Stared-At-Part-2-Its-Implications-for-Theories-of-Vision.pdf.

70. Parthasarathy A. *Vedanta Treatise.* 2d ed. Vedanta Life Institute; 1984.

71. Sheldrake R. *The Sense of Being Stared At: And Other Aspects of the Extended Mind.* Cornerstone Digital; 2013.

72. Sheldrake R. *The Science Delusion: Freeing the Spirit of Enquiry.* Coronet; 2012.

73. Sheldrake R. *A New Science of Life: The Hypothesis of Formative Causation.* 3d ed. Icon; 2009.

74. Frenkel O. A phenomenology of the "placebo effect": Taking meaning from the mind to the body. *J Med Philos.* Feb 2008;33(1):58–79. https://doi.org/10.1093/jmp/jhm005.

75. Meissner K. The placebo effect and the autonomic nervous sy~~for an intimate relationship. *Philos Trans R Soc Lond B Biol Sci.* Jun 27 2011;366(1572):1808–1817. https://doi.org/10.1098/rstb.2010.0403.

76. Kemmerer D, Miller L, Macpherson MK, Huber J, Tranel D. An investiga~~of semantic similarity judgments about action and non-action verbs in Parkinson's disease: Implications for the Embodied Cognition Framework. *Front Hum Neurosci.* 2013;7:146. https://doi.org/10.3389/fnhum.2013.00146.

77. Fuchs T, Schlimme JE. Embodiment and psychopathology: A phenomeno-logical perspective. *Curr Opin Psychiatry.* Nov 2009;22(6):570–575. https://doi.org/10.1097/YCO.0b013e3283318e5c.

78. Arandia IR, Di Paolo EA. Placebo from an enactive perspective. *Frontiers in Psychology.* 2021;12(660118). https://doi.org/10.3389/fpsyg.2021.660118.

79. Naro A, Maggio MG, Latella D, et al. Does embodied cognition allow a better management of neurological diseases? A review on the link between cognitive language processing and motor function. *Appl Neuropsychol Adult.* Mar 8 2021:1–12. https://doi.org/10.1080/23279095.2021.1890595.

80. Morris DB. Placebo, pain, and belief: A biocultural model. In Harrington A, ed. *The Placebo Effect: An Interdisciplinary Exploration*, 187–207. Harvard University Press; 1997.

81. Moerman DE. Editorial: Meaningful placebos—Controlling the uncontrollable. *N Engl J Med* Jul 14 2011;365(2):171–172. https://doi.org/10.1056/NEJMe1104010.

82. Humphrey N, Skoyles J. The evolutionary psychology of healing: A human success story. *Curr Biol.* 2012 Sep 11;22(17):R695-98. https://doi.org/10.1016/j.cub.2012.06.018.

Chapter 7. Placebo and Nocebo Effects Don't Add Up

1. Frank JD, Frank JB. *Persuasion and Healing: A Comparative Study of Psycho-therapy.* 3d ed. Johns Hopkins University Press; 1991.

2. Beecher HK. The powerful placebo. *J Am Med Assoc.* Dec 24 1955;159(17):1602–1606. https://doi.org/10.1001/jama.1955.02960340022006.

3. Hulshof TA, Zuidema SU, Gispen-de Wied CC, et al. Run-in periods and clinical outcomes of antipsychotics in dementia: A meta-epidemiological study of placebo-controlled trials. *Pharmacoepidemiol Drug Saf* 2020;29(2):125–133. https://doi.org/10.1002/pds.4903.

4. Grünbaum A. The placebo concept in medicine and psychiatry. *Psychol Med.* Feb 1986;16(1):19–38. https://doi.org/10.1017/s0033291700002506.

5. Hughes JR, Gulliver SB, Amori G, et al. Effect of instructions and nicotine on smoking cessation, withdrawal symptoms and self-administration of nicotine gum. *Psychopharmacology (Berl)* 1989;99(4):486–91. https://doi.org/10.1007/BF00589896.

6. Aronson JK. Concentration-effect and dose-response relations in clinical pharmacology. *Br J Clin Pharmacol.* Mar 2007;63(3):255–257. http://doi.org/10.1111/j.1365-2125.2007.02871.x.

7. Uhlenhuth EH, Rickels K, Fisher S, Park LC, Lipman RS, Mock J. Drug, doctor's verbal attitude and clinic setting in the symptomatic response to pharmacotherapy. *Psychopharmacologia*. 1966;9(5):392–418. https://doi.org/10.1007/BF00406450.

8. Boussageon R, Howick J, Baron R, Naudet F, Falissard B, Harika-Germaneau G, Wassouf I, Gueyffier F, Jaafari N, Blanchard C. How do they add up? The interaction between the placebo and treatment effect: A systematic review. *Br J Clin Pharmacol*. 2022 Aug;88(8):3638–3656. https://doi.org/10.1111/bcp.15345.

9. Marchant J. Strong placebo response thwarts painkiller trials. Nature (2015). https://doi.org/10.1038/nature.2015.18511.

10. Mossman SA, Mills JA, Walkup JT, et al. The impact of failed antidepressant Trials on outcomes in children and adolescents with anxiety and depression: A systematic review and meta-analysis. *J Child Adolesc Psychopharmacol* 2021;31(4):259–267. https://doi.org/10.1089/cap.2020.0195.

11. Hammami MM, Al-Gaai EA, Alvi S, Hammami MB. Interaction between drug and placebo effects: A cross-over balanced placebo design trial. *Trials*. 2010 Nov 19;11:110. https://doi.org/10.1186/1745-6215-11-110.

12. Cartwright N. *Nature's Capacities and Their Measurement*. Clarendon; 1989.

13. Mill JS. A system of logic, ratiocinative and inductive: Being a connected view of the principles of evidence and the methods of scientific investigation. In *Collected Works of John Stuart Mill*. University of Toronto Press; 1843[1973]. https://doi.org/10.1017/CBO9781139149839.

Chapter 8. Blinding

1. Jefferson T, *Letters of Thomas Jefferson*. Ed. Irwin F. Sanbornton. Bridge Press; 1975.

2. Hill ABS, Hill ID. *Bradford Hill's Principles of Medical Statistics*. 12th ed. Edward Arnold; 1991.

3. Straus SE, Richardson WS, Glasziou P, Haynes RB. *Evidence-Based Medicine: How to Practice and Teach EBM*. 3d ed. Elsevier: Churchill Livingstone; 2005.

4. Armitage P, Berry G, Matthews JNS. *Statistical Methods in Medical Research*. 4th ed. Blackwell Science; 2002.

5. Greenhalgh T. *How to Read a Paper: The Basics of Evidence-Based Medicine*. 3d ed. BMJ Books/Blackwell Pub.; 2006.

6. 21 CFR 314.126: Applications for FDA Approval to Market a New Drug. Accessed May 23, 2006. http://www.accessdata.fda.gov/scripts/cdrh/cfdocs/cfcfr/CFRSearch.cfm?fr=314.126

7. Bland M. *An Introduction to Medical Statistics*. 3d ed. Oxford University Press; 2000.

8. Jadad A. *Randomized Controlled Trials*. BMJ Books; 1998.

9. Hróbjartsson A, Gøtzsche P. Is the placebo powerless? An analysis of clinical trials comparing placebo with no treatment. *N Engl J Med* 2001;344(21):1594–1602. http://doi.org/10.1056/NEJM200105243442106.

10. Bailly A. *Rapport des commissaires chargés par le Roi, de l'examen du magnétisme animale.* Imprimerie Royale; 1784. https://gallica.bnf.fr/ark:/12148/bpt6k6367286z .texteImage.

11. *The Reports of the Royal Commission of 1784 on Mesmer's System of Animal Magnetism: and Other Contemporary Documents.* Trans. I. M. L. Donaldson. 2014. https://www.rcpe.ac.uk/sites/default/files/files/the_royal_commission_on _animal_-_translated_by_iml_donaldson_1.pdf.

12. Mesmerism. In Carroll RT. The *Skeptic's Dictionary.* Accessed February 11, 2020. http://skepdic.com/mesmer.html.

13. Robertson D. The discovery of hypnosis—Braid's lost manuscript, "On hypnotism" (1860): A brief communication. *Int J Clin Exp Hypn.* Apr 2009;57(2):127–132. https://doi.org/10.1080/00207140802665344.

14. Stolberg M. Inventing the randomized double-blind trial: The Nuremberg salt test of 1835. *J R Soc Med.* Dec 2006;99(12):642–643. https://doi.org/10.1258 /jrsm.99.12.642.

15. Neuprez A, Delcour JP, Fatemi F, et al. Patients' expectations impact their satisfaction following total hip or knee arthroplasty. *PLoS One.* 2016;11. https://doi .org/10.1371/journal.pone.0167911.

16. Tilbury C, Haanstra TM, Verdegaal SHM, et al. Patients' pre-operative general and specific outcome expectations predict postoperative pain and function after total knee and total hip arthroplasties. *Scand J Pain.* Jul 26 2018;18(3):457–466. https://doi.org/10.1515/sjpain-2018-0022.

17. Hayden JA, Wilson MN, Riley RD, Iles R, Pincus T, Ogilvie R. Individual recovery expectations and prognosis of outcomes in non-specific low back pain: Prognostic factor review. *Cochrane Database Syst Rev.* Nov 25 2019;2019(11). https://doi.org/10.1002/14651858.CD011284.pub2.

18. Ferrari R, Louw D. Correlation between expectations of recovery and injury severity perception in whiplash-associated disorders. *J Zhejiang Univ Sci B.* Aug 2011;12(8):683–6. https://doi.org/10.1631/jzus.B1100097.

19. Whitford HS, Olver IN. When expectations predict experience: The influence of psychological factors on chemotherapy toxicities. *J Pain Symptom Manage.* Jun 2012;43(6):1036–1050. https://doi.org/10.1016/j.jpainsymman.2011.06.026.

20. Karlowski TR, Chalmers TC, Frenkel LD, Kapikian AZ, Lewis TL, Lynch JM. Ascorbic acid for the common cold. A prophylactic and therapeutic trial. *JAMA.* Mar 10 1975;231(10):1038–1042.

21. Moncrieff J, Wessely S, Hardy R. Active placebos versus antidepressants for depression. *Cochrane Database Syst Rev.* 2004;(1):CD003012. http://doi.org/10.1002 /14651858.CD003012.pub2.

22. Noseworthy JH, Ebers GC, Vandervoort MK, Farquhar RE, Yetisir E, Roberts R. The impact of blinding on the results of a randomized, placebo-controlled multiple sclerosis clinical trial. *Neurology.* Jan 1994;44(1):16–20. http://doi.org/10 .1212/wnl.44.1.16.

23. Moustgaard H, Clayton GL, Jones HE, et al. Impact of blinding on estimated treatment effects in randomised clinical trials: Meta-epidemiological study. *BMJ*. Jan 21 2020;368:l6802. https://doi.org/10.1136/bmj.l6802.

24. Page MJ, Higgins JP, Clayton G, Sterne JA, Hróbjartsson A, Savović J. Empirical evidence of study design biases in randomized trials: Systematic review of meta-epidemiological studies. *PLoS One*. 2016;11(7):e0159267. https://doi.org /10.1371/journal.pone.0159267.

25. Dechartres A, Trinquart L, Faber T, Ravaud P. Empirical evaluation of which trial characteristics are associated with treatment effect estimates. *J Clin Epidemiol*. Sep 2016;77:24–37. https://doi.org/10.1016/j.jclinepi.2016.04.005.

26. Saltaji H, Armijo-Olivo S, Cummings GG, Amin M, da Costa BR, Flores-Mir C. Influence of blinding on treatment effect size estimate in randomized controlled trials of oral health interventions. *BMC Med Res Methodol*. May 18 2018;18(1):42. https://doi.org/10.1186/s12874-018-0491-0.

27. Armijo-Olivo S, Fuentes J, da Costa BR, Saltaji H, Ha C, Cummings GG. Blinding in physical therapy trials and its association with treatment effects: A meta-epidemiological study. *Am J Phys Med Rehabil*. Jan 2017;96(1):34–44. https:// doi.org/10.1097/PHM.0000000000000521.

28. Hróbjartsson A, Thomsen AS, Emanuelsson F, et al. Observer bias in randomised clinical trials with binary outcomes: systematic review of trials with both blinded and non-blinded outcome assessors. *BMJ*. Feb 27 2012;344:e1119. https://doi.org/10.1136/bmj.e1119.

29. Hróbjartsson A, Thomsen AS, Emanuelsson F, et al. Observer bias in randomized clinical trials with measurement scale outcomes: A systematic review of trials with both blinded and nonblinded assessors. *CMAJ*. Mar 5 2013;185(4):E201–11. https://doi.org/10.1503/cmaj.120744.

30. Hróbjartsson A, Thomsen AS, Emanuelsson F, et al. Observer bias in randomized clinical trials with time-to-event outcomes: systematic review of trials with both blinded and non-blinded outcome assessors. *Int J Epidemiol*. Jun 2014;43(3):937–948. https://doi.org/10.1093/ije/dyt270.

31. Hróbjartsson A, Emanuelsson F, Skou Thomsen AS, Hilden J, Brorson S. Bias due to lack of patient blinding in clinical trials: A systematic review of trials randomizing patients to blind and nonblind sub-studies. *Int J Epidemiol*. Aug 2014;43(4):1272–1283. https://doi.org/10.1093/ije/dyu115.

32. Savović J, Jones HE, Altman DG, et al. Influence of reported study design characteristics on intervention effect estimates from randomized, controlled trials. *Ann Intern Med*. 2012 Sep 18;157(6):429–438. https://doi.org/10.7326/0003 -4819-157-6-201209180-00537.

33. Hróbjartsson A, Forfang E, Haahr MT, Als-Nielsen B, Brorson S. Blinded trials taken to the test: An analysis of randomized clinical trials that report tests for the success of blinding. *Int J Epidemiol*. Jun 2007;36(3):654–663. https://doi.org /10.1093/ije/dym020.

34. Bello S, Wei M, Hilden J, Hróbjartsson A. The matching quality of experimental and control interventions in blinded pharmacological randomised clinical trials: A methodological systematic review. *BMC Med Res Methodol.* 2016;16:18. https://doi.org/10.1186/s12874-016-0111-9.

35. Ney PG, Collins C, Spensor C. Double blind: double talk or are there ways to do better research? *Med Hypotheses.* Oct 1986;21(2):119–126. https://doi.org /10.1016/0306-9877(86)90001-0.

36. Senn SJ. Controversies concerning randomization and additivity in clinical trials. *Stat Med.* Dec 30 2004;23(24):3729–3753. http://doi.org/10.1002/sim.2074.

37. Moher D, Schulz KF, Altman D. The CONSORT statement: revised recommendations for improving the quality of reports of parallel-group randomized trials. *JAMA* 2001;285(15):1987–1891. http://doi.org/jsc00437.

38. Schulz KF, Altman DG, Moher D. CONSORT 2010 statement: Updated guidelines for reporting parallel group randomised trials. *PLoS Med* 2010;7(3): e1000251. https://doi.org/10.1371/journal.pmed.1000251.

39. Webster RK, Bishop F, Collins GS, et al. Measuring the success of blinding in placebo-controlled trials: Should we be so quick to dismiss it? *J Clin Epidemiol* 2021. https://doi.org/10.1016/j.jclinepi.2021.02.022.

40. Sackett DL. The sins of expertness and a proposal for redemption. *BMJ* 2000;320(7244):1283.

41. Shapiro S. Widening the field of vision. *BMJ Rapid Responses* February 19, 2004. https://www.bmj.com/rapid-response/2011/10/30/widening-field-vision.

42. Sackett DL. Turning a blind eye: Why we don't test for blindness at the end of our trials. *BMJ.* May 8 2004;328(7448):1136. https://doi.org/10.1136/bmj.328 .74327.37952.631667.EE.

43. Webster RK, Bishop F, Collins GS, et al. Measuring the success of blinding in placebo-controlled trials: Should we be so quick to dismiss it? *J Clin Epidemiol* 2021. https://doi.org/10.1016/j.jclinepi.2021.02.022.

44. Torgerson DJ, Sibbald B. Understanding controlled trials. What is a patient preference trial? *BMJ.* Jan 31 1998;316(7128):360. https://doi.org/10.1136/bmj .316.7128.360.

Part III. Why Every Doctor Needs to Be a Shaman

1. Moerman DE, Jonas WB. Deconstructing the placebo effect and finding the meaning response. *Ann Intern Med.* Mar 19 2002;136(6):471–476. http://doi.org/10 .7326/0003-4819-136-6-200203190-00011.

Chapter 9. The Ethical Requirement to Prescribe More Placebos and Avoid Nocebo Effects in Practice

1. Gipps R. Doctors should be shamans and perhaps they are. *Philosophical Perspectives in Clinical Psychology* (blog). March 10, 2020. https://clinicalphilosophy .blogspot.com/2020/03/doctors-should-be-shamans.html.

2. Kleisiaris CF, Sfakianakis C, Papathanasiou IV. Health care practices in ancient Greece: The Hippocratic ideal. *J Med Ethics Hist Med*. 2014;7:6.

3. Bok S. The ethics of giving placebos. *Sci Am*. Nov 1974;231(5):17–23. http://www.jstor.org/stable/24950213.

4. Caldwell JG, Price EV, Schroeter AL, Fletcher GF. Aortic regurgitation in the Tuskegee study of untreated syphilis. *J Chronic Dis*. Mar 1973;26(3):187–194. https://doi.org/10.1016/0021-9681(73)90089-1.

5. Corbie-Smith G, Thomas SB, Williams MV, et al. Attitudes and beliefs of African Americans toward participation in medical research. *J Gen Intern Med* 1999;14(9):537–46. https://doi.org/10.1046/j.1525-1497.1999.07048.x.

6. Rich BA. A placebo for the pain: A medico-legal case analysis. *Pain Med* 2003;4(4):366–372. https://doi.org/10.1111/j.1526-4637.2003.03046.x.

7. Wendler D, Miller FG. Deception in the pursuit of science. *Arch Intern Med*. Mar 22 2004;164(6):597–600. https://doi.org/10.1001/archinte.164.6.597.

8. Kaptchuk TJ, Friedlander E, Kelley JM, et al. Placebos without deception: A randomized controlled trial in irritable bowel syndrome. *PLoS One*. 2010;5(12):e15591. https://doi.org/.1371/journal.pone.0015591.

9. Park LC, Covi L. Nonblind placebo trial: An exploration of neurotic patients' responses to placebo when its inert content is disclosed. *Arch Gen Psychiatry*. Apr 1965;12:336–345. https://doi.org/10.1001/archpsyc.1965.01720340008002.

10. Aulas JJ, Rosner I. Effets de la prescription d'un placebo "annoncé." [Efficacy of a non-blind placebo prescription]. *L'Encephale*. Jan–Feb 2003;29(1):68–71. https://doi.org/ENC-02-2003-29-1-0013-7006-101019-ART60.

11. Bergmann JF, Chassany O, Gandiol J, et al. A randomised clinical trial of the effect of informed consent on the analgesic activity of placebo and naproxen in cancer pain. *Clin Trials Metaanal*. 1994;29:41–47.

12. Dahan R, Caulin C, Figea L, Kanis JA, Caulin F, Segrestaa JM. Does informed consent influence therapeutic outcome? A clinical trial of the hypnotic activity of placebo in patients admitted to hospital. *Br Med J (Clin Res Ed)*. Aug 9 1986;293(6543):363–364. https://doi.org/10.1136/bmj.293.6543.363.

13. Kirsch I, Weixel LJ. Double-blind versus deceptive administration of a placebo. *Behav Neurosci*. 1988 Apr;102(2):319–323. https://doi.org.10.1037//0735-7044.102.2.319.

14. Pollo A, Amanzio M, Casadio C, Maggi G, Benedetti F. Response expectancies in placebo analgesia and their clinical relevance. *Pain*. 2001;93(1):77–84. https://doi.org/10.1016/S0304-3959(01)00296-2.

15. Sandler AD, Bodfish JW. Open-label use of placebos in the treatment of ADHD: A pilot study. *Child Care Health Dev*. 2008 Jan;34(1):104–110. https://doi.org/10.1111/j.1365-2214.2007.00797.x.

16. Lembo A, Kelley JM, Nee J, et al. Open-label placebo vs double-blind placebo for irritable bowel syndrome: A randomized clinical trial. *Pain* 2021;162(9):2428–2835. https://doi.org10.1097/j.pain.0000000000002234.

17. Nurko S, Saps M, Kossowsky J, et al. Effect of open-label placebo on children and adolescents with functional abdominal pain or irritable bowel syndrome: A randomized clinical trial. *JAMA Pediatr* 2022;176(4):349–356. https://doi.org /10.1001/jamapediatrics.2021.5750

18. Flowers KM, Patton ME, Hruschak VJ, et al. Conditioned open-label placebo for opioid reduction after spine surgery: a randomized controlled trial. *Pain* 2021;162(6):1828–1839. https://doi.org/10.1097/j.pain.0000000000002185.

19. Charlesworth JEG, Petkovic G, Kelley JM, et al. Effects of placebos without deception compared with no treatment: A systematic review and meta-analysis. *J Evid Based Med*. May 2017;10(2):97–107. https://doi.org/10.1111/jebm.12251.

20. General Medical Council. *Good Medical Practice*. October 30, 2019. https:// www.gmc-uk.org/ethical-guidance/ethical-guidance-for-doctors/good-medical -practice.

21. British Medical Association. British Medical Association. Accessed October 13, 2020. https://www.bma.org.uk/?query=placebo

22. American Medical Association. *Code of Medical Ethics: Use of Placebo in Clinical Practice*. Accessed October 13, 2020. https://www.ama-assn.org/delivering -care/ethics/use-placebo-clinical-practice.

23. Moerman D., personal communication with author.

24. Uusitalo S, Howick J. Philosophy of too much medicine conference report. *J Eval Clin Pract*. Oct 2018;24(5):1011–1012. https://doi.org/10.1111/jep.13000.

25. Gabriel M, Sharma V. Antidepressant discontinuation syndrome. *CMAJ*. May 29 2017;189(21):e747. https://doi.org/10.1503/cmaj.160991.

26. Diclofenac. *Drugs.com*. Accessed October 8, 2019. https://www.drugs.com /diclofenac.html.

27. Finestone HM, Conter DB. Acting in medical practice. *Lancet* 1994;344(8925): 801–2. https://doi.org/10.1016/s0140-6736(94)92349-3

28. American Medical Association. *Code of Medical Ethics*. Accessed October 30, 2019. https://www.ama-assn.org/about/publications-newsletters/ama-principles -medical-ethics.

29. Larson EB, Yao X. Clinical empathy as emotional labor in the patient-physician relationship. *JAMA*. Mar 2 2005;293(9):1100–1106. https://doi.org /10.1001/jama.293.9.1100.

30. Case GA, Brauner DJ. Perspective: The doctor as performer: A proposal for change based on a performance studies paradigm. *Acad Med*. Jan 2010;85(1):159–163. https://doi.org/10.1097/ACM.0b013e3181c427eb.

31. Eisenberg A, Rosenthal S, Schlussel YR. Medicine as a performing art: What we can learn about empathic communication from theater arts. *Acad Med*. Mar 2015;90(3):272–6. https://doi.org/10.1097/ACM.0000000000000626.

32. Enthoven WT, Roelofs PD, Deyo RA, van Tulder MW, Koes BW. Non-steroidal anti-inflammatory drugs for chronic low back pain. *Cochrane Database Syst Rev*. Feb 10 2016;2:CD012087. https://doi.org/10.1002/14651858.CD012087.

33. Saragiotto BT, Machado GC, Ferreira ML, Pinheiro MB, Abdel Shaheed C, Maher CG. Paracetamol for low back pain. *Cochrane Database Syst Rev.* Jun 7 2016;(6):CD012230. https://doi.org/10.1002/14651858.CD012230.

34. Derry S, Wiffen PJ, Moore RA, et al. Oral nonsteroidal anti-inflammatory drugs (NSAIDs) for cancer pain in adults. *Cochrane Database Syst Rev.* Jul 12 2017;7:CD012638. https://doi.org/10.1002/14651858.CD012638.pub2.

35. Derry S, Moore RA, Gaskell H, McIntyre M, Wiffen PJ. Topical NSAIDs for acute musculoskeletal pain in adults. *Cochrane Database Syst Rev.* 2015;6:CD007402. https://doi.org/10.1002/14651858.CD007402.pub3.

36. Howick J. *Doctor You: Revealing the Science of Self-Healing.* Hodder & Stoughton; 2017.

37. Rief W, Shedden-Mora MC, Laferton JA, et al. Preoperative optimization of patient expectations improves long-term outcome in heart surgery patients: Results of the randomized controlled PSY-HEART trial. *BMC Med* 2017;15(1):4. https://doi.org/10.1186/s12916-016-0767-3.

38. Newman DH (2008). *Hippocrates' Shadow.* New York: Scribner.

Chapter 10. Fewer Placebos and Nocebos in Trials

1. Enkin M. Commentary on Howick: Questioning the methodological superiority of 'placebo' over 'active' controlled trials. *Am J Bioeth.* 2009; 9:9. https://doi.org/10.1080/15265160903098622.

2. Kirsch I. Are drug and placebo effects in depression additive? *Biol Psychiatry.* Apr 15 2000;47(8):733–735. https://doi.org/10.1016/s0006-3223(00)00832-5.

3. McCullough AJ, O'Connor JF. Alcoholic liver disease: Proposed recommendations for the American College of Gastroenterology. *Am J Gastroenterol.* Nov 1998;93(11):2022–2036. https://doi.org/10.1111/j.1572-0241.1998.00587.x

4. Boetticher NC, Peine CJ, Kwo P, et al. A randomized, double-blinded, placebo-controlled multicenter trial of etanercept in the treatment of alcoholic hepatitis. *Gastroenterology.* Dec 2008;135(6):1953–60. https://doi.org/10.1053/j.gastro.2008.08.057.

5. World Medical Association. *Declaration of Helsinki: Ethical Principles for Research Involving Human Subjects*, Part II: Medical Research Combined with Professional Care (Clinical Research), para. 3. October 1996. https://www.wma.net/wp-content/uploads/2018/07/DoH-Oct1996.pdf.

6. Batra S, Howick J. Empirical evidence against placebo controls. *J Med Ethics.* 2017;43:707–713. https://doi.org/10.1136/medethics-2016-103970.

7. Berwaerts J, Liu Y, Gopal S, et al. Efficacy and safety of the 3-month formulation of paliperidone palmitate vs placebo for relapse prevention of schizophrenia: A randomized clinical trial. *JAMA Psychiatry.* Aug 2015;72(8):830–839. https://doi.org/10.1001/jamapsychiatry.2015.0241.

8. Kishimoto T, Agarwal V, Kishi T, Leucht S, Kane JM, Correll CU. Relapse prevention in schizophrenia: A systematic review and meta-analysis of

second-generation antipsychotics versus first-generation antipsychotics. *Mol Psychiatry*. Jan 2013;18(1):53–66. https://doi.org/10.1038/mp.2011.143.

9. Leucht S, Barnes TR, Kissling W, Engel RR, Correll C, Kane JM. Relapse prevention in schizophrenia with new-generation antipsychotics: a systematic review and exploratory meta-analysis of randomized, controlled trials. *Am J Psychiatry*. Jul 2003;160(7):1209–1222. https://doi.org/10.1176/appi.ajp.160.7.1209.

10. Eggermont AM, Chiarion-Sileni V, Grob JJ, et al. Adjuvant ipilimumab versus placebo after complete resection of high-risk stage III melanoma (EORTC 18071): A randomised, double-blind, phase 3 trial. *Lancet Oncol*. May 2015;16(5): 522–530. https://doi.org/10.1016/S1470-2045(15)70122-1.

11. Mocellin S, Pasquali S, Rossi CR, Nitti D. Interferon alpha adjuvant therapy in patients with high-risk melanoma: A systematic review and meta-analysis. *J Natl Cancer Inst*. Apr 7 2010;102(7):493–501. https://doi.org/10.1093/jnci/djq009.

12. Valente DS, Steffen N, Carvalho LA, Borille GB, Zanella RK, Padoin AV. Preoperative use of dexamethasone in rhinoplasty: A randomized, double-blind, placebo-controlled clinical trial. JAMA Facial Plast Surg. May–Jun 2015;17(3):169–173. https://doi.org/10.1001/jamafacial.2014.1574.

13. Hatef DA, Ellsworth WA, Allen JN, Bullocks JM, Hollier LH, Jr., Stal S. Perioperative steroids for minimizing edema and ecchymosis after rhinoplasty: A meta-analysis. *Aesthet Surg J*. Aug 2011;31(6):648–657. https://doi.org /10.1177/1090820X11416110.

14. Senn SJ, Chalmers I. Giving and taking: Ethical treatment assignment in controlled trials. *J R Soc Med*. 2021 Nov;114(11):525–530. https://doi.org /10.1177/01410768211049972.

15. Fraser A. *King Charles II*. Weidenfeld and Nicolson; 1979.

16. The Cardiac Arrhythmia Suppression Trial II Investigators. Effect of the antiarrhythmic agent moricizine on survival after myocardial infarction. *N Engl J Med*. Jul 23 1992;327(4):227–233. https://doi.org/10.1056/NEJM199207233270403.

17. Moore TJ. *Deadly Medicine: Why Tens of Thousands of Heart Patients Died in America's Worst Drug Disaster*. Simon & Schuster; 1995.

18. Smith R. Where is the wisdom . . . ? *BMJ*. Oct 5 1991;303(6806):798–799. https://doi.org/10.1136/bmj.303.6806.798.

19. Ellis J, Mulligan I, Rowe J, Sackett DL. Inpatient general medicine is evidence based. *Lancet*. Aug 12 1995;346(8972):407–410. https://www.thelancet .com/pdfs/journals/lancet/PIIS0140-6736(95)92781-6.pdf.

20. Gill P, Dowell AC, Neal RD, Smith N, Heywood P, Wilson AE. Evidence based general practice: A retrospective study of interventions in one training practice. *BMJ*. Mar 30 1996;312(7034):819–821. https://doi.org/10.1136/bmj.312.7034.819.

21. Imrie R, Ramey DW. The evidence for evidence-based medicine. *Complement Ther Med*. Jun 2000;8(2):123–126. https://doi.org/10.1054/ctim.2000.0370.

22. Ellenberg SS, Temple R. Placebo-controlled trials and active-control trials in the evaluation of new treatments, part 2: Practical issues and specific cases.

Ann Intern Med. Sep 19 2000;133(6):464–470. https://doi.org/10.7326/0003-4819 -133-6-200009190-00015.

23. Temple R, Ellenberg SS. Placebo-controlled trials and active-control trials in the evaluation of new treatments, part 1: Ethical and scientific issues. *Ann Intern Med.* Sep 19 2000;133(6):455–463. https://doi.org /10.7326/0003-4819-133-6-200009190-00014.

24. International Conference on Harmonisation of Technical Requirements for Registration of Pharmaceuticals for Human Use. *ICH Harmonised Tripartite Guideline: Choice of Control Group and Related Issues in Clinical Trials, E 10.* Step 4 version, July 20, 2000. https://database.ich.org/sites/default/files/E10_Guideline.pdf.

25. Temple R, Ellenberg SS. Placebo-controlled trials and active-control trials in the evaluation of new treatments, part 1: Ethical and scientific issues. *Ann Intern Med.* Sep 19 2000;133(6):455–463. https://doi.org/10.7326/0003-4819-133-6 -200009190-00014.

26. Max MB. Divergent traditions in analgesic clinical trials. *Clin Pharmacol Ther.* Sep 1994;56(3):237–241. https://ascpt.onlinelibrary.wiley.com/doi/pdf/10 .1038/clpt.1994.130.

27. Motamed C, Mazoit X, Ghanouchi K, et al. Preemptive intravenous morphine-6-glucuronide is ineffective for postoperative pain relief. *Anesthesiology.* Feb 2000;92(2):355–360. https://doi.org/10.1097/00000542-200002000-00015.

28. Yusuf S, Peto R, Lewis J, Collins R, Sleight P. Beta blockade during and after myocardial infarction: An overview of the randomized trials. *Prog Cardiovasc Dis.* Mar–Apr 1985;27(5):335–371. https://doi.org/10.1016/s0033-0620(85)80003-7.

29. Tramer MR, Reynolds DJ, Moore RA, McQuay HJ. When placebo controlled trials are essential and equivalence trials are inadequate. *BMJ.* Sep 26 1998;317(7162): 875–80. https://doi.org/10.1136/bmj.317.7162.875.

30. Healy D. Serotonin and depression. *BMJ.* Apr 21 2015;350:h1771. https://doi .org/10.1136/bmj.h1771.

31. Moncrieff J, Wessely S, Hardy R. Active placebos versus antidepressants for depression. *Cochrane Database Syst Rev.* 2004;(1):CD003012. https://doi.org /10.1002/14651858.CD003012.pub2.

32. Kirsch I, Sapirstein G. Listening to Prozac but hearing placebo: A meta- analysis of antidepressant medication. Prevention & Treatment. June 26 1998 1998;1(2). https://doi.org/10.1037/1522-3736.1.1.12a.

33. Kirsch I, Moore T. The emperor's new drugs: An analysis of antidepressant medication data submitted to the U.S. Food and Drug Administration. *Prevention & Treatment.* 15 July 2002 2002;5. https://doi.org/10.1037/1522-3736.5.1.523a.

34. Healy D. *Let Them Eat Prozac.* New York University Press; 2004.

35. Healy D. Did regulators fail over selective serotonin reuptake inhibitors? *BMJ.* Jul 8 2006;333(7558):92–95. https://doi.org/10.1136/bmj.333.7558.92.

36. Hopewell S, Loudon K, Clarke MJ, Oxman AD, Dickersin K. Publication bias in clinical trials due to statistical significance or direction of trial results.

Cochrane Database Syst Rev. 2009;(1):MR000006. https://doi.org/10.1002/14651858. MR000006.pub3

37. De Angelis C, Drazen JM, Frizelle FA, et al. Clinical trial registration: A statement from the International Committee of Medical Journal Editors. *N Engl J Med.* 2004 Sep 16;351(12):1250–1251. https://doi.org/10.1056 /NEJMe048225.

38. Howick J. Exploring the asymmetrical relationship between the power of finance bias and evidence. *Perspect Biol Med.* 2019;62(1):159–187. https://doi.org /10.1353/pbm.2019.0009.

39. Leopold SS, Warme WJ, Fritz Braunlich E, Shott S. Association between funding source and study outcome in orthopaedic research. *Clin Orthop Relat Res.* Oct 2003;(415):293–301. https://doi.org/10.1097/01.blo.0000093888.12372.d9.

40. Yaphe J, Edman R, Knishkowy B, Herman J. The association between funding by commercial interests and study outcome in randomized controlled drug trials. *Fam Pract.* Dec 2001;18(6):565–568. https://doi.org/10.1093/fampra/18.6.565.

41. Moerman DE. Cultural variations in the placebo effect: Ulcers, anxiety, and blood pressure. *Med Anthropol Q.* 2000 Mar;14(1):51–72. https://doi.org/10.1525 /maq.2000.14.1.51.

42. Patel SM, Stason WB, Legedza A, et al. The placebo effect in irritable bowel syndrome trials: A meta-analysis. *Neurogastroenterol Motil.* Jun 2005;17(3):332–340. https://doi.org/10.1111/j.1365-2982.2005.00650.x.

43. Stebbings R, Findlay L, Edwards C, et al. "Cytokine storm" in the phase I trial of monoclonal antibody TGN1412: Better understanding the causes to improve preclinical testing of immunotherapeutics. *J Immunol.* 2007 Sep 1;179(5):3325–3331. https://doi.org/10.4049/jimmunol.179.5.3325.

44. World Medical Association. When are placebo controlled trials ethically acceptable? November 3, 2020. https://www.wma.net/news-post/when-are-placebo -controlled-trials-ethically-acceptable/

45. Svobodova, M., Jacob, N., Hood, K. et al. Developing principles for sharing information about potential trial intervention benefits and harms with patients: Report of a modified Delphi survey. *Trials* 23, 863 (2022). https://doi.org/10.1186 /s13063-022-06780-1

46. Goldenberg MJ. Placebo orthodoxy and the double standard of care in multinational clinical research. *Theor Med Bioeth.* Feb 2015;36(1):7–23. https://doi .org/10.1007/s11017-015-9317-9.

Chapter 11. Public Health, Surgery, and Alternative Medicine

1. Chapman SAO. Wind Turbine Syndrome: A communicated disease. *Journal & Proceedings of the Royal Society of New South Wales.* 2018;15(151):39–44. https://www .royalsoc.org.au/images/pdf/journal/151-1-Chapman.pdf.

2. Khan S, Holbrook A, Shah BR. Does Googling lead to statin intolerance? *Int J Cardiol* 2018;262:25–27. https://doi.org/10.1016/j.ijcard.2018.02.085.

3. Marlow LL, Faull OK, Finnegan SL, Pattinson KTS. Breathlessness and the brain: The role of expectation. *Curr Opin Support Palliat Care*. Sep 2019;13(3):200–210. https://doi.org/10.1097/SPC.0000000000000441.

4. Howick J, Kelly P, Kelly M. Establishing a causal link between social relationships and health using the Bradford Hill Guidelines. *SSM Popul Health*. Aug 2019;8:100402. https://doi.org/10.1016/j.ssmph.2019.100402.

5. Howick J. Exploring the asymmetrical relationship between the power of finance bias and evidence. *Perspect Biol Med*. 2019;62(1):159–187. https://doi.org /10.1353/pbm.2019.0009.

6. Healy D. *Let Them Eat Prozac*. New York University Press; 2004.

7. Healy D. Serotonin and depression. *BMJ*. Apr 21 2015;350:h1771. https://doi .org/10.1136/bmj.h1771.

8. Moncrieff, J., Cooper, R.E., Stockmann, T. et al. The serotonin theory of depression: A systematic umbrella review of the evidence. *Mol Psychiatry* 2022 Jul 20. https://doi.org/10.1038/s41380-022-01661-0.

9. Miller, Abby. Lilly Airs Depression-Treatment Infomercial. June 15, 1999. Accessed November 17, 2022. https://www.dmnews.com/lilly-airs-depressiontreatment -infomercial/

10. Productions T. Prozac Super Bowl Spec Commercial. Accessed September 21, 2021. https://www.youtube.com/watch?v=sFVW_t2xVjo.

11. Block AE. Costs and benefits of direct-to-consumer advertising: The case of depression. *Pharmacoeconomics*. 2007;25(6):511–521. https://doi.org/10.2165/00019053 -200725060-00006.

12. Piller C. The war on 'prediabetes' could be a boon for pharma—but is it good medicine? *Science*, March 7, 2019. https://www.sciencemag.org/news/2019/03/war -prediabetes-could-be-boon-pharma-it-good-medicine.

13. Yudkin JS, Montori VM. The epidemic of pre-diabetes: The medicine and the politics. *BMJ*. Jul 15 2014;349:g4485. https://doi.org/10.1136/bmj.g4485.

14. Richter B, Hemmingsen B, Metzendorf MI, Takwoingi Y. Development of type 2 diabetes mellitus in people with intermediate hyperglycaemia. *Cochrane Database Syst Rev*. Oct 29 2018;10:CD012661. https://doi.org/10.1002/14651858. CD012661.pub2.

15. Mahase E. NICE lowers treatment threshold for high blood pressure. *BMJ*. Aug 29 2019;366:l5315. https://doi.org/10.1136/bmj.l5315.

16. Howick J. *Doctor You: Revealing the Science of Self-Healing*. Hodder & Stoughton; 2017.

17. Yusuf S, Bosch J, Dagenais G, et al. Cholesterol lowering in intermediate-risk persons without cardiovascular disease. *N Engl J Med*. May 26 2016;374(21):2021–2031. https://doi.org/10.1056/NEJMoa1600176.

18. Stead M, Angus K, Langley T, et al. Mass media to communicate public health messages in six health topic areas: A systematic review and other reviews of the evidence. *NIHR Journals Library*; 2019 Apr. http://doi.org/10.3310/phr07080.

19. Tuttle AH, Tohyama S, Ramsay T, et al. Increasing placebo responses over time in U.S. clinical trials of neuropathic pain. *Pain.* Dec 2015;156(12):2616–2626. https://doi.org/10.1097/j.pain.0000000000000333.

20. Chaput de Saintonge DM, Herxheimer A. Harnessing placebo effects in health care. *Lancet.* Oct 8 1994;344(8928):995–8. https://doi.org/10.1016/s0140-6736(94)91647-0.

21. Stanger-Hall KF, Hall DW. Abstinence-only education and teen pregnancy rates: Why we need comprehensive sex education in the U.S. *PLoS One.* 2011;6(10):e24658. https://doi.org/10.1371/journal.pone.0024658.

22. Livingston KE. Cingulate cortex isolation for the treatment of psychoses and psychoneuroses. *Res Publ Assoc Res Nerv Ment Dis* 1953; 31: 374–378.

23. Beecher HK. Surgery as placebo: A quantitative study of bias. *JAMA.* Jul 1 1961;176:1102–1107. https://doi.org/10.1001/jama.1961.63040260007008.

24. Cobb LA, Thomas GI, Dillard DH, Merendino KA, Bruce RA. An evaluation of internal-mammary-artery ligation by a double-blind technic. *N Engl J Med.* May 28 1959;260(22):1115–1118. https://doi.org/10.1056/NEJM195905282602204.

25. Dimond EG, Kittle CF, Crockett JE. Comparison of internal mammary artery ligation and sham operation for angina pectoris. *Am J Cardiol.* Apr 1960;5:483–486. https://doi.org/10.1016/0002-9149(60)90105-3.

26. Buchbinder R, Osborne RH, Ebeling PR, et al. A randomized trial of vertebroplasty for painful osteoporotic vertebral fractures. *N Engl J Med.* Aug 6 2009;361(6):557–568. https://doi.org/10.1056/NEJMoa0900429.

27. Miller FG, Kallmes DF, Buchbinder R. Vertebroplasty and the placebo response. *Radiology.* Jun 2011;259(3):621–625. https://doi.org/10.1148/radiol.11102412.

28. Martin DJ, Rad AE, Kallmes DF. Prevalence of extravertebral cement leakage after vertebroplasty: Procedural documentation versus CT detection. *Acta Radiol.* Jun 1 2012;53(5):569–572. https://doi.org/10.1258/ar.2012.120222.

29. Sisodia GB. Methods of predicting vertebral body fractures of the lumbar spine. *World J Orthop.* 2013;4(4):241–247. https://doi.org/10.5312/wjo.v4.i4.241.

30. Howick, J., Lyness, Emily, Albury, Charlotte, Smith, Kirsten, Dambha-Miller, Hajira, Ratnapalan, Mohana, Vennik, Jane, Hughes, Stephanie, Bostock, Jennifer, Morrison, Leanne, Mallen, Christian D., Everitt, Hazel, Dean, Sue, Levett-Jones, Tracy, Ivynian, Serra, Little, Paul and Bishop, Felicity (2020) Anatomy of positive messages in healthcare consultations: component analysis of messages within 22 randomised trials. *European Journal for Person Centered Healthcare*, 7 (4), 656–664.

31. Harris I. *Surgery, the Ultimate Placebo: A Surgeon Cuts through the Evidence.* NewSouth; 2016.

32. Sinno H, Prakash S. Complements and the wound healing cascade: An updated review. *Plast Surg Int.* 2013;2013:146764. https://doi.org/10.1155/2013/146764.

33. Hayden JA, van Tulder MW, Malmivaara A, Koes BW. Exercise therapy for treatment of non-specific low back pain. *Cochrane Database Syst Rev.* 2005;(3): CD000335. https://doi.org/10.1002/14651858.CD000335.pub2.

34. Macklin R. The ethical problems with sham surgery in clinical research. *N Engl J Med.* Sep 23 1999;341(13):992–996. https://doi.org/10.1056/NEJM199909233411312.

35. Horng S, Miller FG. Is placebo surgery unethical? *N Engl J Med.* Jul 11 2002;347(2):137–139. https://doi.org/10.1056/NEJMsb021025.

36. Howick J. Questioning the methodologic superiority of 'placebo' over 'active' controlled trials. *Am J Bioeth.* Sep 2009;9(9):34–48. https://doi.org/10.1080/15265160903090041.

37. Howick J. *The Philosophy of Evidence-Based Medicine.* Wiley-Blackwell; 2011.

38. Howick J, Koletsi D, Pandis N, et al. The quality of evidence for medical interventions does not improve or worsen: A metaepidemiological study of Cochrane reviews. *J Clin Epidemiol.* Oct 2020;126:154–159. https://doi.org/10.1016/j.jclinepi.2020.08.005.

39. Beard DJ, Campbell MK, Blazeby JM, et al. Considerations and methods for placebo controls in surgical trials. *Lancet.* 2020;395(10226):828–838. https://doi.org/10.1016/S0140-6736(19)33137-X.

40. Beard DJ, Campbell MK, Blazeby JM, et al. Placebo comparator group selection and use in surgical trials: The ASPIRE project including expert workshop. *Health Technol Assess.* Sep 2021;25(53):1–52. https://doi.org/10.3310/hta25530.

41. Reichenbach S, Rutjes AW, Nuesch E, Trelle S, Juni P. Joint lavage for osteoarthritis of the knee. *Cochrane Database Syst Rev.* May 12 2010;(5):CD007320. https://doi.org/10.1002/14651858.CD007320.pub2.

42. Laupattarakasem W, Laopaiboon M, Laupattarakasem P, Sumananont C. Arthroscopic debridement for knee osteoarthritis. *Cochrane Database Syst Rev.* Jan 23 2008;(1):CD005118. https://doi.org/10.1002/14651858.CD005118.pub2.

43. Khan M, Evaniew N, Bedi A, Ayeni OR, Bhandari M. Arthroscopic surgery for degenerative tears of the meniscus: A systematic review and meta-analysis. *CMAJ.* Oct 7 2014;186(14):1057–1064. https://doi.org/10.1503/cmaj.140433.

44. Shah NV, Solow M, Kelly JJ, et al. Demographics and rates of surgical arthroscopy and postoperative rehabilitative preferences of arthroscopists from the Arthroscopy Association of North America (AANA). *J Orthop.* Jun 2018;15(2): 591–595. https://doi.org/10.1016/j.jor.2018.05.033.

45. Hamilton DF, Howie CR. Knee arthroscopy: Influence of systems for delivering healthcare on procedure rates. *BMJ.* Sep 24 2015;351:h4720. https://doi.org/10.1136/bmj.h4720.

46. Probst P, Grummich K, Harnoss JC, et al. Placebo-controlled trials in surgery: A systematic review and meta-analysis. *Medicine* (Baltimore). Apr 2016;95(17):e3516. https://doi.org/10.1097/MD.0000000000003516.

47. Jefferson T, Jones M, Doshi P, Spencer EA, Onakpoya I, Heneghan CJ. Oseltamivir for influenza in adults and children: Systematic review of clinical

study reports and summary of regulatory comments. *BMJ.* 2014;348:g2545. https://doi.org/10.1136/bmj.g2545.

48. Furlan AD, van Tulder M, Cherkin D, et al. Acupuncture and dry-needling for low back pain: An updated systematic review within the framework of the Cochrane collaboration. *Spine.* Apr 15 2005;30(8):944–963. https://doi.org /10.1097/01.brs.0000158941.21571.01.

49. Sell S. Quarter of GPs spend half their time on paperwork. January 24, 2012. *GP Online.* https://www.gponline.com/quarter-gps-spend-half-time-paperwork /article/1113043.

50. NCCAM. *The Use of Complementary and Alternative Medicine in the United States;* 2007.

51. Posadzki P, Watson L, Alotaibi A, et al. Prevalence of use of complementary and alternative medicine (CAM) by patients/consumers in the UK: systematic review of surveys. Clin Med 2013;13(2):126–31. http://doi.org/10.7861/clinmedicine .13-2-126.

Chapter 12. The Next Placebo Revolution

1. Howick J, Mittoo S, Abel L, Halpern J, Mercer SW. A price tag on clinical empathy? Factors influencing its cost-effectiveness. *J R Soc Med.* Oct 2020;113(10): 389–393. https://doi.org/10.1177/0141076820945272.

2. Hoy D, Bain C, Williams G, et al. A systematic review of the global prevalence of low back pain. *Arthritis Rheum.* Jun 2012;64(6):2028–37. https://doi.org/10.1002 /art.34347.

3. World Bank. *The Global Burden of Disease: Generating Evidence, Guiding Policy: Europe and Central Asia Regional Edition.* Institute for Health Metrics and Evaluation, University of Washington, and the Human Development Network, the World Bank; 2013.

4. World Bank. *The Global Burden of Disease: Generating Evidence, Guiding Policy.* Institute for Health Metrics and Evaluation, University of Washington, and the Human Development Network, the World Bank; 2013.

5. World Bank. *The Global Burden of Disease: Generating Evidence, Guiding Policy: Middle East and North America Edition.* Institute for Health Metrics and Evaluation, University of Washington, and the Human Development Network, the World Bank; 2013.

6. Gaskin DJ, Richard P. The economic costs of pain in the United States. *J Pain.* Aug 2012;13(8):715–724. https://doi.org/10.1016/j.jpain.2012.03.009.

7. Maniadakis N, Gray A. The economic burden of back pain in the UK. *Pain.* Jan 2000;84(1):95–103. https://doi.org/10.1016/S0304-3959(99)00187-6.

8. Gustavsson A, Bjorkman J, Ljungcrantz C, et al. Socio-economic burden of patients with a diagnosis related to chronic pain: Register data of 840,000 Swedish patients. *Eur J Pain.* Feb 2012;16(2):289–299. https://doi.org/10.1016/j.ejpain .2011.07.006.

9. Raftery MN, Ryan P, Normand C, Murphy AW, de la Harpe D, McGuire BE. The economic cost of chronic noncancer pain in Ireland: Results from the PRIME study, part 2. *J Pain*. Feb 2012;13(2):139–45. https://doi.org/10.1016/j.jpain.2011.10.004.

10. Breivik H, Eisenberg E, O'Brien T, Openminds. The individual and societal burden of chronic pain in Europe: The case for strategic prioritisation and action to improve knowledge and availability of appropriate care. *BMC Public Health*. 2013;13:1229. https://doi.org/10.1186/1471-2458-13-1229.

11. Deyo RA, Weinstein JN. Low back pain. *N Engl J Med*. Feb 1 2001;344(5):363–370. https://doi.org/10.1056/NEJM200102013440508.

12. Hollingworth W, Todd CJ, King H, et al. Primary care referrals for lumbar spine radiography: Diagnostic yield and clinical guidelines. *Br J Gen Pract*. Jun 2002;52(479):475–480.

13. Agingan R. Doctors paying patients in ancient China. *xHistory Unveiled*. October 13, 2014. Accessed November 10, 2021. https://xhistoryunveiledx .wordpress.com/2014/10/13/doctors-paying-patients-in-ancient-china/.

14. Taleb N. *Skin in the Game: Hidden Asymmetries in Daily Life*. Random House; 2018.

15. NHS Digital. *Quality and Outcomes Framework*. Accessed July 1, 2022. https://qof.digital.nhs.uk/.

16. What is value-based healthcare? *NEJM Catalyst*. January 1, 2017. https:// catalyst.nejm.org/doi/full/10.1056/CAT.17.0558.

17. Thistlethwaite J, Gilbert J, Anderson E. Interprofessional education important for transition to interprofessional collaboration. *Med Educ*. 2022 May;56(5):585. https://doi.org/10.1111/medu.14730.

18. Keroack MA. System integration: Managing complexity to advance health care value. *NEJM Catalyst Innovations in Care Delivery* Sep 15 2021. 2021;2(10) https://doi.org/10.1056/CAT.21.0243.

19. The Rockefeller Foundation. Peterborough Social Impact Bond reduces reoffending by 8.4%; Investors on course for payment in 2016. Accessed September 13, 2021. https://www.rockefellerfoundation.org/report/peterborough-social -impact-bond-reduces-reoffending-by-8-4-investors-on-course-for-payment-in -2016/.

20. The King's Fund. Myth four: the NHS has too many managers. Accessed September 13, 2021. https://www.kingsfund.org.uk/projects/health-and-social -care-bill/mythbusters/nhs-managers.

21. The King's Fund. Key facts and figures about the NHS. Accessed September 13, 2021. https://www.kingsfund.org.uk/audio-video/key-facts-figures-nhs.

22. Sell S. Quarter of GPs spend half their time on paperwork. January 24, 2012. *GP Online*. https://www.gponline.com/quarter-gps-spend-half-time-paperwork /article/1113043.

23. Health Service Journal. 'More time' on admin than patients. September 25, 2013. https://www.hsj.co.uk/home/more-time-on-admin-than-patients/5063644 .article

24. Himmelstein DU, Campbell T, Woolhandler S. Health care administrative costs in the United States and Canada, 2017. *Ann Intern Med.* Jan 21 2020;172(2): 134–142. https://doi.org/10.7326/M19-2818.

Appendix 1. Adolf Grünbaum's Model and a Reply to Its Critics

1. Grünbaum A. The placebo concept in medicine and psychiatry. *Psychol Med.* Feb 1986;16(1):19–38. https://doi.org/10.1017/s0033291700002506.

2. Greenwood JD. Placebo control treatments and the evaluation of psychotherapy: A reply to Grünbaum and Erwin. *Philosophy of Science.* 1997;64(September): 497–510. https://www.jstor.org/stable/188322.

3. Hróbjartsson A. What are the main methodological problems in the estimation of placebo effects? *J Clin Epidemiol.* May 2002;55(5):430–435. https://doi.org /10.1016/s0895-4356(01)00496-6.

4. Walach H. Placebo controls: historical, methodological and general aspects. *Philos Trans R Soc Lond B Biol Sci.* Jun 27 2011;366(1572):1870–1878. https://doi.org /10.1098/rstb.2010.0401.

5. Waring D. Paradoxical drug response and the placebo effect: A discussion of Grünbaum's definitional scheme. *Theor Med Bioeth.* 2003;24(1):5–17. https://doi.org /10.1023/a:1022988413047.

6. Hauben M, Aronson JK. Paradoxical reactions: Under-recognized adverse effects of drugs. *Drug Saf.* 2006;29(10):970. https://doi.org/10.2165/00002018 -200629100-00120.

7. Mitchall J, Stanimirovic R, Klein B, Vella-Brodrick D. A randomised controlled trial of a self-guided internet intervention promoting well-being. *Computers in Human Behavior.* 2009;25(3):749–760. https://doi.org/10.1016/j.chb .2009.02.003.

8. Bolier L, Haverman M, Westerhof GJ, Riper H, Smit F, Bohlmeijer E. Positive psychology interventions: A meta-analysis of randomized controlled studies. *BMC Public Health.* 2013;13:119. https://doi.org/10.1186/1471-2458-13-119.

9. Hyland ME, Whalley B, Geraghty AW. Dispositional predictors of placebo responding: A motivational interpretation of flower essence and gratitude therapy. *J Psychosom Res.* Mar 2007;62(3):331–340. https://doi.org/10.1016/j.jpsychores .2006.10.006.

Appendix 2. Binary Outcomes May Underestimate Placebo Effects

1. Greene PJ, Wayne PM, Kerr CE, et al. The powerful placebo: Doubting the doubters. *Adv Mind Body Med.* Fall 2001;17(4):298–307; discussion 312–318.

2. Scharf HP, Mansmann U, Streitberger K, et al. Acupuncture and knee osteoarthritis: A three-armed randomized trial. *Ann Intern Med.* Jul 4 2006;145(1):12–20. https://doi.org/10.7326/0003-4819-145-1-200607040-00005.

3. Wolfe F. Determinants of WOMAC function, pain and stiffness scores: Evidence for the role of low back pain, symptom counts, fatigue and depression in

osteoarthritis, rheumatoid arthritis and fibromyalgia. *Rheumatology (Oxford)*. Apr 1999;38(4):355–361. https://doi.org/10.1093/rheumatology/38.4.355.

4. Goldsmith CH, Boers M, Bombardier C, Tugwell P. Criteria for clinically important changes in outcomes: Development, scoring and evaluation of rheumatoid arthritis patient and trial profiles. OMERACT Committee. *J Rheumatol*. Mar 1993;20(3):561–5.

5. Olsen MF, Bjerre E, Hansen MD, et al. Pain relief that matters to patients: systematic review of empirical studies assessing the minimum clinically important difference in acute pain. *BMC Med*. Feb 20 2017;15(1):35. https://doi.org/10.1186/s12916 H>016-0775 H>3.

Appendix 4. Balanced Placebo Design

1. Senn SJ. Controversies concerning randomization and additivity in clinical trials. *Stat Med*. Dec 30 2004;23(24):3729–3753. https://doi.org/10.1002/sim.2074.

Appendix 5. The Nocebo Effect as a Smokescreen in the Great Statin Debate

1. Vinogradova Y, Coupland C, Brindle P, Hippisley-Cox J. Discontinuation and restarting in patients on statin treatment: Prospective open cohort study using a primary care database. *BMJ*. Jun 28 2016;353:i3305. https://doi.org/10.1136/bmj.i3305.

2. Yusuf S. Why do people not take life-saving medications? The case of statins. *Lancet*. Sep 3 2016;388(10048):943–5. https://doi.org/10.1016/S0140-6736(16)31532-X.

3. Matthews A, Herrett E, Gasparrini A, et al. Impact of statin related media coverage on use of statins: Interrupted time series analysis with UK primary care data. *BMJ*. Jun 28 2016;353:i3283. https://doi.org/10.1136/bmj.i3283.

4. Gupta A, Thompson D, Whitehouse A, Collier T, Dahlof B, Poulter N, Collins R, Sever P; ASCOT Investigators. Adverse events associated with unblinded, but not with blinded, statin therapy in the Anglo-Scandinavian Cardiac Outcomes Trial-Lipid-Lowering Arm (ASCOT-LLA): A randomised double-blind placebo-controlled trial and its non-randomised non-blind extension phase. *Lancet*. 2017 Jun 24;389(10088):2473–2481. https://doi.org/10.1016/S0140-6736(17)31075-9.

5. Herrett E, Williamson E, Beaumont D, et al. Study protocol for statin web-based investigation of side effects (StatinWISE): A series of randomised controlled N-of-1 trials comparing atorvastatin and placebo in UK primary care. *BMJ Open*. Dec 1 2017;7(12):e016604. https://doi.org/10.1136/bmjopen-2017-016604.

6. Wood FA, Howard JP, Finegold JA, et al. N-of-1 trial of a statin, placebo, or no treatment to assess side effects. *N Engl J Med*. Nov 26 2020;383(22):2182–2184. https://doi.org/10.1056/NEJMc2031173.

7. Collins R, Reith C, Emberson J, et al. Interpretation of the evidence for the efficacy and safety of statin therapy. *Lancet*. Nov 19 2016;388(10059):2532–2561. https://doi.org/10.1016/S0140-6736(16)31357-5.

7. Kirsch I. Hidden administration as ethical alternatives to the balanced placebo design. *Prevention & Treatment.* 23 June 2003;6. https://doi.org/10.1037/1522-3736.6.1.65c.

Appendix 6. Why We Need to Measure Blinding Success

1. Devereaux PJ, Manns BJ, Ghali WA, et al. Physician interpretations and textbook definitions of blinding terminology in randomized controlled trials. *JAMA.* Apr 18 2001;285(15):2000–2003. http://doi.org/10.1001/jama.285.15.2000.

2. Moher D, Schulz KF, Altman D. The CONSORT statement: Revised recommendations for improving the quality of reports of parallel-group randomized trials. *JAMA.* Apr 18 2001;285(15):1987–1891. https://doi.org/10.1186/1471-2288-1-2.

3. Webster RK, Bishop F, Collins GS, et al. Measuring the success of blinding in placebo-controlled trials: Should we be so quick to dismiss it? *J Clin Epidemiol.* Mar 1 2021. https://doi.org/10.1016/j.jclinepi.2021.02.022.

4. Boutron I, Estellat C, Ravaud P. A review of blinding in randomized controlled trials found results inconsistent and questionable. *J Clin Epidemiol.* Dec 2005;58(12):1220–1226. https://doi.org/10.1016/j.jclinepi.2005.04.006.

5. Bang H, Ni L, Davis CE. Assessment of blinding in clinical trials. *Controlled Clinical Trials.* 2004/04/01/ 2004;25(2):143–156. https://doi.org/10.1016/j.cct.2003.10.016.

6. James KE, Bloch DA, Lee KK, Kraemer HC, Fuller RK. An index for assessing blindness in a multi-centre clinical trial: Disulfiram for alcohol cessation—a VA cooperative study. *Stat Med.* Jul 15 1996;15(13):1421–34. https://doi.org/10.1002/(SICI)1097-0258(19960715)15:13<1421::AID-SIM266>3.0.CO;2-H

7. Gill J, Prasad V. Testing for blinding in sham-controlled studies for procedural interventions: The third-party video method. *CMAJ : Canadian Medical Association Journal / journal de l'Association medicale canadienne.* Mar 11 2019;191(10):e272–e273. https://doi.org/10.1503/cmaj.181590.

8. Hróbjartsson A, Forfang E, Haahr MT, Als-Nielsen B, Brorson S. Blinded trials taken to the test: An analysis of randomized clinical trials that report tests for the success of blinding. *Int J Epidemiol.* Jun 2007;36(3):654–63. https://doi.org/10.1093/ije/dym020.

9. Fergusson D, Glass KC, Waring D, Shapiro S. Turning a blind eye: The success of blinding reported in a random sample of randomised, placebo controlled trials. *BMJ (Clinical research ed).* 2004;328(7437):432. https://doi.org/10.1136/bmj.328.74327.37952.631667.EE.

10. Savović J, Jones HE, Altman DG, et al. Influence of reported study design characteristics on intervention effect estimates from randomized, controlled trials. *Ann Intern Med.* 2012 Sep 18;157(6):429–438. https://doi.org/10.7326/0003-4819-157-6-201209180-00537.

11. Hróbjartsson A, Emanuelsson F, Skou Thomsen AS, Hilden J, Brorson S. Bias due to lack of patient blinding in clinical trials: A systematic review of trials

randomizing patients to blind and nonblind sub-studies. *Int J Epidemiol.* Aug 2014;43(4):1272–1283. https://doi.org/10.1093/ije/dyu115.

12. Bello S, Wei M, Hilden J, Hróbjartsson A. The matching quality of experimental and control interventions in blinded pharmacological randomised clinical trials: A methodological systematic review. *BMC Med Res Methodol.* 2016;16:18. https://doi.org/10.1186/s12874-016-0111-9.

13. Page MJ, Higgins JP, Clayton G, Sterne JA, Hróbjartsson A, Savović J. Empirical evidence of study design biases in randomized trials: Systematic review of meta-epidemiological studies. *PLoS One.* 2016;11(7):e0159267. https://doi.org/10.1371/journal.pone.0159267.

14. Dechartres A, Trinquart L, Faber T, Ravaud P. Empirical evaluation of which trial characteristics are associated with treatment effect estimates. *J Clin Epidemiol.* Sep 2016;77:24–37. https://doi.org/10.1016/j.jclinepi.2016.04.005.

15. Saltaji H, Armijo-Olivo S, Cummings GG, Amin M, da Costa BR, Flores-Mir C. Influence of blinding on treatment effect size estimate in randomized controlled trials of oral health interventions. *BMC Med Res Methodol.* May 18 2018;18(1):42. https://doi.org/10.1186/s12874-018-0491-0.

16. Armijo-Olivo S, Fuentes J, da Costa BR, Saltaji H, Ha C, Cummings GG. Blinding in physical therapy trials and its association with treatment effects: A meta-epidemiological study. *Am J Phys Med Rehabil.* Jan 2017;96(1):34–44. https://doi.org/10.1097/PHM.0000000000000521.

17. Hróbjartsson A, Thomsen AS, Emanuelsson F, et al. Observer bias in randomised clinical trials with binary outcomes: Systematic review of trials with both blinded and non-blinded outcome assessors. *BMJ.* Feb 27 2012;344:e1119. https://doi.org/10.1136/bmj.e1119.

18. Hróbjartsson A, Thomsen AS, Emanuelsson F, et al. Observer bias in randomized clinical trials with measurement scale outcomes: A systematic review of trials with both blinded and nonblinded assessors. *CMAJ.* Mar 5 2013;185(4):e201–e211. https://doi.org/10.1503/cmaj.120744.

19. Hróbjartsson A, Thomsen AS, Emanuelsson F, et al. Observer bias in randomized clinical trials with time-to-event outcomes: Systematic review of trials with both blinded and non-blinded outcome assessors. *Int J Epidemiol.* Jun 2014;43(3):937–948. https://doi.org/10.1093/ije/dyt270.

20. Moustgaard H, Clayton GL, Jones HE, et al. Impact of blinding on estimated treatment effects in randomised clinical trials: Meta-epidemiological study. *BMJ.* Jan 21 2020;368:l6802. https://doi.org/10.1136/bmj.l6802.

22. Tack M. Problems with the MetaBLIND study: An examination of data on blinding patients in trials with patient-reported outcomes. *Journal of Health Psychology.* 2021;0(0). https://doi.org/10.1177/13591053211059391.

23. Howick J. Re: Impact of blinding on estimated treatment effects in randomised clinical trials: Meta-epidemiological study. https://www.bmj.com/content/368/bmj.l6802/rapid-responses. 7 Feb 2020. Accessed November 22, 2022.

24. Webster RK, Bishop F, Collins GS, Evers AWM, Hoffmann T, Knottnerus JA, Lamb SE, Macdonald H, Madigan C, Napadow V, Price A, Rees JL, Howick J. Measuring the success of blinding in placebo-controlled trials: Should we be so quick to dismiss it? *J Clin Epidemiol.* 2021 Jul;135:176–181. https://doi.org/10.1016/j.jclinepi.2021.02.022.

25. Kinnersley P, Phillips K, Savage K, et al. Interventions to promote informed consent for patients undergoing surgical and other invasive healthcare procedures. *Cochrane Database Syst Rev.* Jul 6 2013;(7):CD009445. https://doi.org/10.1002/14651858.CD009445.pub2.

26. Stacey D, Legare F, Lewis K, et al. Decision aids for people facing health treatment or screening decisions. *Cochrane Database Syst Rev.* Apr 12 2017;4:CD001431. https://doi.org/10.1002/14651858.CD001431.pub5.

27. Wong PKK, Christie L, Johnston J, Bowling A, Freeman D, Joshua F, Bird P, Chia K, Bagga H. How well do patients understand written instructions? Health literacy assessment in rural and urban rheumatology outpatients. *Medicine* (Baltimore). 2014 Nov;93(25):e129. https://doi.org/10.1097/MD.0000000000000129.

28. Garden AL, Merry AF, Holland RL, Petrie KJ. Anaesthesia information: What patients want to know. *Anaesth Intensive Care.* 1996 Oct;24(5):594–598. https://doi.org/10.1177/0310057X9602400516.

Appendix 7. An Open Letter to the World Medical Association

1. World Medical Association, *Declaration of Helsinki: Recommendations Guiding Physicians in Biomedical Research Involving Human Subjects.* October 1996. https://www.wma.net/wp-content/uploads/2018/07/DoH-Oct1996.pdf.

2. World Medical Association. *Declaration of Helsinki: Ethical Principles for Medical Research Involving Human Subjects.* Accessed July, 7 2022. https://www.wma.net/policies-post/wma-declaration-of-helsinki-ethical-principles-for-medical-research-involving-human-subjects/.

3. Howick J. Questioning the methodologic superiority of 'placebo' over 'active' controlled trials. *Am J Bioeth.* Sep 2009;9(9):34–48. https://doi.org/10.1080/15265160903090041.

4. Howick J. Reviewing the unsubstantiated claims for the methodological superiority of 'placebo' over 'active' controlled trials: Reply to open peer commentaries. *Am J Bioeth.* 2009;9(9):W5–W7.

5. Batra S, Howick J. Empirical evidence against placebo controls. *J Med Ethics.* 2017 Aug 9:medethics-2016-103970. https://doi.org/10.1136/medethics-2016-103970.

Appendix 8. More on Noninferiority Trials

1. Group EIBS. Failure of extracranial-intracranial arterial bypass to reduce the risk of ischemic stroke: Results of an international randomized trial. *N Engl J Med.* Nov 7 1985;313(19):1191–1200. https://doi.org/10.1056/NEJM198511073131904.

2. Sackett DL, Spitzer WO, Gent M, Roberts RS. The Burlington randomized trial of the nurse practitioner: Health outcomes of patients. *Ann Intern Med*. Feb 1974;80(2):137–142. https://doi.org/10.7326/0003-4819-80-2-137.

3. Ellenberg SS, Temple R. Placebo-controlled trials and active-control trials in the evaluation of new treatments, part 2: Practical issues and specific cases. *Ann Intern Med*. Sep 19 2000;133(6):464–470. https://doi.org/10.7326/0003-4819-133-6-200009190-00015.

4. Lesaffre E, Bluhmki E, Wang-Clow F, et al. The general concepts of an equivalence trial, applied to ASSENT-2, a large-scale mortality study comparing two fibrinolytic agents in acute myocardial infarction. *Eur Heart J*. Jun 2001;22(11):898–902. https://doi.org/10.1053/euhj.2000.2323.

5. Senn SJ. Active control equivalence studies. In: Everitt BS, Palmer CR, eds. *Encyclopaedic Companion to Medical Statistics*. Hodder Arnold; 2005:19–22.

6. Piaggio G, Elbourne DR, Altman DG, Pocock SJ, Evans SJ. Reporting of noninferiority and equivalence randomized trials: an extension of the CONSORT statement. *JAMA*. Mar 8 2006;295(10):1152–1160. https://doi.org/10.1001/jama.2012.87802.

7. Morgan SG, Bassett KL, Wright JM, et al. "Breakthrough" drugs and growth in expenditure on prescription drugs in Canada. *BMJ*. Oct 8 2005;331(7520):815–816. https://doi.org/10.1136/bmj.38582.703866.AE.

8. Greene WL, Concato J, Feinstein AR. Claims of equivalence in medical research: Are they supported by the evidence? *Ann Intern Med*. May 2 2000;132(9):715–22. https://doi.org/10.7326/0003-4819-132-9-200005020-00006.

9. Armitage P, Berry G, Matthews JNS. *Statistical Methods in Medical Research*. 4th ed. Ed. PArmitage, G Berry, JNS Matthews. Blackwell Science; 2002.

10. Hwang IK, Morikawa T. Design issues in noninferiority/equivalence trials. *Drug Information Journal*. 1999;33:1205–1218. https://doi.org/10.1177/009286159903300042.

11. Blackwelder WC. "Proving the null hypothesis" in clinical trials. *Controlled Clinical Trials*. 1982;3:345–353. https://doi.org/10.1016/0197-2456(82)90024-1.

12. International Conference on Harmonisation of Technical Requirements for Registration of Pharmaceuticals for Human Use. *ICH Harmonised Tripartite Guideline: Choice of Control Group and Related Issues in Clinical Trials*, E 10. Step 4 version, July 20, 2000. https://database.ich.org/sites/default/files/E10_Guideline.pdf.

13. Howson C, Urbach P. *Scientific Reasoning: The Bayesian Approach*. 2d ed. Open Court; 1993.

14. Anderson JA. The ethics and science of placebo-controlled trials: Assay sensitivity and the Duhem-Quine thesis. *J Med Philos*. 2006 Feb;31(1):65–81. https://doi.org/10.1080/03605310500499203.

Tables and figures are indicated by page numbers in bold.

Charles II (king of England), 165–66
Chaucer, 22–23
cholesterol-lowering agents, 62. *See also* statins
clinical trials. *See* trials
Cochrane, Archie, 83
Cochrane Handbook, 87, 94
Colloca, Luana, 107
communication: in clinical trials, 177–78; doctor–patient, 12–13, 42–48, 197–98, 201–2, 203, 207; nocebo effects and, 152–54; in public health messaging, 181–82, 184–85
compassionate care. *See* empathic care
conditioning, 107
confidence intervals, 246–47
consultation, as component of treatment, 48, 69
contagiousness of placebo and nocebo effects, 114
context effect, 55–56
core (characteristic) features, 75–77, 213–14, 217–18, 225, **75**
cost of placebos, 176
costs of empathic care, 204–5, 207–8
covert treatment groups, 104, 232
Covi, Uno, 150
COVID-19 public health messaging, 181–82
COVID-19 vaccine trials, 60, 61
Crick, Francis, 116–17
cumulative effects, 101

deception, 38, 148–50; placebos and, 4, 20, 22, 147
Declaration of Helsinki, 162, 163, 164, 167, 177, 179–80, 240–41
depression, 64–66, 75–76, 182–83, 214, 243
developing nations, placebo-controlled trials in, 175–77
diagnosis, effect on expectations, 41
Di Blasi, Zelda, 6, 55
diclofenac, 155
doses, comparison of, 78
double-blinding, 61, 132, 138–39, 236, 237
double dummy trials, 65
dramatic effects, treatments and, 141, 191–92

drugs: additives in, 54, 75, 76, 216; comparing, 142; as controls in trials, 162; interaction with placebos, 126; shared properties with placebos, 101; types of: biosimilar, 40, 41; generic, 40; imitation, 242, 243

effect size, 173–74, 237
effect strength, 124
Ellenberg, Susan, 167, 168, 169–73
embodied cognition, 118–19
empathic care, 12–13, 43–45, 204–5, 207–8
empathy, 48, 157–58, 198, 201
enactivism, 118–19
endorphins, 65–66, 101, 102
Engel, George, 39
enteric nervous system, 117
environment, 30, 48–50, 199, 201
equations for interactions, 229
equivalence, 243, 244–46, **246**
Ernest (Dr.), story of, 152–53
errors (type I and type II) 247–50, **249**
ethics, 3, 152–56, 240–41; clinical trials and 36, 65, 177–78; deception and 20–21, 148–50; placebo-controlled trials and, 166–67, 168, 175–77, 180, 211; placebo surgery and 192; proven/ effective treatments and, 162, 163–64; use of placebos and, 145, 147, 158–59
ethics committees, 177–78
evolution, healing and, 120–21
exercise, 64–66, 78
expectancy, 89, 93, 105–6, 142, 185, 219–23
expectations: effect of, 51, 126–27, 136–39; surgery and, 188–89, 203
expectations, negative, 35, 103, 105, 108
expectations, positive, 104, 172, 221–23
extended minds, 118–19

faith, 59. *See also* beliefs
false positives and negatives, 247
fear and public health messaging, 185–86
feed and breed response (rest and digest), 112–13.
fight-or-flight response, 111–13. *See also* stress hormones
finasteride, 105
Franklin, Benjamin, 134–35

Freud, Sigmund, 123–24
fringe science, perception of placebo
    research as, 4–5, 6
furosemide, 66–67

General Medical Council (UK), 158
generic nocebo (Grünbaum's model), 224
generic placebo (Grünbaum's model), 214,
    224
genes, placebo effects on, 103
genki (behavior), 156–58
global effects of placebos 100, 103, 110–11,
    121
global perspective of the mind, 119–20
global responses in the body, 113
Gordon, Newton, 101, 102
Gøtzsche, Peter, 6, 26, 84–94, 132–33;
    critique of, 87–90, 93–94
Greenwood, John, 216–17, 219
Grünbaum, Adolf, 24; definition of
    placebos, 74–77; model of therapeutic
    theory, **75**, 213–26, **214**, **224**; modified
    version of his model, 223–26

harm, surgery and, 188, 191
harmful intervention (Grünbaum's
    model), 224
Hawthorne Effect, 91–92
Haygarth, John, 58–59
healing, 128; body's natural capacity
    for, 82–83, 120–21; environment and,
    49–50; wound-healing cascade and,
    190, 194
health care, 9; continuity of, 45–46; costs
    of, 208–9, 210–11; empathic care in,
    12–13, 43–45, 208; fee for service model
    of, 209, 210; value-based model of,
    209–10
health governor, 121
Helping Dad principles (empathic care),
    implementation of, 207–8
heterogeneity, 87–88, 98
Hill, Austin Bradford, 132
homeopathy, 59, 135–36
honest/open-label placebos, 105–6,
    150–51, 160
hospitalization, placebo effect of, 49
hospitals, cost of, 207

Howick, Jeremy, 11, 12–13, 154–55
Hróbjartsson, Asbjørn, 6, 84–94, 132–33;
    critique of, 87–90, 93–94
Hughes, John, 124–25
Human, Delon, 177
Humphrey, Nicholas, 121
hypotheses, alternative and null, 244,
    245, **246**, **249**. See also assay sensitivity
hypothesis tests, **249**

ICH E10 Guidelines, 245
imagination, 134–35
immune system, 112, 113–114, 120–21
inadvertent placebo (Grünbaum's model)
    215
inappropriate placebo controls, 62–63,
    72–73, 78
incidental features (non-characteristic),
    75, 76–77, 213, 214, 215, 217–18, 224–25
informed consent, 148, 149, 225
ingredients, inactive, 54
ingredients in placebos, 72–73
intentional placebo (Grünbaum's model),
    214–15, 224
interactions, 67, 229–30, 231, 234–35, **230**;
    measuring of, 124–27; placebos and,
    123, 127–28, 131
interconnectivity of placebo responses,
    114–15. See also global effects of
    placebos
interdisciplinary approach, 7, 15
interdisciplinary research, 9
International Conference on Harmonisa-
    tion, 167–68
interprofessionalism, 210
interventions 38, 63–72, 218
irritable bowel syndrome, 105–6
Italian doctor, story of the, 20–21

Jacobson, Lenore, 52
John Henry Effect, 91–92

Kaptchuk, Ted, 4–5, 7, 48
Kennedy, W. P., 35
Kirsch, Irving, 7, 70–71, 88
knee osteoarthritis, 90
knee surgery, 63, 186–88, 193
Kuhn, Thomas, 5–6